A 21st CENTURY SYSTEM FOR EVALUATING VETERANS FOR DISABILITY BENEFITS

Committee on Medical Evaluation of Veterans for Disability Compensation

Board on Military and Veterans Health

Michael McGeary, Morgan A. Ford, Susan R. McCutchen, and David K. Barnes, *Editors*

INSTITUTE OF MEDICINE
OF THE NATIONAL ACADEMIES

THE NATIONAL ACADEMIES PRESS
Washington, D.C.
www.nap.edu

THE NATIONAL ACADEMIES PRESS 500 Fifth Street, N.W. Washington, DC 20001

NOTICE: The project that is the subject of this report was approved by the Governing Board of the National Research Council, whose members are drawn from the councils of the National Academy of Sciences, the National Academy of Engineering, and the Institute of Medicine. The members of the committee responsible for the report were chosen for their special competences and with regard for appropriate balance.

This study was supported by Contract No. V101 (93) P-2136 between the National Academy of Sciences and United States Department of Veterans Affairs. Any opinions, findings, conclusions, or recommendations expressed in this publication are those of the author(s) and do not necessarily reflect the view of the organizations or agencies that provided support for this project.

Library of Congress Cataloging-in-Publication Data

A 21st century system for evaluating veterans for disability benefits / Committee on Medical Evaluation of Veterans for Disability Compensation, Board on Military and Veterans Health ; Michael McGeary . . . [et al.], editors.
p. ; cm.
Includes bibliographical references.
ISBN-13: 978-0-309-10631-3 (pbk. : alk. paper)
ISBN-10: 0-309-10631-1 (pbk. : alk. paper) 1. Disabled veterans—United States. 2. Disability retirement—United States. 3. Military pensions—United States. I. McGeary, Michael G. H. II. Institute of Medicine (U.S.). Committee on Medical Evaluation of Veterans for Disability Compensation. III. Title: Twenty-first century system for evaluating veterans for disability benefits.
UB373.A113 2007
362.4086′97—dc22

2007027713

Additional copies of this report are available from the National Academies Press, 500 Fifth Street, N.W., Lockbox 285, Washington, DC 20055; (800) 624-6242 or (202) 334-3313 (in the Washington metropolitan area); Internet, http://www.nap.edu.

For more information about the Institute of Medicine, visit the IOM home page at: **www.iom.edu.**

Printed in the United States of America.

The serpent has been a symbol of long life, healing, and knowledge among almost all cultures and religions since the beginning of recorded history. The serpent adopted as a logotype by the Institute of Medicine is a relief carving from ancient Greece, now held by the Staatliche Museen in Berlin.

Suggested citation: IOM (Institute of Medicine). 2007. *A 21st Century System For Evaluating Veterans For Disability Benefits*. Washington, DC: The National Academies Press.

"Knowing is not enough; we must apply.
Willing is not enough; we must do."
—Goethe

INSTITUTE OF MEDICINE
OF THE NATIONAL ACADEMIES

Advising the Nation. Improving Health.

THE NATIONAL ACADEMIES

Advisers to the Nation on Science, Engineering, and Medicine

The **National Academy of Sciences** is a private, nonprofit, self-perpetuating society of distinguished scholars engaged in scientific and engineering research, dedicated to the furtherance of science and technology and to their use for the general welfare. Upon the authority of the charter granted to it by the Congress in 1863, the Academy has a mandate that requires it to advise the federal government on scientific and technical matters. Dr. Ralph J. Cicerone is president of the National Academy of Sciences.

The **National Academy of Engineering** was established in 1964, under the charter of the National Academy of Sciences, as a parallel organization of outstanding engineers. It is autonomous in its administration and in the selection of its members, sharing with the National Academy of Sciences the responsibility for advising the federal government. The National Academy of Engineering also sponsors engineering programs aimed at meeting national needs, encourages education and research, and recognizes the superior achievements of engineers. Dr. Charles M. Vest is president of the National Academy of Engineering.

The **Institute of Medicine** was established in 1970 by the National Academy of Sciences to secure the services of eminent members of appropriate professions in the examination of policy matters pertaining to the health of the public. The Institute acts under the responsibility given to the National Academy of Sciences by its congressional charter to be an adviser to the federal government and, upon its own initiative, to identify issues of medical care, research, and education. Dr. Harvey V. Fineberg is president of the Institute of Medicine.

The **National Research Council** was organized by the National Academy of Sciences in 1916 to associate the broad community of science and technology with the Academy's purposes of furthering knowledge and advising the federal government. Functioning in accordance with general policies determined by the Academy, the Council has become the principal operating agency of both the National Academy of Sciences and the National Academy of Engineering in providing services to the government, the public, and the scientific and engineering communities. The Council is administered jointly by both Academies and the Institute of Medicine. Dr. Ralph J. Cicerone and Dr. Charles M. Vest are chair and vice chair, respectively, of the National Research Council.

www.national-academies.org

COMMITTEE ON MEDICAL EVALUATION OF VETERANS FOR DISABILITY COMPENSATION

LONNIE R. BRISTOW (*Chair*), Former President, American Medical Association, Walnut Creek, CA
GUNNAR B. J. ANDERSSON, Professor and Chair, Department of Orthopedic Surgery, Rush University Medical Center
JOHN F. BURTON, JR., Professor Emeritus, School of Management and Labor Relations, Rutgers University
LYNN H. GERBER, Director of the Center for Chronic Illness and Disability, College of Nursing and Health Science, George Mason University
SID GILMAN, William J. Herdman Distinguished University Professor, Director, Michigan Alzheimer's Disease Research Center, Department of Neurology, University of Michigan
HOWARD H. GOLDMAN, Professor of Psychiatry, School of Medicine, University of Maryland
SANDRA GORDON-SALANT, Professor, Department of Hearing and Speech Sciences, University of Maryland
JAY S. HIMMELSTEIN, Assistant Chancellor for Health Policy, Director, Center for Health Policy and Research, School of Medicine, University of Massachusetts
ANA E. NÚÑEZ, Associate Professor, College of Medicine and Institute for Women's Health and Leadership, Drexel University
JAMES W. REED, Chief of Endocrinology, Grady Memorial Hospital, Professor of Medicine and Associate Chair of Medicine for Clinical Research, Morehouse School of Medicine
DENISE G. TATE, Professor, Director of Research, Division of Rehabilitation Psychology and Neuropsychology, Department of Physical Medicine and Rehabilitation, University of Michigan
BRIAN M. THACKER, Regional Director, Congressional Medal of Honor Society, Wheaton, MD
DENNIS TURK, Professor of Anesthesiology and Pain Research, Department of Anesthesiology, School of Medicine, University of Washington
RAYMOND JOHN VOGEL, President, RJ VOGEL and Associates, Mt. Pleasant, SC
REBECCA A. WASSEM, Professor of Nursing, College of Nursing, University of Utah
EDWARD H. YELIN, Professor of Medicine, Institute for Health Policy Studies, University of California, San Francisco

Project Staff

MICHAEL McGEARY, Study Director
MORGAN A. FORD, Program Officer
SUSAN R. McCUTCHEN, Research Associate
REINE Y. HOMAWOO, Senior Program Assistant
FREDERICK (RICK) ERDTMANN, Director, Board on Military and Veterans Health and Medical Follow-up Agency
PAMELA RAMEY-McCRAY, Administrative Assistant
ANDREA COHEN, Financial Associate
WILLAM McLEOD, Senior Librarian
DAVID K. BARNES, Consultant
ROBERT J. EPLEY, Consultant
MARK GOODIN, Copy Editor

Reviewers

This report has been reviewed in draft form by individuals chosen for their diverse perspectives and technical expertise, in accordance with procedures approved by the NRC's Report Review Committee. The purpose of this independent review is to provide candid and critical comments that will assist the institution in making its published report as sound as possible and to ensure that the report meets institutional standards for objectivity, evidence, and responsiveness to the study charge. The review comments and draft manuscript remain confidential to protect the integrity of the deliberative process. We wish to thank the following individuals for their review of this report:

Dan G. Blazer, Duke University Medical Center
Gerard N. Burrow, Dean Emeritus, Yale University School of Medicine
Molly Carnes, Departments of Medicine, Psychiatry, and Industrial & Systems Engineering and UW Center for Women's Health Research, University of Wisconsin, Madison
Bruce M. Gans, Kessler Institute for Rehabilitation
Allen Heinemann, Department of Physical Medicine and Rehabilitation, Feinberg School of Medicine, Northwestern University
J. Gary Hickman, Former Director, Compensation and Pension Service, Department of Veterans Affairs
Richard T. Johnson, The Johns Hopkins University School of Medicine and Bloomberg School of Public Health and The Johns Hopkins Hospital
Arthur T. Meyerson, New York University School of Medicine

Peter B. Polatin, Department of Anesthesiology and Pain Management, University of Texas Southwestern Medical Center
Bonnie Rogers, Occupational Health Nursing Program, School of Public Health, University of North Carolina
Lewis P. Rowland, The Neurological Institute of New York, Columbia University Medical Center
Marc Swiontkowski, Department of Orthopaedic Surgery, University of Minnesota
Alvin J. Thompson, Emeritus Clinical Professor, University of Washington School of Medicine
John D. Worrall, College of Arts and Sciences, Rutgers University

Although the reviewers listed above have provided many constructive comments and suggestions, they were not asked to endorse the conclusions or recommendations nor did they see the final draft of the report before its release. The review of this report was overseen by **Harold J. Fallon**, Dean Emeritus, School of Medicine, University of Alabama at Birmingham, and **Paul D. Stolley**, Adjunct Professor, School of Medicine, University of Maryland. Appointed by the National Research Council and Institute of Medicine, respectively, they were responsible for making certain that an independent examination of this report was carried out in accordance with institutional procedures and that all review comments were carefully considered. Responsibility for the final content of this report rests entirely with the authoring committee and the institution.

Preface

As McCullough reports in his Pulitzer Prize winning book, *1776*, Nathaniel Greene, one of George Washington's most stalwart generals, wrote to John Adams on May 24, 1776, "that if Congress were to provide support for those soldiers maimed or killed, this in itself would increase enlistments and 'inspire those engaged with as much courage as any measure that can be fixed upon.'" The scope of the concern for our servicemen and servicewomen has increased since then, of course, but there has been one unwavering constant: the desire of a nation to honor those who serve in our armed forces and to compensate for sacrifices incurred during military service.

Just prior to America's entry into World War II, it was a common sight to see individuals with wooden "peg-legs" or eye patches covering an empty orbit. These were usually veterans of World War I. Our country's entry into World War II had an enormous cost in life and treasure, but one of the more positive spin offs was a galvanizing of the field of bioengineering, leading to the development of improved prosthetics, along with a concern about the potential for rehabilitation. Over the subsequent years (and several wars) since then, we have progressed figuratively, and often literally, with the development of functioning prostheses and other assistive devices.

This IOM Committee on Medical Evaluation of Veterans for Disability Compensation notes in its report that our nation's veterans benefits program has not kept a similar pace of progress in understanding disability. If one steps back in order to gain a multi-dimensional perspective, it could be argued that there is more emphasis being placed on the "dis" aspect of the word "disability" and less on the "ability" potential within the same word. The original concern for the sacrifices made by those who serve our nation's colors had it genesis in the Revolutionary War, when loss of limbs, eyes, or other body parts sharply reduced a person's ability to support himself. This emphasis on anatomical loss persisted through the 19th century, was codified in the Rating Schedule developed to implement the War Risk Insurance Act of 1917, and retained with modifications in subsequent Rating Schedules, including the current one when it was developed in 1945. The architecture put in place at that time has been updated from time to time in a piecemeal manner, and some sections are largely the same as in 1945. There has been resistance to change the familiar and comfortable status quo, which is understandable, but this should not stand in the way of our ability to evaluate and compensate for disability based on up-to-date medical knowledge of impairment and function.

As the understanding of what constitutes disability has evolved, so has the ability to recognize and quantify the contributory components. The questions posed by the commission to this IOM committee reflect the uncertainties created by a lack of clear statement of purpose for the program, the use of an evaluation tool that has not kept pace with the changing dynamics of the likely losses incurred by our servicemen and servicewomen, and the changing economics of the workforce in America, as well as the changing social context into which our veterans return.

I deeply appreciate the willingness of the members of the committee that produced this report to serve in this timely effort to improve the system for compensating veterans for injuries and illnesses suffered while in military service. It was an important assignment. With members of the military being injured in combat nearly every day, the system of evaluating and rating disability should be as up to date as medical knowledge of impairment and its effects on a person's functioning and quality of life permits. It also should have the capacity to keep pace with the constant advances in our understanding of the impacts of injuries and diseases that do not entail visible losses, for example, traumatic brain injury and posttraumatic stress disorder. The committee worked diligently to assess the current system and to develop the recommendations in this report. I thank the members for the time they spent in, and between, meetings to formulate the findings and recommendations. I also greatly appreciate the efforts of the staff and consultants who provided key assistance and support to the committee.

It is hoped this report will provide insight into how best to serve the needs of our men and women who left a civilian environment as individuals and entered into one in which they were trained to work and fight as a group, and who have experienced disability as a result. They have now returned to a society where the emphasis is again on them functioning as individuals, and our VA programs must facilitate that transition.

Since the preface (above) was drafted initially, the importance of ensuring an adequate system of veterans benefits has escalated sharply. Since the committee's first meeting in May 2006, the U.S. military has continued to suffer steady casualties in Operation Enduring Freedom in Afghanistan and Operation Iraqi Freedom (OEF/OIF). Nearly 1.5 million servicemembers have been deployed to OEF/OIF. Of these, nearly 700,000 have separated from active duty and become veterans—some of them grievously wounded, physically or mentally, or both. This set of events has only heightened the need for a thorough review of the Schedule for Rating Disabilities, which contains the criteria used to evaluate the disabling effects of military service on servicemembers who are wounded, sickened, or otherwise injured. Additionally, the VA Rating Schedule is used by the military in their disability decision-making system, which has a slightly different primary focus, that of determining potential fitness for return to duty.

Recognition of the importance of ensuring an adequate system of veterans benefits also has escalated sharply. In February 2007, the *Washington Post* published a series of articles about problems facing injured service members being treated as outpatients at Walter Reed Army Hospital while on medical hold and awaiting a decision by the military on their disability status. The *Post*'s series resulted in a number of investigations, from a multitude of sponsors, of the adequacy of the military and VA systems of care and benefits.

While these inquiries are important and no doubt will result in needed changes, I do not think they will change the recommendations in this report, except perhaps to increase the impetus for implementing them. The VA claims process was largely shaped by the needs of veterans of World War II. It struggled to meet the needs of veterans of Vietnam and, more recently, of the first Gulf War. The current Rating Schedule is not as up to date as it should be in areas affecting many veterans. The musculoskeletal and neurological sections of the Rating Schedule have not been comprehensively updated since 1945, and other important sections, such as the one addressing mental disorders, have not been updated for more than 10 years. This is why the committee is recommending a complete overhaul of the Rating Schedule and establishment of a process for keeping it up to date. The committee is also recommending that the revisions be based in part on information about the effects of veterans' impairments on their ability to function in society (including, but not limited to, employment) and their quality of life. This is in part because we now know that degree of impairment, on which most of the current Rating Schedule is based, does not always correlate with today's understanding of degree of disability. Also, we have a better understanding of how to measure functional limitations.

Finally, some of the signature injuries incurred in OEF/OIF (e.g., closed head traumatic brain injury [TBI], posttraumatic stress disorder [PTSD]) are not visible or subject to a laboratory test and, instead, must be evaluated in terms of their functional consequences. Similarly, it is difficult to determine the disability resulting from multiple impairments (e.g., combinations of TBI, amputation, paralysis, loss of vision or hearing, PTSD, and depression) without referring to their net effect on a veteran's functional capacity.

The committee respectfully hopes we have made the case for substantial change to be made and that our nation will respond to the challenge promptly and positively. Our veterans deserve no less.

Lonnie R. Bristow, M.D.
Chair

Acknowledgments

The committee and staff wish to thank many individuals for the information and views they provided during the course of the study. We particularly appreciate the support, guidance, and data we received from Rick Surratt, Ray Wilburn, Jim Wear, Steve Riddle, Jacqueline Garrick, and Kathleen Greve, Veterans' Disability Benefits Commission. Marcelle Habibion, Department of Veterans Affairs' (VA's) contracting officer's technical representative for the commission, was very helpful both by facilitating responses from the knowledgeable individuals to the many requests made by the committee, and in explaining VA operations and procedures and offering guidance as appropriate, particularly in facilitating the arrangement of site visits. George T. Fitzelle, VA Program Evaluation Service, was instrumental in arranging meetings with staff from the CNA Corporation, who are working with the commission on surveys and data analyses and who assisted the committee by coordinating their activities with ours.

VA staff (in alphabetical order) greatly assisted the committee by taking time out of their busy schedules to speak with and provide information about VA operations for the committee. These individuals included Mark Bologna, Daniel J. Cunningham, and Susan Perez from the Office of Performance Analysis and Integrity, Veterans Benefits Administration (VBA). Staff who helped further the committee's understanding of VBA's Compensation and Pension Service operations and the Veterans Health Administration's compensation and pension examination process by making presentations to and answering questions from the committee, or by providing information, included Dr. Steven H. Brown, Ed Davenport, Catherine Dischner, Bradley B. Flohr, Kurt Hessling, Janice Jacobs, Dr. Patrick C. Joyce, Bradley

G. Mayes, Dr. Vicki Milton, Thomas J. Pamperin, Stephen C. Simmons, and Mike Wells. VBA's Vocational Rehabilitation and Employment Service staff who provided information and spoke with the committee included Bill Borom and Fred Steier.

James P. Terry, chairman, and Steven L. Keller, senior deputy vice chairman, Board of Veterans' Appeals, provided information and spoke with the committee about the board's procedures. Betty Moseley Brown, associate director, Center for Women Veterans, offered valuable input about the center's programs and procedures. The committee learned about the military disability program from Al Bruner, assistant director, Officer and Enlisted Personnel Management (Separation/Retirement), Office of the Under Secretary of Defense for Personnel and Readiness; Paul D. Williamson, president, Naval Physical Evaluation Board; and Lt. Col. Melissa J. Applegate, USAF, assistant director, Military Compensation, Office of the Under Secretary of Defense for Personnel and Readiness.

Dr. Elena M. Andresen, professor and chief, Epidemiology Division, Department of Health Services Research, Management and Policy, University of Florida Health Sciences Center, discussed defining and measuring quality of life. The committee also heard from Dr. Alan M. Jette, director, Health and Disability Research Institute, Boston University, about conceptualizing and measuring disability. Dr. William Narrow, American Psychiatric Institute for Research and Education and American Psychiatric Association (APA) Office of Research, gave an overview of DSM-V, the next edition of APA's *Diagnostic and Statistical Manual of Mental Disorders.* Similarly, Dr. Robert D. Rondinelli gave an overview of the next edition of the American Medical Association's *Guides to the Evaluation of Permanent Impairment.*

The committee wishes to thank individuals who were instrumental in arranging committee and staff site visits to several VBA regional offices and other facilities to enhance their understanding of actual operations. VA staff who worked with us in gaining approvals and making initial arrangements included Shana Brown, Central Office, and Beth McCoy, Office of Field Operations, Washington, DC. VA staff who hosted site visits included Joe Beaudoin and Earl Hutchinson, Veterans Service Center, Boston, MA; Judy Bilicki, Veterans Service Center, Detroit, MI; Paul Black, Veterans Service Center, San Antonio, TX; Mary L. Glenn and George C. Wolohojian, Veterans Service Center, Baltimore, MD; Larry Jordan, Veterans Service Center, Columbia, SC; Bill Kabel, Veterans Service Center, Atlanta, GA; Vickie Orlando and Pat Wicks, Veterans Service Center, Salt Lake City, UT; Jaime Ramirez and Frank M. Tejeda, [VA] Outpatient Clinic, San Antonio, TX; and Uli Willimon, Veterans Service Center, Oakland, CA.

Other individuals provided information about and represented the views of service and state organizations that work extensively with veterans.

These included Peter S. Gaytan, The American Legion; David Houppert, Vietnam Veterans of America; Sidney A. Lee, African American PTSD Association; Pat Rowe Kerr, Missouri Veterans Commission; Jerry Manar, National Veterans Service, Veterans of Foreign Wars; Leonard J. Selfon, United Spinal Association; and Rick Surratt, Disabled American Veterans.

We would like to thank Dr. Eric Christensen, Dr. Joyce McMahon, Dr. Laurie May, and Elizabeth Schaefer of the CNA Corporation; and Cynthia A. Bascetta, Dr. Carol D. Petersen, and Robert E. Robertson of the Government Accountability Office for their contributions as well.

We also received thoughtful comments from members of the public, including Dr. Craig Bash and John King.

Throughout the course of the study, the committee received several public comments that shed light on issues of concern. Committee and staff wish to thank those who followed our study's progress and took the time to make comments that served to heighten our awareness of important issues to consider during the deliberations.

Finally, the committee wants to acknowledge the expert support of the IOM staff and consultants: Michael McGeary, study director; David K. Barnes and Robert Epley, consultants; Rick Erdtmann, board director; Morgan A. Ford, program officer; Susan R. McCutchen, research associate; Reine Y. Homawoo, senior program assistant; William McLeod, senior librarian (The National Academies); Andrea Cohen, financial associate; Pamela Ramey-McCray, administrative assistant; and Mark Goodin, copy editor.

Contents

Tables, Figures, and Boxes

TABLES

FIGURES

BOXES

Abbreviations and Acronyms

ADLs	Activities of daily living
ALS	Amyotrophic lateral sclerosis
AMA	American Medical Association
AMIE	Automated Medical Information Exchange
APA	American Psychiatric Association
ASIA	American Spinal Injury Association
BDD	Benefits Delivery at Discharge
BDN	Benefits Delivery Network
BVA	Board of Veterans' Appeals
C&P	Compensation and Pension
CAPRI	Compensation and Pension Record Interchange
CAVC	(U.S.) Court of Appeals for Veterans Claims
CDC	Centers for Disease Control and Prevention
CFR	Code of Federal Regulations
CHAMPVA	Civilian Health & Medical Program of the Department of Veterans Affairs
CHPR	Center for Health Policy and Research of the University of Massachusetts
CHTW	Coming Home to Work program
CM	Clinical Modification
CPEP	Compensation and Pension Examination Program
CPI	Claims Process Improvement
CT	Computerized tomography

CY	Calendar year
DIC	Dependency and Indemnity Compensation
DoD	Department of Defense
DOL	Department of Labor
DOL-VETS	Department of Labor Veteran's Employment and Training Services
DRO	Decision review officer
DSM-IV	*Diagnostic and Statistical Manual of Mental Disorders*, 4th Edition (1994)
DSM-IV-TR	*Diagnostic and Statistical Manual of Mental Disorders*, 4th Edition, Text Revision 2000)
DTAP	Disabled Transition Assistance Program
DVOP	Disabled Veterans Outreach Program
ECAB	Employee's Compensation Appeals Board of the Department of Labor
ECVARS	*E*Conomic *VA*lidation of the *R*ating *S*chedule
EP	End product
FECA	Federal Employee Compensation Act
FERS	Federal Employee Retirement System
FEV_1	Forced expiratory volume in one second
FTE	Full-time equivalent
FY	Fiscal year
GAF	Global Assessment of Functioning
GAO	Government Accountability Office (formerly the General Accounting Office)
GWOT	Global War on Terrorism
HIV	Human immunodeficiency virus
HRQOL	Health-related quality of life
IADLs	Instrumental activities of daily living (see ADLs)
ICD-9	*International Classification of Diseases*, 9th Revision
ICD-9-CM	*International Classification of Diseases*, 9th Revision, Clinical Modification
ICD-10	*International Statistical Classification of Diseases and Related Health Problems*, 10th Revision
ICD-10-CM	*International Statistical Classification of Diseases and Related Health Problems*, 10th Revision, Clinical Modification

ICD-11	*International Statistical Classification of Diseases and Related Health Problems*, 11th Revision
ICF	*International Classification of Functioning, Disability and Health*
IEEP	Individualized extended evaluation plans
IU	Individual unemployability
LVER	Local veterans' employment representative
MEB	Medical Evaluation Board
METS	Metabolic equivalents of task
mg/dL	Milligrams per deciliter
M.P.H.	Master of public health
MRI	Magnetic resonance imaging
NAPA	National Academy of Public Administration
NASI	National Academy of Social Insurance
NCHS	National Center for Health Statistics
NIH	National Institutes of Health
NIMH	National Institute of Mental Health
NOD	Notice of disagreement
NOS	Not otherwise specified
OEF	Operation Enduring Freedom
OIF	Operation Iraqi Freedom
OIG	[VA] Office of Inspector General
OPM	Office of Personnel Management
PA	Physician's assistant
PA&I	Office of Performance Analysis and Integrity
PEB	Physical Evaluation Board
Ph.D.	Doctor of philosophy
P.L.	Public law
POW	Prisoner of war
PRTF	Psychiatric Review Technique Form
PTSD	Posttraumatic stress disorder
QOL	Quality of life
QR	Quality rating; quality review
QTC	QTC Medical Group, Inc.
QUERI	Quality Enhancement Research Initiative
RBA 2000	Rating Board Automation 2000

RO	Regional office
RVSR	Rating veterans service representative
SCI	Spinal cord injury
SF-36	Short Form 36
SMR	Service medical record
SOC/SSOC	Statement of case/Supplemental statement of case
SOFAS	Social and Occupational Assessment Scale
SSA	Social Security Administration
SSDI	Social Security Disability Insurance
SSI	Supplemental Security Income
STAR	Statistical Technical Accuracy Review
TAP	Transition Assistance Program
TBI	Traumatic brain injury
U.S.C.	United States Code
VA	Department of Veterans Affairs
VACO	VA central office
VARO	VA regional office
VBA	Veterans Benefits Administration
VCAA	Veterans Claim Assistance Act (of 2000)
VERIS	Veterans Examination Request Information System
VHA	Veterans Health Administration (VA)
VISN	Veterans Integrated Service Network
VLJ	Veterans law judge
VR	Vocational rehabilitation
VRC	Vocational rehabilitation counselor
VR&E	Vocational Rehabilitation and Employment (Service)
VRECC	Vocational rehabilitation and employment case coordinators
VSC	Veterans service center
VSO	Veterans service organization
VSR	Veterans service representative
WHO	World Health Organization

Summary

ABSTRACT: *The Department of Veterans Affairs (VA) compensates veterans for injuries and diseases acquired or aggravated during military service. Currently (2007), the amount of monthly compensation to a veteran without dependents ranges from $115 for a 10 percent rating to $2,471 for a 100 percent rating. Approximately 2.8 million veterans are receiving compensation totaling about $30 billion a year (dependents and survivors receive another $5 billion a year). The rating is determined using the VA Schedule for Rating Disabilities (Rating Schedule), which has criteria based mostly on degree of impairment—i.e., loss of body structures and systems. This report recommends that VA comprehensively update the entire Rating Schedule and establish a regular process for keeping it up to date. VA should dedicate staff to maintaining the Rating Schedule and reestablish an external advisory committee of medical and other disability experts to assist in the updating process. The report also recommends that the current statutory purpose of VA's disability compensation program—to compensate for average loss of earning capacity—should be expanded to compensate for nonwork disability and loss of quality of life as well as average loss of earning capacity. VA should investigate how well the rating levels correspond to average loss of earnings and adjust rating criteria to ensure that as ratings increase, average loss of earnings also increases (vertical equity), and that the same ratings are associated with similar average losses of earnings across body systems (horizontal equity). VA should also apply measures of* *functional limitations, such as activities of daily living and instrumental activities of daily living, and determine if the Rating Schedule accounts for them (i.e., as limitations on ability to engage in usual life activities increase, ratings tend to increase). If not, VA should incorporate functional criteria in rating criteria or develop a separate mechanism for compensating for functional limitations beyond work disability. The methodology for measuring quality of life (QOL) is not as well developed as it is for measuring functional limitations. Accordingly, VA initially should engage in research and development efforts to create measures valid for the veteran population before determining if the Rating Schedule compensates for QOL (i.e., as quality of life diminishes, ratings generally increase) and, if it does not, develop a mechanism for compensating for loss of QOL clearly beyond loss in earnings or limitations in daily life. The report also addresses a number of other topics, for example, use of computer-based templates to improve disability examinations; better training of examiners and raters; adoption of commonly used diagnostic classification systems; comprehensive needs assessment of veterans separating from military service for health care, vocational rehabilitation, educational, and other benefits and services provided by VA; involvement of vocational expertise in determining individual unemployability; and research to improve the rating process (e.g., analyze the validity and reliability of the Rating Schedule, evaluate training and certification programs, and assess the extent to which compensation and ancillary benefits meet the needs of veterans).*

INTRODUCTION

The Institute of Medicine (IOM) was asked by the Veterans' Disability Benefits Commission to study and recommend improvements in the medical evaluation and rating of veterans for the benefits provided by the Department of Veterans Affairs (VA) to compensate for illnesses or injuries incurred in or aggravated by military service. The main topics examined in this report by the committee formed to undertake the study are VA's "Schedule for Rating Disabilities"—usually referred to as the "Rating Schedule"—and the development of medical information in the evaluation of veterans claiming disability and the use of that information in the rating process.

Compensation for service-connected disability is a monthly cash benefit made to veterans who are disabled due to an illness or injury that occurred during service or was aggravated by service. Raters use the Rating Schedule to determine degree of disability, ranging in 10 percent increments from 0 to 100 percent, and a veteran's benefit level is tied to his or her rating. Benefits in 2007 range from $115 a month for a 10 percent rating to $2,471 for a 100 percent rating (plus additional amounts for dependents of those with 30 percent ratings or higher).

The statutory purpose of disability benefits is to compensate veterans for "the average impairments of earning capacity resulting from such injuries in civil occupations." VA program policies clearly reflect a grateful nation. They include deciding in favor of the veteran if there is reasonable doubt; assisting the veteran in gathering evidence; identifying conditions that might be compensable even if the veteran does not claim them; and presumption of service connection for certain conditions. A disability rating also entitles a veteran to ancillary services, such as vocational rehabilitation and employment services, and higher ratings provide access to more benefits, such as free health care. The compensation is tax exempt, and there are annual cost-of-living adjustments.

It is important that the tool used to determine the rating—the Rating Schedule—be as effective as possible in fulfilling the purpose of the compensation program. Is it valid and reliable in determining degree of disability? Is it up to date, and are there adequate arrangements for keeping it up to date? Are there better ways of evaluating disability? This report addresses these and related questions and makes recommendations for improvements.

IMPAIRMENT, DISABILITY, AND QUALITY OF LIFE

The statutory purpose of the cash benefits currently provided to veterans with disabilities is to compensate for the work disability ("average impairment in earning capacity") resulting from service-related injuries and diseases. In practice, Congress and VA have implicitly recognized consequences in addition to work disability of impairments suffered by veterans in the Rating Schedule and other ways. Modern concepts of disability include work disability, nonwork disability, and quality of life (QOL), although not all of the tools used to operationalize the evaluation of this broader concept of disability are well developed. The Rating Schedule currently emphasizes impairment and limitations or loss of specific body structures and functions, which may not predict disability well. However, the Rating Schedule could be revised to include factors that are more directly related to disability, such as activities of daily living and other whole-person-level functional limitations. It also may be possible to develop procedures to measure and compensate for loss of QOL. Revising the Rating Schedule would be greatly assisted by a clearer definition of the purpose of compensation.

Recommendation 3-1.[1] The purpose of the current veterans disability compensation program as stated in statute currently is to compensate for average impairment in earning capacity, that is, work disability. This is an unduly restrictive rationale for the program and is inconsistent with current models of disability. The veterans disability compensation program should compensate for three consequences of service-connected injuries and diseases: work disability, loss of ability to engage in usual life activities other than work, and loss in quality of life. (Specific recommendations on approaches to evaluating each consequence of service-connected injuries and diseases are in Chapter 4.)

The committee is aware that adopting Recommendation 3-1 would be difficult and costly. Legislative endorsement would be very helpful, if not required. If the recommendation is adopted, the Rating Schedule and the procedures needed to implement it will need to be revised to reflect the expanded purposes for disability benefits endorsed by the committee. This can be done in phases, after appropriate research and analysis and pilot projects to study the feasibility of changes. This issue is addressed in Chapters 4 and 5.

Expanding the bases for veterans disability compensation also has cost implications. There will be start-up costs incurred in developing the instruments for evaluating degree of functional limitation and loss of QOL, transitional costs such as training, and possibly greater compensation costs (if functional or QOL deficits are greater on average than are accounted for using the current impairment ratings). Although the committee was not asked to consider costs in recommending improvements in medical evaluation of veterans for disability benefits, the issue is addressed at the end of Chapter 4.

In addition, if disability compensation is considered in the larger context of veterans benefits, in conjunction with today's views on the rights of individuals with disabilities to live as full a life as possible, it is possible to envision a more comprehensive evaluation of a veteran's needs—including medical, educational, vocational, and compensation. Currently, the assessment process is piecemeal and fragmented. Either the veteran must receive a rating to access related services, such as health care and vocational rehabilitation and employment services, or the other service, such as education, is separate. This issue is addressed in Chapter 6.

[1]Recommendations used throughout the Summary and the rest of the report are numbered according to the chapter in which they appear and the order in which they appear in that chapter. Thus Recommendation 3-1, which is the first recommendation in the report, is the first recommendation to appear in Chapter 3. See Box S-1 for all of the recommendations, categorized according to the committee's specific tasks.

THE RATING SCHEDULE

Updating the Rating Schedule

It is important for the Rating Schedule to be as up to date as possible in current medical approaches and terminology to serve veterans with disabilities most effectively. This ensures that the criteria in the Rating Schedule are based on concepts and terms used by medical personnel who provide medical evidence, and that evolving understanding of, or recognition of, new disabling conditions is reflected.

Currently, the Rating Schedule is out of date medically. It has been more than 10 years since many body systems were comprehensively updated, and some have not been updated for much longer. The Rating Schedule should be revised to remove ambiguous criteria and obsolete conditions and language, reflect current medical practice, and include medical advances in diagnosis and classification of new conditions.

VA should expeditiously undertake a comprehensive revision of the Rating Schedule and establish a formal process to revise it approximately every 10 years. Several body systems could be revised each year on a staggered basis to make this feasible. VA will need to increase its staff capacity to update and revise the Rating Schedule. The process would also benefit from external advice from medical, rehabilitation, and vocational experts, and the veteran community.

Recommendation 4-1. VA should immediately update the current Rating Schedule, beginning with those body systems that have gone the longest without a comprehensive update, and devise a system for keeping it up to date. VA should reestablish a disability advisory committee to advise on changes in the Rating Schedule.

Revising the Rating Schedule to Improve the Relationship Between Ratings and Earnings Losses

The formal purpose of the Rating Schedule is to compensate for loss of earning capacity. Loss of earning capacity is more a legal or economic than a medical concept. In practice, the best proxy for earning capacity is actual earnings. There is no current evidence on the relationship between the Rating Schedule's severity ratings and average loss of earnings of veterans with disabilities. Findings were mixed when VA last looked at this in 1971. Since that time, substantial social and technological changes have occurred (e.g., passage of the Americans with Disabilities Act, advances in assistive devices) that make it easier for people with disabilities to work. A comparison study should be done using a nationally representative sample of veterans with and without disabilities. The rating criteria could be adjusted accordingly to achieve vertical equity (i.e., the higher the rating, the lower the earnings on average) and horizontal equity (i.e., average earnings at any given rating level are the same across conditions).

Recommendation 4-2. VA should regularly conduct research on the ability of the Rating Schedule to predict actual loss in earnings. The accuracy of the Rating Schedule to predict such losses should be evaluated using the criteria of horizontal and vertical equity.

Recommendation 4-3. VA should conduct research to determine if inclusion of factors in addition to medical impairment, such as age, education, and work experience, improves the ability of the Rating Schedule to predict actual losses in earnings.

Recommendation 4-4. VA should regularly use the results from research on the ability of the Rating Schedule to predict actual losses in earnings to revise the rating system, either by changing the rating criteria in the Rating Schedule or by adjusting the amounts of compensation associated with each rating degree.

Revising the Rating Schedule to Improve the Relationship Between Ratings and Limitations on Ability to Engage in Usual Life Activities

The lives of veterans with service-connected injuries and diseases can be changed in many ways from what their lives might have been had they not become limited by the effects of those injuries or diseases, which can affect even those veterans who can work. It is possible that the Rating Schedule, when updated, will compensate for consequences in addition to work disability even though it is intended to compensate for loss of earning capacity. This is an empirical question that VA should address by developing a functional limitation scale (or adapting an existing scale) to a sample of veterans with and without disabilities, and determining if it would lead to different ratings than would the Rating Schedule. If it is found that functional measures capture disability not captured by the Rating Schedule, VA should decide how to compensate for it.

Recommendation 4-5. VA should compensate for nonwork disability, defined as functional limitations on usual life activities, to the extent that the Rating Schedule does not, either by modifying the Rating Schedule criteria to take account of the degree of functional limitation or by developing a separate mechanism.

Revising the Rating Schedule to Improve the Relationship Between Ratings and Losses in Quality of Life

The purpose of the current Rating Schedule is to compensate for work disability, not for losses in quality of life. Therefore, it is likely that the relationship between ratings under the current Rating Schedule and the QOL measures are not particularly close, which creates an empirical question that should be addressed. If research shows a disparity between the Rating Schedule and loss of QOL measures, VA should develop a way to compensate for the loss not compensated by the Rating Schedule. This could be done by adapting the Rating Schedule to be used for both work disability and loss in quality of life, or there could be separate Rating Schedules for these two consequences of service-related injuries and diseases.

Recommendation 4-6. VA should determine the feasibility of compensating for loss of quality of life by developing a tool for measuring quality of life validly and reliably in the veteran population, conducting research on the extent to which the Rating Schedule already accounts for loss in quality of life, and if it does not, developing a procedure for evaluating and rating loss of quality of life of veterans with disabilities.

THE MEDICAL EXAMINATION AND DISABILITY RATING PROCESS

Medical Evaluation Process

Nearly every veteran applying for disability compensation is examined by a physician or other clinician (e.g., audiologist) working for or under contract to VA. Investigations of the claims process in the 1990s showed that incompleteness and lateness of such compensation and pension (C&P) examinations were a serious problem. The Veterans Benefits Administration (VBA) and the Veterans Health Administration (VHA) have worked to improve this process, but more needs to be done and stronger measures need to be taken to implement the improved procedures that have been developed.

Need for Regular Updating of Examination Worksheets/Templates

VA does not systematically update the C&P examination worksheets and some—developed as long ago as 10 years—are seriously out of date.

Recommendation 5-1. VA should develop a process for periodic updating of the disability examination worksheets. This process should be

part of, or closely linked to, the process recommended above for updating and revising the Schedule for Rating Disabilities. There should be input from the disability advisory committee recommended above (see Recommendation 4-1).

Requiring the Use of the Examination Templates

Use of the worksheets is not required and many examiners do not use them. Use of the online templates has increased rapidly, presumably because of their ease of use. VA is considering a mandate that the latter be used, although that is not the case currently.

Recommendation 5-2. VA should mandate the use of the online templates that have been developed for conducting and reporting disability examinations.

Assessing and Improving Quality and Consistency of Examinations

Quality assurance of medical examinations and ratings currently is process oriented—meaning, focused on whether the information provided on the examination form was complete and timely, not whether it was correct. A sample of ratings is reviewed substantively, but the results are not systematically analyzed for general problems or consistency.

Recommendation 5-3. VA should establish a recurring assessment of the substantive quality and consistency, or inter-rater reliability, of examinations performed with the templates and, if the assessment finds problems, take steps to improve quality and consistency, for example, by revising the templates, changing the training, or adjusting the performance standards for examiners.

The Rating Process

Quality of Rating Decisions

VBA's quality assurance program, STAR, implemented in 1998, has improved the accuracy rate from 80 percent in FY 2002 to 88 percent in FY 2006. The sample is only large enough to determine the aggregate accuracy rate of regional offices. It does not assess accuracy at the body system or diagnostic code level, and it does not measure consistency across regional offices.

There are many sources of variability in decision making that, if not addressed and reduced to the extent possible, make it unlikely that veterans with similar disabilities are being treated similarly. Variability cannot be totally eliminated, but sources of variability that can be controlled, such as training, guidelines, and rater qualifications, should be addressed.

Recommendation 5-4. The rating process should have built-in checks or periodic evaluations to ensure inter-rater reliability as well as the accuracy and validity of rating across impairment categories, ratings, and regions.

Better Access to Medical Expertise

Few raters have medical backgrounds. They are required to review and assess medical evidence provided by treating physicians and VHA examining physicians and determine percentage of disability, but VBA does not have medical consultants or advisers to support the raters. Medical advisers would also improve the process of deciding what medical examinations and tests are needed to sufficiently prepare a case for rating.

Recommendation 5-5. VA raters should have ready access to qualified health-care experts who can provide advice on medical and psychological issues that arise during the rating process (e.g., interpreting evidence or assessing the need for additional examinations or diagnostic tests).

Medical consultants to adjudicators could come from VHA or outside contractors, or VBA could hire health-care providers as part of its own staff.

Training of Examiners and Adjudicators

VBA has a training program and is implementing a certification program for raters and, with VHA, is implementing a training and certification program for medical examiners. The training should be more intensive, and the training program should be rigorously evaluated.

Recommendation 5-6. Educational and training programs for VBA raters and VHA examiners should be developed, mandated, and uniformly implemented across all regional offices with standardized performance objectives and outcomes. These programs should make use of advances in adult education techniques. External consultants should serve as advisors to assist in the development and evaluation of the educational and training programs.

MEDICAL CRITERIA FOR ANCILLARY BENEFITS

Currently, VA requires a disability rating for access to other benefits that are meant to help a veteran realize his or her potential in civilian life. The process is not ideal, because it requires the veteran to establish his or her disability, which may take months or sometimes years, before he or she is eligible for benefits from available services—such as health care, vocational rehabilitation, and adaptive vehicles and housing—that could improve his or her economic situation and quality of life. There are also practical advantages to conducting a comprehensive evaluation of newly separating servicemembers that includes a determination of rehabilitation and vocational needs as well as compensation needs.

Recommendation 6-1. VA and the Department of Defense should conduct a comprehensive multidisciplinary medical, psychosocial, and vocational evaluation of each veteran applying for disability compensation at the time of service separation.

VA does not systematically assess the needs of veterans or evaluate its ancillary service programs. Many ancillary benefits, such as clothing allowances, automobile grants, and adaptive housing, arose piecemeal in response to circumstances of the time they were adopted. It might be that these programs could be changed to better serve veterans or that there are unaddressed needs. However, it is not possible to judge their appropriateness because the thresholds that have been set for ancillary benefits requirements were not based on research on who benefits or who benefits most from the services in terms of rating level.

Recommendation 6-2. VA should sponsor research on ancillary benefits and obtain input from veterans about their needs. Such research could include conducting intervention trials to determine the effectiveness of ancillary services in terms of increased functional capacity and enhanced health-related quality of life.

The current 12-year limit on eligibility for vocational rehabilitation services is a policy decision with no medical basis, although there may be administrative convenience or fiscal control reasons. There are types of employment and training requirements that do not realistically adhere to a 12-year deadline. For example, emerging assistive and workplace technologies (e.g., computing) may provide training or retraining opportunities for veterans with disabilities through continuing education of various kinds. New types of work may also emerge for which veterans with disabilities could be trained.

Recommendation 6-3. The concept underlying the extant 12-year limitation for vocational rehabilitation for service-connected veterans should be reviewed and, when appropriate, revised on the basis of current employment data, functional requirements, and individual vocational rehabilitation and medical needs.

The percentage of entitled veterans applying for vocational rehabilitation and employment (VR&E) services is relatively low. In FY 2005, about 40,000 veterans applied for VR&E services and were accepted. Of those deemed eligible, between a quarter and a third have not completed the program in recent years. VA should explore ways to increase participation in this program.

Recommendation 6-4. VA should develop and test incentive models that would promote vocational rehabilitation and return to gainful employment among veterans for whom this is a realistic goal.

INDIVIDUAL UNEMPLOYABILITY

Individual unemployability (IU) is a way for VA to compensate veterans at the 100 percent rate who are unable to work because of their service-connected disability, although their rating according to the Rating Schedule does not reach 100 percent. IU is based on an evaluation of the individual veteran's capacity to engage in a substantially gainful occupation, which is defined as the inability to earn more than the federal poverty level, rather than on the schedular evaluation, which is based on the average impairment of earnings concept.

Vocational Assessment in IU Evaluation

Currently, VA's policy is to consider vocational and other factors, but the process for obtaining and assessing vocational evaluations is weak. Raters have disability evaluation reports from medical professionals and other medical records to analyze, but they do not have comparable functional capacity or vocational evaluations from vocational experts. Raters must determine the veteran's ability to engage in normal work activities from medical reports and from information in the two-page application for IU and the one-page report from employers, neither of which asks about functional limitations. Raters do not receive training in vocational assessment.

Recommendation 7-1. In addition to medical evaluations by medical professionals, VA should require vocational assessment in the deter-

mination of eligibility for individual unemployability benefits. Raters should receive training on how to interpret findings from vocational assessments for the evaluation of individual unemployability claims.

IU Eligibility Thresholds

Currently, to be eligible for IU, a veteran must have a rating of 60 percent for one impairment or 70 percent for more than one impairment, as long as one of them is rated 40 percent. The basis for these threshold percentages is not known; they were adopted in 1941. Having a threshold makes obvious administrative sense, as long as it is not so high that many people with lower ratings who are legitimately unemployable are excluded. What that threshold should be, and the extent to which the current threshold requirements reflect actual unemployability, are not known.

Recommendation 7-2. VA should monitor and evaluate trends in its disability program and conduct research on employment among veterans with disabilities.

Age of IU Recipients

As noted in the discussion of ancillary benefits, VA does not systematically assess the economic situation of the veteran population and its needs. VA does not know, therefore, the reasons for the rapid increase in the number of IU beneficiaries, and whether it indicates a need to address special employment or medical needs of older veterans.

Recommendation 7-3. VA should conduct research on the earnings histories of veterans who initially applied for individual unemployability benefits past the normal age of retirement for benefits under the Old Age, Survivors, and Disability Insurance Program under the Social Security Act.

Factors Considered in IU Evaluation

Congress has made a policy decision not to put an age limit on eligibility for IU. It is true that individuals are able and willing to work, and do work, into their 70s and 80s, and they should not be barred from receiving IU if disability forces them to quit. But age should still be considered a factor contributing to unemployability, in conjunction with other vocational factors that also reduce an individual's likelihood of getting or keeping a job, such as minimal education, lack of skills, and employment history (e.g., manual labor).

Recommendation 7-4. Eligibility for individual unemployability should be based on the impacts of an individual's service-connected disabilities, in combination with education, employment history, and the medical effects of that individual's age on his or her potential employability.

Employment of IU Recipients

Under the current system, a veteran on IU is permitted to engage in substantially gainful employment for up to 12 months before IU benefits are terminated, after which his or her payments drop back to their scheduler rating of 60, 70, 80, or 90 percent. Disability compensation amounts do not increase in direct proportion to disability rating percentages. The largest dollar increase in payment is between the 90 percent ($1,483 per month) and 100 percent ($2,471 per month) rating, which means that a veteran terminated from IU after working a year will have his or her monthly payments drop by 40 to 64 percent, depending on the scheduler rating. This poses a sudden "cash cliff" that may deter some veterans from trying to reenter the workforce. Most cash support programs try to provide incentives to work by using some sort of sliding scale to ease the transition from being a beneficiary to being ineligible.

Recommendation 7-5. VA should implement a gradual reduction in compensation to individual unemployability recipients who are able to return to substantial gainful employment rather than abruptly terminate their disability payments at an arbitrary level of earnings.

OTHER DIAGNOSTIC CLASSIFICATION SYSTEMS AND RATING SCHEDULES

Alternative Diagnostic Classification Codes

Having the same diagnostic categories for the disability compensation program as VHA and other health-care providers—*International Classification of Diseases* (ICD) and *Diagnostic and Statistical Manual of Mental Disorders* (DSM)—would facilitate communication and understanding of a veteran's health problems. The rater would be better able to relate information in medical records to the Rating Schedule if the diagnostic categories were the same. It would also help the program keep up with advances in medical understanding, because the ICD and the DSM undergo regular revision and periodic comprehensive revisions. This would help avoid the present situation in which some currently identified conditions are not in the Rating Schedule. Another advantage of using ICD codes would be the reduction in the rate of use of analogous codes.

Use of common diagnostic categories also would allow VA program managers and researchers to compare populations and trends that would help in program planning and in epidemiological and health services research. VA's diagnostic codes are unique and do not allow comparisons of trends in disabilities in populations served by VHA or the Department of Defense or research normed to the veteran population.

Recommendation 8-1. VA should adopt a new classification system using the *International Classification of Diseases* (ICD) and the *Diagnostic and Statistical Manual of Mental Disorders* (DSM) codes. This system should apply to all applications, including those that are denied. During the transition to ICD and DSM codes, VA can continue to use its own diagnostic codes, and subsequently track and analyze them comparatively for trends affecting veterans and for program planning purposes. Knowledge of an applicant's ICD or DSM codes should help raters, especially with the task of properly categorizing conditions.

AMA *Guides* Impairment Rating System

The AMA *Guides to the Evaluation of Permanent Impairment* is superior to the current Rating Schedule in two important respects. The *Guides* uses current medical concepts, terminology, and tests, and is updated regularly; however, it is not designed to measure disability, only impairment, and it is also designed for use by physicians. The *Guides*, designed to measure degree of permanent impairment, not degree of ability to work (which is to be determined by government agencies or insurance companies), tends to have lower ratings than the Rating Schedule. The *Guides* do not determine percentage of impairment from mental disorders.

Recommendation 8-2. Considering some of the unique conditions relevant for disability following military activities, it would be preferable for VA to update and improve the Rating Schedule on a regular basis rather than adopt an impairment schedule developed for other purposes.

SERVICE CONNECTION ON AGGRAVATION AND SECONDARY BASES

Compensation for Aggravation of Preservice Disability and Allen Aggravation Claims

Determination of aggravation is an individualized clinical judgment.

Recommendation 9-1. VA should seek the judgment of qualified experts, supported by findings from current peer-reviewed literature, as guidance for adjudicating both aggravation of preservice disability and Allen aggravation claims. Judgment could be provided by VHA examiners, perhaps from VA centers of excellence, who have the appropriate expertise for evaluating the condition(s) in question in individual claims.

Secondary Service Connection

Like aggravation, secondary service connection involves individualized clinical judgment, but clinical judgment should be informed by the state of knowledge of causation in the condition being evaluated.

Recommendation 9-2. VA should guide clinical evaluation and rating of claims for secondary service connection by adopting specific criteria for determining causation, such as those cited above (e.g., temporal relationship, consistency of research findings, strength of association, specificity, plausible biological mechanism). VA should also provide and regularly update information to compensation and pension examiners about the findings of epidemiological, biostatistical, and disease mechanism research concerning the secondary consequences of disabilities prevalent among veterans.

CONCLUSION

Some important cross-cutting themes emerged from the committee's study. VA does not devote adequate resources to systematic analysis of how well it is providing its services (process analysis) or how much the lives of veterans are being improved (outcome analysis), the knowledge of which, in turn, would enable VA to improve the effectiveness and impacts of its benefit programs and services.

VBA does not have a program of research oriented toward understanding and improving the effectiveness of its benefit programs. Research efforts in the areas of applied process research, clinical outcomes, and economic outcomes should be undertaken.

VA is missing the opportunity to take a more veteran-centered approach to service provision across its benefits programs. VA has the services needed to maximize the potential of veterans with disabilities, but they are not actively coordinated and thus are not as effective as they could be. The disability compensation evaluation process provides an opportunity to assess the needs of veterans with disabilities for the other services VA provides, such as vocational rehabilitation, employment services, and specialized

BOX S-1
Summary of Tasks and Associated Recommendations

TASK 1. *How well do the medical criteria in the VA Rating Schedule and VA rating regulations enable assessment and adjudication of the proper levels of disability to compensate both for the impact on quality of life and impairment in earnings capacity? Provide an analysis of the descriptions associated with each condition's rating level that considers progression of severity of condition as it relates to quality-of-life impairment and impairment in average earnings capacity.*

Recommendation 3-1. The purpose of the current veterans disability compensation program as stated in statute currently is to compensate for average impairment in earning capacity, that is, work disability. This is an unduly restrictive rationale for the program and is inconsistent with current models of disability. The veterans disability compensation program should compensate for three consequences of service-connected injuries and diseases: work disability, loss of ability to engage in usual life activities other than work, and loss in quality of life. (Specific recommendations on approaches to evaluating each consequence of service-connected injuries and diseases are in Chapter 4.)

Recommendation 4-1. VA should immediately update the current Rating Schedule, beginning with those body systems that have gone the longest without a comprehensive update, and devise a system for keeping it up to date. VA should reestablish a disability advisory committee to advise on changes in the Rating Schedule.

Recommendation 4-2. VA should regularly conduct research on the ability of the Rating Schedule to predict actual loss in earnings. The accuracy of the Rating Schedule to predict such losses should be evaluated using the criteria of horizontal and vertical equity.

Recommendation 4-3. VA should conduct research to determine if inclusion of factors in addition to medical impairment, such as age, education, and work experience, improves the ability of the Rating Schedule to predict actual losses in earnings.

Recommendation 4-4. VA should regularly use the results from research on the ability of the Rating Schedule to predict actual losses in earnings to revise the rating system, either by changing the rating criteria in the Rating Schedule or by adjusting the amounts of compensation associated with each rating degree.

Recommendation 4-5. VA should compensate for nonwork disability, defined as functional limitations on usual life activities, to the extent that the Rating Schedule does not, either by modifying the Rating Schedule criteria to take account of the degree of functional limitation or by developing a separate mechanism.

Recommendation 4-6. VA should determine the feasibility of compensating for loss of quality of life by developing a tool for measuring quality of life validly and reliably in the veteran population, conducting research on the extent to which the Rating Schedule already accounts for loss in quality of life, and if it does not, developing a procedure for evaluating and rating loss of quality of life of veterans with disabilities.

TASK 2. *Certain criteria and/or levels of disability are required for entitlement to ancillary and special purpose benefits. To what extent, if any, do the required thresholds need to change? Determine from a medical perspective at what disability rating level a veteran's medical or vocational impairment caused by disability could be improved by various special benefits such as adapted housing, automobile grants, clothing allowance, and vocational rehabilitation. Consideration should be given to existing and additional benefits.*

Recommendation 6-1. VA and the Department of Defense should conduct a comprehensive multidisciplinary medical, psychosocial, and vocational evaluation of each veteran applying for disability compensation at the time of service separation.

Recommendation 6-2. VA should sponsor research on ancillary benefits and obtain input from veterans about their needs. Such research could include conducting intervention trials to determine the effectiveness of ancillary services in terms of increased functional capacity and enhanced health-related quality of life.

Recommendation 6-3. The concept underlying the extant 12-year limitation for vocational rehabilitation for service-connected veterans should be reviewed and, when appropriate, revised on the basis of current employment data, functional requirements, and individual vocational rehabilitation and medical needs.

Recommendation 6-4. VA should develop and test incentive models that would promote vocational rehabilitation and return to gainful employment among veterans for whom this is a realistic goal.

TASK 3. *Analyze the current application of the Individual Unemployability (IU) extra-schedular benefit to determine whether the VASRD descriptions need to more accurately reflect a veteran's ability to participate in the economic marketplace. Propose alternative medical approaches, if any, to IU that would more appropriately reflect individual circumstances in the determination of benefits. For the population of disabled veterans, analyze the cohort of IU recipients. Examine the base rating level to identify patterns. Determine if the VASRD description of conditions provide a barrier to assigning the base disability rating level commensurate with the veteran's vocational impairment.*

Recommendation 7-1. In addition to medical evaluations by medical professionals, VA should require vocational assessment in the determination of eligibility for individual unemployability benefits. Raters should receive training on how to interpret findings from vocational assessments for the evaluation of individual unemployability claims.

BOX S-1 Continued

Recommendation 7-2. VA should monitor and evaluate trends in its disability program and conduct research on employment among veterans with disabilities.

Recommendation 7-3. VA should conduct research on the earnings histories of veterans who initially applied for individual unemployability benefits past the normal age of retirement for benefits under the Old Age, Survivors, and Disability Insurance Program under the Social Security Act.

Recommendation 7-4. Eligibility for individual unemployability should be based on the impacts of an individual's service-connected disabilities, in combination with education, employment history, and the medical effects of that individual's age on his or her potential employability.

Recommendation 7-5. VA should implement a gradual reduction in compensation to individual unemployability recipients who are able to return to substantial gainful employment rather than abruptly terminate their disability payments at an arbitrary level of earnings.

TASK 4. *What are the advantages and disadvantages of adopting universal medical diagnostic codes rather than using a unique system? Compare and contrast the advantages/disadvantages of VA Schedule for Rating Disabilities and the* American Medical Association *Guides to the Evaluation of Permanent Impairment.*

Recommendation 8-1. VA should adopt a new classification system using the *International Classification of Diseases* (ICD) and the *Diagnostic and Statistical Manual of Mental Disorders* (DSM) codes. This system should apply to all applications, including those that are denied. During the transition to ICD and DSM codes, VA can continue to use its own diagnostic codes, and subsequently track and analyze them comparatively for trends affecting veterans and for program planning purposes. Knowledge of an applicant's ICD or DSM codes should help raters, especially with the task of properly categorizing conditions.

Recommendation 8-2. Considering some of the unique conditions relevant for disability following military activities, it would be preferable for VA to update and improve the Rating Schedule on a regular basis rather than adopt an impairment schedule developed for other purposes.

TASK 5. *From a medical perspective, analyze the current VA practice of assigning service connection on "secondary" and "aggravation" bases. In "secondary" claims, determine what medical principles and practices should be applied in determining whether a causal relationship exists between two conditions. In "aggravation" claims, determine what medical principles and practices should be applied in determining* *whether a preexisting disease was increased due to military service or was increased due to the natural process of the disease.*

Recommendation 9-1. VA should seek the judgment of qualified experts, supported by findings from current peer-reviewed literature, as guidance for adjudicating both aggravation of preservice disability and Allen aggravation claims. Judgment could be provided by VHA examiners, perhaps from VA centers of excellence, who have the appropriate expertise for evaluating the condition(s) in question in individual claims.

Recommendation 9-2. VA should guide clinical evaluation and rating of claims for secondary service connection by adopting specific criteria for determining causation, such as those cited above (e.g., temporal relationship, consistency of research findings, strength of association, specificity, plausible biological mechanism). VA should also provide and regularly update information to compensation and pension examiners about the findings of epidemiological, biostatistical, and disease mechanism research concerning the secondary consequences of disabilities prevalent among veterans.

TASK 6. *Compare and contrast the role of healthcare professionals in the claims/appeals process in VA and DoD, Social Security, and federal employee disability benefits programs. What skills, knowledge, training, and certification are required of the persons performing the examinations and assigning the ratings?*

Recommendation 5-1. VA should develop a process for periodic updating of the disability examination worksheets. This process should be part of, or closely linked to, the process recommended above for updating and revising the Schedule for Rating Disabilities. There should be input from the disability advisory committee recommended above (see Recommendation 4-1).

Recommendation 5-2. VA should mandate the use of the online templates that have been developed for conducting and reporting disability examinations.

Recommendation 5-3. VA should establish a recurring assessment of the substantive quality and consistency, or inter-rater reliability, of examinations performed with the templates and, if the assessment finds problems, take steps to improve quality and consistency, for example, by revising the templates, changing the training, or adjusting the performance standards for examiners.

Recommendation 5-4. The rating process should have built-in checks or periodic evaluations to ensure inter-rater reliability as well as the accuracy and validity of rating across impairment categories, ratings, and regions.

Recommendation 5-5. VA raters should have ready access to qualified health-care experts who can provide advice on medical and psychological issues that arise during the rating process (e.g., interpreting evidence or assessing the need for additional examinations or diagnostic tests).

BOX S-1 Continued

Recommendation 5-6. Educational and training programs for VBA raters and VHA examiners should be developed, mandated, and uniformly implemented across all regional offices with standardized performance objectives and outcomes. These programs should make use of advances in adult education techniques. External consultants should serve as advisors to assist in the development and evaluation of the educational and training programs.

Appendix D. The Role of Medical Personnel in Selected Disability Benefit Programs.

1

Introduction

The story of the Cuban missile crisis is well known. In the summer of 1962, in response to evidence of a significant increase in shipments from the Soviet Union to Cuba, President Kennedy ordered Air Force U-2 reconnaissance flights over Cuba. These reconnaissance missions produced evidence of ballistic missile and nuclear storage facility construction. On October 22, President Kennedy addressed the nation about the situation in Cuba and, in the end, the world breathed a long sigh of relief at the conclusion of the missile crisis, as a potentially catastrophic war was narrowly avoided.

Less well known, perhaps, is the personal story of Air Force Major Rudolph Anderson, one of the U-2 pilots who flew those reconnaissance missions. On October 27, five days after President Kennedy's address to the nation, Major Anderson flew yet another reconnaissance mission over Cuba. He died when his U-2 jet was shot down by a Soviet-supplied surface-to-air missile, and became the sole U.S. military casualty of the Cuban missile crisis.

The following day, in a personal letter to Major Anderson's widow, Frances, President Kennedy expressed his shock over the loss of her husband's life. The President described the kind of sacrifice Major Anderson made by giving his life in service to his country, and referred to it as "the source of our freedom." Kennedy went on to say, "On behalf of a grateful nation, I wish to convey to you and your children the sincere gratitude of all the people."

Other presidents have used similar words on many occasions, dating back to the days of the Revolutionary War. However, in his letter to Mrs. Anderson, President Kennedy eloquently expressed the entire country's feeling of indebtedness to veterans and their families who sacrifice on behalf of our nation.

It is impossible to undertake any responsible assessment of a veterans assistance program without starting here—with an understanding and acknowledgment that these programs are but one way (and, sometimes, an inadequate way) that a "grateful nation" attempts to repay its indebtedness to those who serve in the military. Any judgment about how these programs perform has to be made through this lens. That is why any comparisons between the veterans disability compensation program and similar disability assistance programs (such as Social Security Disability Insurance, workers' compensation, or private disability retirement programs) are bound to fall short. The standard is just not the same.

Of course, this does not mean that the veterans disability compensation program is perfect or that it should not be held to high standards of performance. Careful and critical assessment of program performance is essential, but it has to be done within the context of the program's unique circumstances.

The following is how the Department of Veterans Affairs (VA), the government agency responsible for veterans programs, expresses the unique circumstances under which a "grateful nation" provides for its veterans (VA, 2006):

> For 230 years, Americans in uniform have set aside their personal aspirations and safety to procure and protect the freedoms established by the Founders of our great nation. Through their service, and, all too often, through their sacrifices, these brave men and women have earned the gratitude and respect of the entire nation.
>
> During the Civil War, President Abraham Lincoln affirmed our nation's commitment ". . . to care for him who shall have borne the battle, and for his widow and his orphan." His eloquent words endured from his century to ours and serve today as the motto of the Department of Veterans Affairs, the federal agency responsible for honoring our debt of gratitude to America's patriots.

PROJECT BACKGROUND

P.L. No. 108-136 (the National Defense Authorization Act of 2004) established the Veterans' Disability Benefits Commission to "carry out a study of the benefits under the laws of the United States that are provided to compensate and assist veterans and their survivors for disabilities and deaths attributable to military service." The law requires the commission to make recommendations to the president and to Congress about (1) the appropriateness of such benefits under the laws in effect on the date of the enactment of the act, (2) the appropriateness of the level of such benefits, and (3) the appropriate standard or standards for determining whether a disability or death of a veteran should be compensated.

The law also requires the commission, in its report, to include an evaluation and assessment of the following:

- the laws and regulations that determine eligibility for disability and death benefits and other assistance for veterans and their survivors;
- the rates of such compensation, including the appropriateness of a schedule for rating disabilities based on average impairment of earning capacity; and
- comparable disability benefits provided to individuals by the federal government, state governments, and the private sector.

In carrying out these tasks, the commission developed a comprehensive set of research questions for study in determining whether the current disability compensation design is appropriate or whether more appropriate alternatives exist. As required by its statutory mandate, the commission consulted with the Institute of Medicine (IOM) on those research questions relating to the medical aspects of contemporary disability compensation policies.

The commission asked IOM to convene two committees of experts to address the following six tasks (with one committee addressing tasks 1 through 5 and the other addressing task 6):

1. Conduct a comprehensive review of VA's "Schedule for Rating Disabilities" (the "Rating Schedule"). Assess whether the schedule is an appropriate, valid, and reliable instrument for evaluating medical impairment and determining degree of disability.
2. Examine adequacy and appropriateness of medical criteria used to qualify veterans for special purpose and ancillary benefits including individual unemployability (IU).
3. Determine if the methods for determining and coding impairments and the methods for determining their severity are medically sound for single and multiple conditions.
4. Assess the medical criteria currently used to qualify veterans for secondary and aggravated service-connected conditions and how to measure and control for the effect of natural disease progression.
5. Assess how medical expertise is used to evaluate veterans throughout the claims process. Comment on the appropriateness of medical credentials and training requirements needed to support the disability evaluation and rating process.
6. Review the current scientific methodology used to support pre-

sumptive compensation decisions. Suggest alternate models that better leverage scientific knowledge for these decisions.

In response to the request, IOM formed the Committee on Evaluation of the Presumptive Disability Decision-Making Process for Veterans to address task 6. That committee's report will be issued separately.

IOM also formed the Committee on Medical Evaluation of Veterans for Disability Compensation (hereafter referred to simply as "the committee") to respond to tasks 1 through 5. The remainder of this report provides the findings, conclusions, and recommendations of that committee.

The committee consists of 16 experts representing disciplines of particular relevance to these tasks, as specified by the commission, including experts in clinical medicine, mental health, disability medicine, legal medicine (disability), physical rehabilitation, private-sector disability programs, veteran health compensation policy, and the veterans health system. In addressing these five tasks, the committee considered specific questions posed for it by the commission. (The original five tasks evolved into six specific study questions, with the exception of task 2, which produced two separate study questions):

- How well do the medical criteria in the Rating Schedule and VA rating regulations enable the assessment and adjudication of the proper levels of disability to compensate both for the impact on quality of life and impairment in earnings capacity? Provide an analysis of the descriptions associated with each condition's rating level that considers progression of severity of condition as it relates to quality-of-life impairment and impairment in average earnings capacity.
- Certain criteria and/or levels of disability are required for entitlement to ancillary and special-purpose benefits. To what extent, if any, do the required thresholds need to change? Determine from a medical perspective at what disability rating level a veteran's medical or vocational impairment caused by disability could be improved by various special benefits (such as adapted housing, automobile grants, clothing allowance, and vocational rehabilitation). Consideration should be given to existing and additional benefits.
- Analyze the current application of the IU benefit to determine whether the Rating Schedule descriptions need to more accurately reflect a veteran's ability to participate in the economic marketplace. For the population of veterans with disabilities, analyze the cohort that has been rated as being unemployable. Examine the base rating level to identify patterns. Determine if the Rating Schedule description of the condition provides a barrier to assigning the base disability rating level commensurate with the veteran's true vocational condition.

- What are the advantages and disadvantages of adopting universal medical diagnostic codes rather than using a unique system? Compare and contrast the advantages and disadvantages of the Rating Schedule and the American Medical Association *Guides to the Evaluation of Permanent Impairment* (AMA *Guides*).
- From a medical perspective, analyze the current VA practice of assigning service connection on "secondary" and "aggravation" bases. In secondary claims, determine what medical principles and practices should be applied in determining whether a causal relationship exists between two conditions. In aggravation claims, determine what medical principles and practices should be applied in determining whether a preexisting disease was increased because of military service or was increased because of the natural process of the disease.
- Compare and contrast the role of medical clinicians in the claims and appeals processes in VA and the Department of Defense (DoD), in Social Security, and in the various federal employee disability benefits programs.

The committee met five times between May 25, 2006, and January 8, 2007. Three of these meetings included sessions open to the public, and the committee heard from a wide range of individuals and organizations with interest or expertise in veterans health and disability, as well as experts in measurement of disability and quality of life.

In addition, members of the committee and staff visited several VA regional offices and a VA medical center to observe compensation claims processing. They spoke with a variety of individuals, including regional office directors and assistant directors, clinicians, veterans service representatives, rating veterans service representatives, and decision review officers.

Agencies, organizations, and other groups who provided data, other information, and statements to the committee included the following (in alphabetical order):

- African American PTSD Association
- American Legion
- American Medical Association
- American Psychiatric Association
- Board of Veterans Appeals
- Department of Veterans Affairs
- Disabled American Veterans
- Missouri Veterans Commission
- Navy Physical Evaluation Board
- Office of the Secretary of Defense

- Veterans' Disability Benefits Commission
- Veterans of Foreign Wars, National Veterans Service
- Vietnam Veterans of America

BRIEF OVERVIEW OF THE VETERANS DISABILITY COMPENSATION PROGRAM

VA administers federal veterans assistance programs. Generally, a veteran must have been discharged from active military service under other than dishonorable conditions to qualify for assistance. Veterans benefits include, but are not limited to

- health care;
- compensation for service-connected disabilities;
- assistive devices and special benefits for service-connected disabilities;
- disability pension;
- education and training;
- vocational rehabilitation;
- home loan guaranty;
- life insurance; and
- burial and memorial benefits.

A variety of stakeholders are involved in these veterans benefit programs, with separate, but interrelated, roles and interests. These include the following:

- Veterans and their dependents and survivors—These are the recipients of veterans benefits, as well as other veterans, dependents, and survivors who wish to receive benefits, but who do not qualify.
- Members of the general public—The public, which funds these programs through the taxes they pay, have a keen interest in ensuring that these programs are efficient, effective, fair, and accurate.
- The legislative branch of the U.S. government—Congress makes the laws that authorize payment of veterans benefits and prescribe the overall program structure.
- The executive branch of the U.S. government—Under the direction of the president, VA administers these programs.
- The judicial branch of the U.S. government—The Court of Appeals for Veterans Claims has jurisdiction over appeals of VA decisions.
- Providers of health-care services to veterans and their families within the VA hospitals and clinics
- Evaluators of impairment and disability (physicians and others)
- VA raters (interpreters of the regulations governing disability)

- Those within VA who resolve the disputes that may arise concerning presence or absence of disability and its extent
- Veterans service organizations and other advocacy groups—Veterans service organizations include groups chartered by Congress or recognized by VA for purposes of representing veterans in claims (such as the American Legion, Vietnam Veterans of America, Veterans of Foreign Wars, Paralyzed Veterans of America, and Disabled American Veterans) and other non-chartered groups. These also include state and local veterans service organizations.

The VA disability compensation program (which is described in much greater detail later in this report) provides a monthly, tax-exempt, cash payment to veterans who are disabled due to an illness or injury that is "service-connected." A disability is "service-connected" if the particular illness or injury that results in disability was incurred while the individual was on active duty in the armed forces of the United States, or if a preexisting illness or injury was made worse (aggravated) during active duty service. A disability is also service connected if, although it was not incurred during active duty service, it was nevertheless either caused or made worse by another service-connected disability (i.e., it is a "secondary" disability).

Determining whether a disability was incurred while an individual was on active duty (i.e., a direct service connection) is relatively straightforward. If a veteran's illness or injury causes disability and it was coincident with (i.e., it occurred or began during) active duty, then direct service connection is established. The concept of "incurred while/during" active duty should not be confused with the medical concept of "caused by." The subtle difference is intentional and undoubtedly represents a manifestation of the nation's gratitude explained earlier. "Incurred while" is an assumption of national responsibility for the risks accepted during service.

Establishing service connection based on aggravation of a preexisting condition or based on a secondary disability is more complex. In the case of a secondary disability, there must be a causal relationship between the veteran's current (secondary) disability and another (primary) service-connected disability. In the case of aggravation of a preexisting condition, service connection is established when there is an increase in disability (i.e., a worsening of the preexisting condition) during the service that is not caused by natural progression of the condition. However, VA applies a presumption of aggravation "unless there is a specific finding that the increase in disability is due to the natural progress of the disease."[1] Such determinations require complex medical judgments, which gave rise to task 4 of the commission's request to IOM, which is concerned with the

[1] 38 CFR 3.306(a).

medical principles and practices that should apply when evaluating secondary or aggravation cases. These issues are discussed in detail in Chapter 9 of this report.

These monthly cash payments are intended to compensate veterans for the loss of earning capacity that results from the disability. However, the amount of compensation is not based on the specific veteran's actual loss of earnings. Rather, it is based on the "average" impairment in earning capacity caused by the disability. Further, although not explicit in the law, the legislative history of the VA disability compensation program is believed to include an implicit congressional intent to compensate veterans for non-economic losses, such as loss or loss of use of a limb or organ that may not affect ability to work but reduces the quality of life of the veteran (VA, 2004).

The amount of compensation is set by law, based on a percentage disability rating (from 0 to 100 percent, in increments of 10 percent). The percentage rating is determined according to the Rating Schedule, which is intended to reflect the relative severity of the disability, meaning impairment of earning capacity. However, there are persistent questions about the extent to which the Rating Schedule compensates for impairment of average earning capacity. As one obvious example, although the disability ratings increase in 10 percent increments, the associated dollar payments do not. There are additional questions. According to the Government Accountability Office, the last comprehensive review of the validity of the Rating Schedule as a measure of loss of earning capacity was performed in the early 1970s (VA, 1971). It measured the difference between the earning capacity of veterans with disabilities and the earnings of veterans without disabilities, controlling for age, education, and region of residence. Of the approximately 700 diagnostic codes studied, almost half (330) overestimated loss of earning capacity and more than 10 percent (75) underestimated loss of earning capacity (GAO, 1997). Given the additional 35 years of medical, social, technological, occupational, and economic changes that have transpired since that study was conducted, one would expect the correlation between the Rating Schedule and actual economic loss to be even more tenuous today. In addition, there has never been a study of the extent to which the Rating Schedule compensates for reduction in quality of life. These issues, which correspond to the commission's task 1, are discussed in detail in Chapter 4 of this report.

When a veteran files a claim for disability compensation (see Figure 1-1 for an overview of the claims application and development process), the disability rating is made by a rating veterans service representative (RVSR) working on a rating team. RVSRs are nonmedical personnel who review veterans' medical records and apply the Rating Schedule based on those records. Generally, an applicant's claim file will include a compensation and pension examination, conducted either by medical personnel at a VA medi-

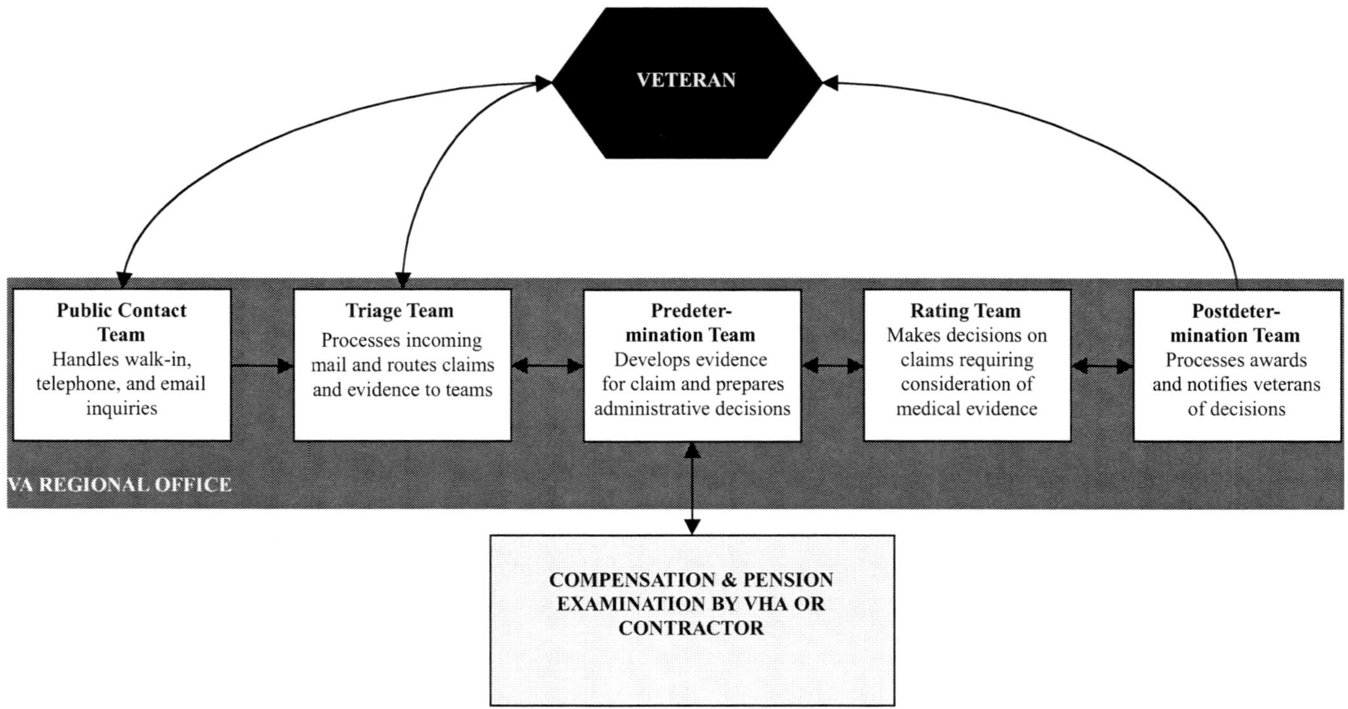

FIGURE 1-1 VA claims application and development process.
NOTE: This process is likely to vary somewhat among regional offices.

cal facility or by a contract examination provider using VA's examination protocols. However, physicians or other health-care professionals are not directly involved in making the rating decisions. Health-care professionals' involvement is generally limited to the examination component of the claim process and, on occasion, to providing opinions on such issues as whether an impairment occurred or was aggravated during service or is a secondary consequence of a service-connected condition. Health-care professionals are not asked for their judgment on the degree of disability resulting from an impairment, and they are not available to advise raters on the meaning of medical evidence while they are deciding a case.

In 2006, Veterans Benefits Administration (VBA) regional offices received over 654,000 claims for disability compensation.[2] Just over 81 percent of these were reopened claims (claims that were initially denied or where the veteran was not satisfied with the disability rating) and the rest were original claims. VBA made decisions on 628,000 claims.[3] It took an average of 177 days to process claims requiring compensation and pension examinations.[4]

A veteran who is dissatisfied with his or her rating decision may file an appeal (see Figure 1-2 for an overview of the appeal process) with the local

[2]FY 2007 budget request for 2000 and 2005 actuals (p. 3D-4), and FY 2008 for 2006 actual and 2007 and 2008 estimates (p. 6B-4) and for 2000–2005 actuals (rounded to nearest 1,000) (p. 6B7).

[3]GAO-07-512T, March 7, 2007:4, for FY 2000–FY 2006.

[4]The average elapsed time (in days) it takes to complete claims that require a disability decision is measured from the date the claim is received by the regional office (RO) to the date the decision is made by the RO, including the following types of claims: original compensation, with 1–7 issues (end product [EP] 110), original compensation, 8 or more issues (EP 010), original service-connected death claims (EP 140), and reopened compensation claims (EP 020).

FIGURE 1-2 VA appeal process. (on facing page)
*NOTE: If a veteran is not satisfied with the decision, he or she can (1) reopen the claim with the regional office, (2) file a motion with the Board of Veterans Appeals (BVA) for reconsideration, (3) file a motion with BVA because there was clear and unmistakable error in BVA's initial decision, or (4) file an appeal with the U.S. Court of Appeals for Veterans Claims.

- NOD (notice of disagreement): A written notice to the regional office that the veteran disagrees with the initial rating decision.
- SOC (statement of case): A detailed explanation of the evidence, laws, and regulations used by the regional office in deciding a claim.
- Form 9 (VA's Substantive Appeal form): A form on which the veteran indicates the benefit he or she wants, any mistakes found on the SOC, and a request for a personal hearing.
- DRO (decision review officer): A regional office staff member responsible for holding post-decisional hearings and processing appeals.

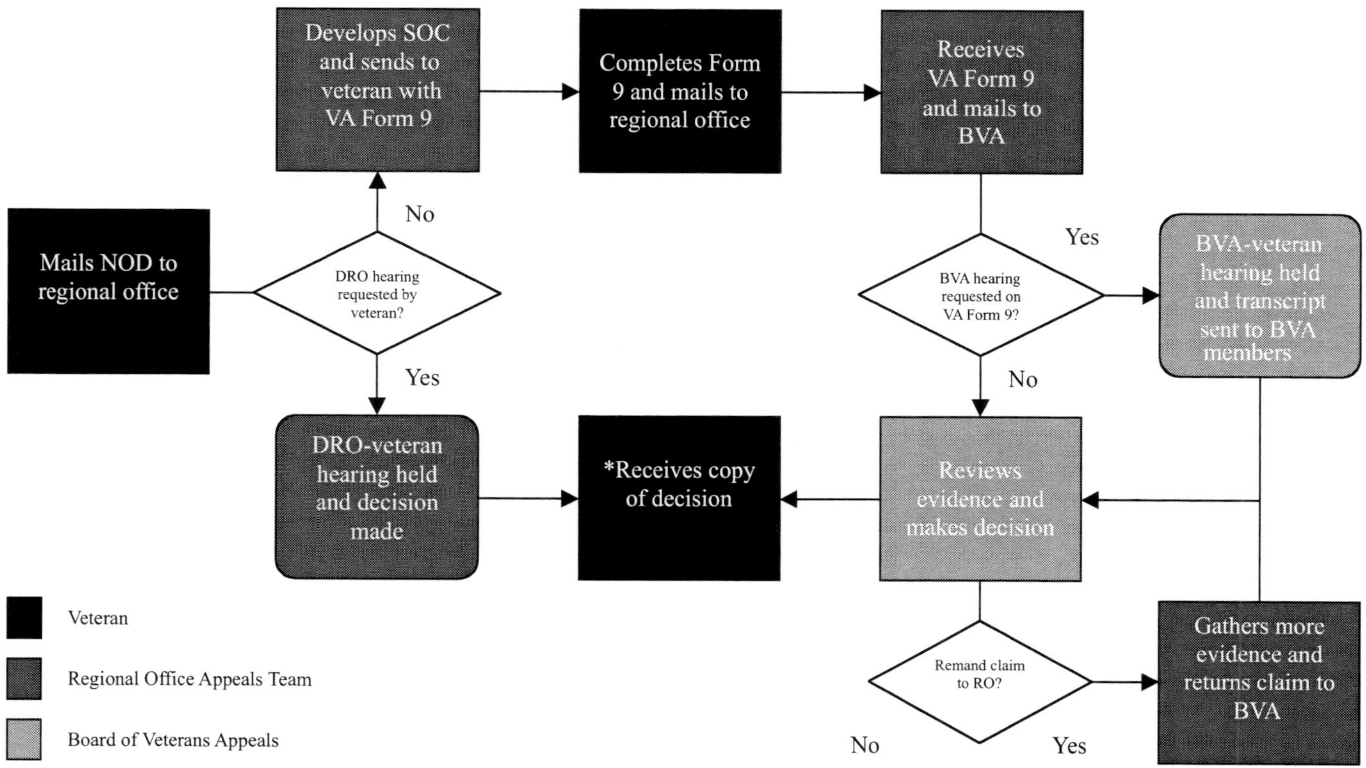
Mails NOD to regional office
DRO hearing requested by veteran?
No
Yes
Develops SOC and sends to veteran with VA Form 9
DRO-veteran hearing held and decision made
Completes Form 9 and mails to regional office
*Receives copy of decision
Receives VA Form 9 and mails to BVA
BVA hearing requested on VA Form 9?
Yes
No
BVA-veteran hearing held and transcript sent to BVA members
Reviews evidence and makes decision
Remand claim to RO?
No
Yes
Gathers more evidence and returns claim to BVA
Veteran
Regional Office Appeals Team
Board of Veterans Appeals

regional office. Members of an appeals team working at the regional office handle these cases. When a veteran requests an appeal, he or she has the option of having an informal hearing with a regional office staff member, called a Decision Review Officer (DRO), for reconsideration of the case. If the DRO decides that the reconsideration upholds the RO's initial decision, the appeal is moved forward for review by an administrative law judge on the Board of Veterans Appeals (BVA). Alternatively, a veteran may choose to skip the regional office hearing step and instead have a hearing with a BVA member, or have no hearing and let the claim go directly to BVA.

In 2006, VA received 101,240 appeals notices (notices of disagreement) and almost 12,000 BVA hearings were held. BVA made a total of 39,000 decisions on appeals. Of these, 19.3 percent were grants, 32 percent were remands, 46.3 percent were denials, and 2.4 percent were other dispositions. The appeals resolution time averaged 657 days.[5]

BVA may request a new medical examination or an independent medical opinion, but health professionals are not involved in making the appeal decision. The absence of direct involvement in the rating process by health-care professionals has raised concerns about the quality and accuracy of the assessments, particularly in cases that involve complex medical judgments (e.g., secondary and aggravation cases and multiple conditions, as discussed above). Such concerns are at the heart of the commission's task 5. Health-care professionals involved in the claims and appeals processes are discussed throughout the remainder of this report, particularly in Chapter 5 and Appendix D.

When a veteran is found to have a ratable disability, a diagnostic code is used to show the basis for the rating and for statistical analysis. These codes do not correspond to any widely used diagnostic coding system, such as the World Health Organization's *International Classification of Diseases* (ICD) or the American Psychiatric Association's *Diagnostic and Statistical Manual of Mental Disorders* (DSM). Adopting such a standardized coding system might help VA organize and analyze data for research, management, and policy development, and match and compare data across program agencies. However, changing to a new coding system could be difficult and costly.

Beyond the issue of impairment coding, there are also widely used and regularly updated disability rating systems, such as the AMA *Guides to the Evaluation of Permanent Impairment*, that could be used instead of the Rating Schedule and might provide for a more valid and reliable assessment process. However, changing over to such a system would be a significant departure from the current process and would require a major overhaul of the VA compensation claim system. These issues give rise to the commission's task 3, and they are addressed in detail in Chapter 8 of this report.

[5]IOM analysis of BVA data.

In addition to regular monthly compensation payments, veterans can also qualify for additional special-purpose and ancillary benefits, including vocational rehabilitation, specially adapted homes, automobile assistance, and clothing allowance. Eligibility for these benefits is based on meeting specific qualification criteria and/or disability rating levels. For example, to qualify for vocational rehabilitation and employment services, a veteran must have a service-connected disability rated at (or likely to be rated at) 20 percent or more, as well as an "employment handicap."[6] To qualify for automobile assistance, a veteran must be rated totally and permanently disabled or have one of a specified list of service-connected impairments: loss or loss of use of one or both hands or feet; permanent impairment of vision of both eyes to a certain degree; or ankylosis of one or both knees, or one or both hips. The commission, as a part of task 2, asked IOM to evaluate whether the qualification criteria for ancillary benefits are appropriate or need to change. These issues are discussed in detail in Chapter 6 of this report.

A veteran with a rating of at least 60 percent for a single disability or 70 percent for a combination of disabilities (provided that one of the disabilities is rated at least 40 percent) can qualify for a 100 percent disability rating and compensation if he or she is unable to secure or retain employment because of the service-connected disabilities. This is known as "individual unemployability" (IU), which is considered to be one of the most controversial of the additional benefits because (1) an IU rating decision is based on an individualized assessment of the applicant's vocational capacity rather than on the standard Rating Schedule concept of average impairment of earning capacity, and (2) the number of veterans granted IU has more than doubled between 2000 and 2006.

Generally (as noted above), the percentage disability rating is based on *average* impairment of earning capacity—not on any specific veteran's actual loss of earning capacity. Consequently, some veterans who have a particular medical condition or conditions that warrant less than a 100 percent rating nevertheless may be totally precluded from engaging in employment because of the actual effects of the condition or conditions. IU allows such an individual to be compensated at 100 percent if he or she is "unable to secure or follow a substantially gainful occupation as a result of service-connected disabilities."[7] Concerns have been raised about a dramatic increase in the number of veterans receiving IU, including a high percentage of individuals receiving the benefit who are beyond the normal age of retirement. There are also concerns about the extent to which the

[6]Employment handicap is defined at 38 CFR § 21.51. The term means an impairment of the veteran's ability to prepare for, obtain, or retain employment consistent with the veteran's abilities, aptitudes, and interests.

[7]38 CFR § 4.16(a).

benefit encourages veterans to return to productive employment through vocational rehabilitation. The IU benefit is also a subject of the commission's task 2, and is addressed in detail in Chapter 7 of this report.

To carry out its work, the committee reviewed known historical and current evidence, including detailed information on the Rating Schedule updates that have been carried out since 1945, and heard from numerous experts in the relevant subject areas. Many committee members visited regional offices in different parts of the country to try to better understand firsthand the operations of the current system, particularly the handling of claims as related to the medical questions they had been asked to address. After carefully considering this body of information, committee members put a great deal of thought into possible scenarios that might more optimally employ the structure of or improve the current system. They discussed possible alternatives to the current system as part of their effort to bring this system into the 21st century, and recommended ways both to enhance the system and to approach future research with an eye on making improvements.

The committee's report characterizes veterans with disabilities in the 21st century (Chapter 2); defines veterans disability (Chapter 3); describes the Rating Schedule's history and current structure (Chapter 4) and the evaluation process (Chapter 5); discusses medical criteria for ancillary benefits (Chapter 6), individual unemployability (Chapter 7), the potential role of other diagnostic classifications (e.g., the ICD and the DSM) and rating schedules (e.g., the AMA *Guides*) (Chapter 8), and service connection on aggravation and secondary bases (Chapter 9); and offers suggestions for building a 21st century disability evaluation system (Chapter 10). Appendix C contains the paper "The Relationship between Impairments and Earnings Losses in Multicondition Studies," which is strategic to part of Chapter 4's discussions. Appendix D compares the role of medical personnel in various disability benefits programs. Acronyms are provided at the front of the report, and the committee charge is found in Appendix B to assist the reader in following the text more easily and in understanding the committee's responses to the tasks assigned by the commission. Appendix A provides biographical sketches of committee members, consultants, and staff.

REFERENCES

GAO (Government Accountability Office). 1997. *VA disability compensation: Disability ratings may not reflect veterans' economic losses*. GAO/HEHS-97-9. http://www.gao.gov/archive/1997/he97009.pdf (accessed February 20, 2007).

VA (Department of Veterans Affairs). 1971. Economic validation of the Rating Schedule. In *Veterans Administration proposed revision of Schedule for Rating Disabilities*. Submitted to the Committee on Veterans' Affairs, U.S. Senate, 93rd Cong., 1st Sess., February 12. Senate Committee Print No. 3. Washington, DC: U.S. Government Printing Office.

VA. 2004. *VA disability compensation program legislative history.* http://www.1888932-2946.ws/vetscommission/e-documentmanager/gallery/Documents/Reference_Materials/LegislativeHistory_12-2004.pdf (accessed February 10, 2007).

VA. 2006. *Federal benefits for veterans and dependents.* http://www.va.gov/opa/vadocs/fedben_pt1.pdf (accessed February 10, 2007).

2

Veterans with Disabilities in the 21st Century

An effective medical evaluation system for a veterans disability compensation program depends in part on the purpose of the program, which is addressed in Chapter 3. The effectiveness of such a system also depends in part on the volume of claims and the types of impairments for which veterans are likely to seek compensation.

The numbers and types of claims submitted to the Department of Veterans Affairs (VA) for disability compensation depend on a number of variables, some of which are demographic. According to the VA secretary, "The number of active duty servicemembers as well as reservists and National Guard members who have been called to active duty to support Operation Enduring Freedom [OEF] and Operation Iraqi Freedom [OIF] is one of the key drivers of new claims activity" (U.S. Congress, House of Representatives, Committee on Veterans' Affairs, 2007a). The VA under secretary for benefits reported in March 2007 that nearly 1.46 million active duty servicemembers and reservists had been deployed to Afghanistan and Iraq, of whom more than 689,000 had returned and been discharged (U.S. Congress, House of Representatives, Committee on Veterans' Affairs, 2007c). Original (i.e., first-time) compensation claims have doubled in recent years from 112,000 in fiscal year (FY) 2000 to 217,000 in FY 2006 (VA, 2007a).

However, original claims constitute only a third of the claims. The remaining two-thirds of compensation claims made each year are from veterans previously determined to have a service-connected disability, most of them veterans of World War II, Korea, and Vietnam.[1] As the population of veterans ages, the Veterans Benefits Administration (VBA) can expect to see a growing percentage of claims for worsening chronic conditions, such as cardiovascular diseases, mental illnesses, and diabetes, and secondary conditions resulting from already service-connected disabilities.[2] This in turn has implications for VA's Schedule for Rating Disabilities (Rating Schedule) and the process for applying it in the rating process. VBA is already reporting higher rates of claims for complications of diabetes.[3] Often, these are more complex claims, requiring a determination that a new impairment, such as kidney or coronary heart disease, is as likely as not caused by the veteran's service-connected diabetes, an issue that is addressed more fully in Chapter 9. If the incidence of a particular condition is likely to increase substantially, VBA might want to review and, if warranted, update the criteria in the Rating Schedule, to ensure that appropriate specialists are available to conduct examinations, and to provide specialized training and information resources to the raters.

Similarly, if a war is under way, VBA can expect to see a new cohort of veterans with wounds and other injuries and diseases encountered in wartime situations. As protective equipment, frontline emergency medicine, and medical evacuation techniques improve, more seriously injured servicemembers will survive at a higher rate. For example, the average time to evacuate a wounded servicemember from the battlefield to stateside care is 3 days, compared with 10 to 14 days during the Persian Gulf War in 1991 and 45 days during the Vietnam War (U.S. Congress, Senate, Defense Appropriations Subcommittee, 2007).

The ratio of wounded to killed in the current wars in Iraq and Afghanistan is 9.1 to 1, compared with 3.2 to 1 in Vietnam and 2.3 to 1 in World War II.[4]

---

[1]According to data provided to the committee by VA, nearly half (48 percent) of the 926,000 service-connected disabilities considered for higher ratings during calendar years 2004–2006 were from reopened claims of veterans of World War II, Korea, and Vietnam, and more than a third (36 percent) of the 4.3 million disabilities considered for service connection (i.e., claimed for the first time) during the same three-year time period were from veterans of the same three wars.

[2]It should be noted that members of the National Guard and reserves called up to serve in Afghanistan and Iraq who were once in the active services may have been granted service-connected disabilities earlier, and they would be considered reopened cases if they apply for injuries suffered during their current active service.

[3]According to VA's budget submission for FY 2008, "VA has started to see increasingly complex medical cases resulting in neuropathies, vision problems, cardiovascular problems, and other issues directly related to diabetes" (VA, 2007a). Nearly a quarter of the veterans currently receiving care from VA have diabetes (U.S. Congress, House of Representatives, Committee on Appropriations, 2007).

[4]Calculated from Department of Defense (DoD) tables (DoD, 2007b). The Iraq and Afghanistan figures are as of February 17, 2007.

The main cause of injury in Iraq has been blasts from roadside bombs, resulting in a characteristic or "signature" set of multi-system injuries likely to result in permanent severe impairments and functional limitations (Scott, 2005).[5] These include brain injury, blinding, hearing and vestibular impairment, nerve and organ damage, burns, and amputation of one or more extremities, some or all of which can happen to one person.[6] Some of these injuries are caused by bomb fragments and flying debris, but some are caused by overpressure from the blast wave. The latter injuries may not be as apparent, such as closed-head brain injury and internal lung and other organ damage. As a VA physician treating these injuries told the Veterans' Disability Benefits Commission, such impairments may be underestimated (Scott, 2005).[7] Given the unprecedented combination of severe injuries distinctive of combat in southwest Asia, VBA may want to reassess the ability of the Rating Schedule and rating process to evaluate blast injuries to the brain and other internal organs and to rate the disability caused by interaction of impairments in multiple body systems.

THE VETERAN POPULATION

There are approximately 24 million living veterans of active duty in the U.S. military. VA expects this number to fall to less than 15 million over the next 25 years, barring a large increase in troop levels (Figure 2-1).[8] As the number of veterans declines, the average age increases. The median age of veterans is 60 years, up from 57 as recently as 2000 (VA, 2001b, 2006b).

---

[5]As of February 10, 2007, 68 percent of the wounded in action in Iraq were injured by an improvised explosive device, landmine, or other explosive device (12,000 of the 18,000 for which the cause of injury was known) (DoD, 2007a).

[6]According to the director of the Polytrauma Rehabilitation Center at the Tampa VA medical center, "A typical patient has TBI [traumatic brain injury], vision and/or hearing loss, pain, wounds, burns and orthopedic problems (including amputations)" (U.S. Congress, House of Representatives, Committee on Veterans' Affairs, 2007b). A Veterans Health Administration handbook on polytrauma rehabilitation procedures notes that TBI often occurs with other injuries, "such as amputation, auditory and visual impairments, SCI [spinal cord injury], PTSD [posttraumatic stress disorder], and other mental health conditions" (VA, 2005a).

[7]The diagnosis of closed-head brain injuries from blasts is based on symptoms such as headaches, decreased memory, inability to concentrate, slower thinking, irritability, anger, depression, and other personality and behavioral changes (DVBIC, 2007). Of the first 433 traumatic brain injury patients seen at Walter Reed Army Medical Center between January 2003 and April 2005, 89 percent had closed-head brain injuries rather than penetrating wounds (Warden, 2006).

[8]Starting in 2008, the projection includes DoD estimates of separations from active duty forecast by the Office of the Actuary of the Department of Defense, based on an assumption that the size of the military will remain about 1.38 million. This projection of the actual number of servicemembers is very uncertain, because it depends on external events and advances in technology that cannot be predicted.

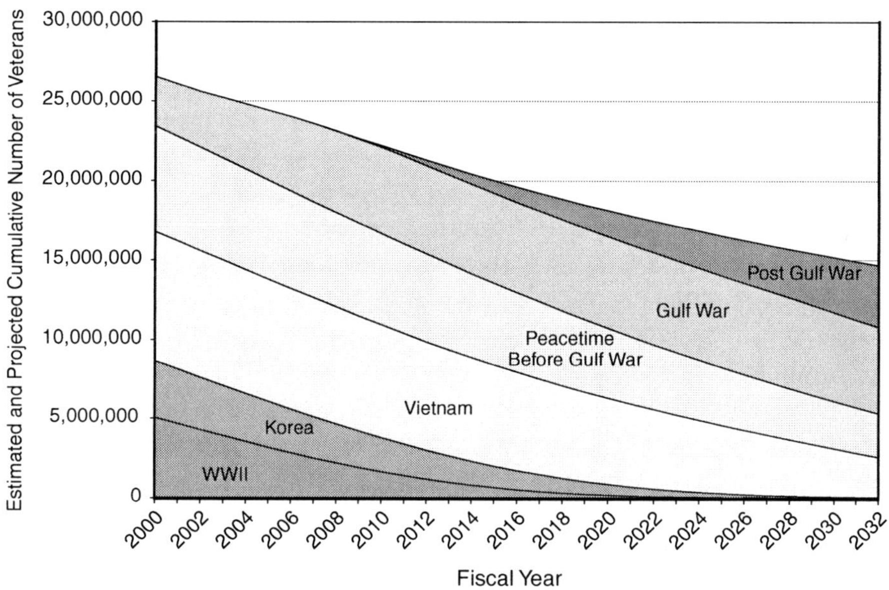

FIGURE 2-1 Estimated and projected cumulative number of veterans by period of service, FY 2000–FY 2032.
NOTES: Veterans of more than one period are counted in the latest period in which they served; for example, veterans who served in WWII, Korea, and Vietnam are counted as part of the Vietnam era service period. Gulf War includes veterans from the beginning of the first Gulf War in 1990 through 2007. Post Gulf War includes new veterans in 2008 and later. This means that individuals who served in OEF/OIF are counted as Gulf War veterans if they separate from service before 2008 and as Post Gulf War veterans if they separate in 2008 or later.
SOURCE: IOM (2007).

The number of veterans ages 65 and older is expected to increase in the near future but begin to decrease within 10 years, from 9.2 million in 2012 to 6.7 million in 2032. They will constitute a larger percentage of living veterans, however, increasing from 39 to 46 percent of the total between 2007 and 2017, before declining slightly to 45 percent in 2032 (Figure 2-2).

VA expects the percentage of women veterans to double during the next 25 years, from the current 7 percent to 14 percent in 2032. The percentage of non-Hispanic white veterans, currently 80 percent of living veterans, is projected to decrease to 71 percent by 2032. The percentages of Hispanic, non-Hispanic black, and other minority veterans would increase in the same time period, from 5 to 9 percent, 10 to 15 percent, and 3 to 5 percent, respectively (IOM, 2007).

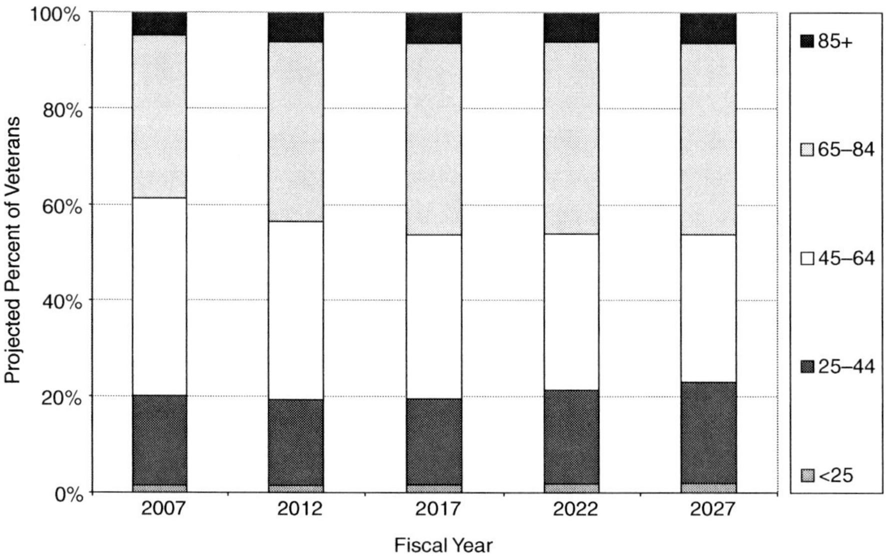

FIGURE 2-2 Projected percentages of veterans by age group, FY 2007–FY 2032.
SOURCE: IOM (2007).

VA does not forecast the number of veterans it expects to apply for or be granted disability benefits beyond the next few years, but experience has shown that more recent veterans tend to apply at higher rates, and that the percentage of veterans service connected for disability compensation has been increasing accordingly. Approximately 12 percent of the veterans who served during the Gulf War era (i.e., since August 1990) had been granted a service-connected disability rating when OEF was launched in Afghanistan in October 2001, compared with 9.5 percent of Vietnam era veterans and 10.4 percent of World War II veterans (VA, 2002). As of the end of May 2006, approximately 105,000 veterans of the current wars in Iraq and Afghanistan had been granted disability compensation—about 18 percent of those who had separated from service at that time (VA, 2006a).[9] Thus the number of veterans service connected for disability compensation is increasing, although the overall number of veterans is decreasing. In FY 2000, when there were 27 million veterans, 2.3 million were receiving disability compensation. The annual number of claims received for service-

[9]If the same percentage of the 34,000 claims then pending were granted compensation as the claims already processed, the percentage of veterans of Iraq and Afghanistan with service-connected disabilities would have been 24 percent.

connected compensation, which was 579,000 in FY 2000, reached 806,000 in FY 2006. In 2008, when VA estimates there will be 23 million veterans (13 percent fewer than in 2000), 2.9 million are expected to be receiving compensation (25 percent more than in 2000).

THE POPULATION OF VETERANS WITH DISABILITIES

In FY 2006, about 2.7 million veterans were receiving $26.5 billion monthly in disability compensation from VA. VA estimates that compensation payments to veterans will increase to about $32.4 billion in FY 2008, when there will be an estimated 2.9 million beneficiaries. Compensation per veteran is expected to average $11,258 in 2008, up from $9,864 in 2006 (VA, 2007a).[10]

Period of Service

Of the 2.3 million veterans with service-connected disabilities at the end of FY 2000, the largest group was Vietnam era veterans, followed by (in descending order) veterans serving in peacetime, World War II, the Gulf War, and the Korean conflict. This composition is expected to change substantially by 2008, when the number of Gulf War veterans is expected to have increased by 160 percent, while the number of World War II and Korean War veterans is expected to fall by 19 and 3 percent, respectively (Figure 2-3). As a result, Gulf War veterans will constitute 29 percent of service-connected beneficiaries in 2008, compared with 14 percent in 2000.

Age

In FY 2005, more than half of the 2.6 million veterans with service-connected disabilities were older than age 55 (Figure 2-4). Most of the rest were between ages 36 and 55. Only 8 percent were ages 35 or younger. The median age was 60 in FY 2006, compared with 59 in FY 2000 (VA, 2006b).

Disability Rating Levels

Each condition for which a veteran receives VA disability compensation is given a rating, expressed as a percentage between 0 and 100 in increments of 10; higher ratings are intended to reflect greater severity than lower

[10]This does not include ancillary benefits, as described in Chapter 6, for which veterans with service-connected disabilities may be eligible.

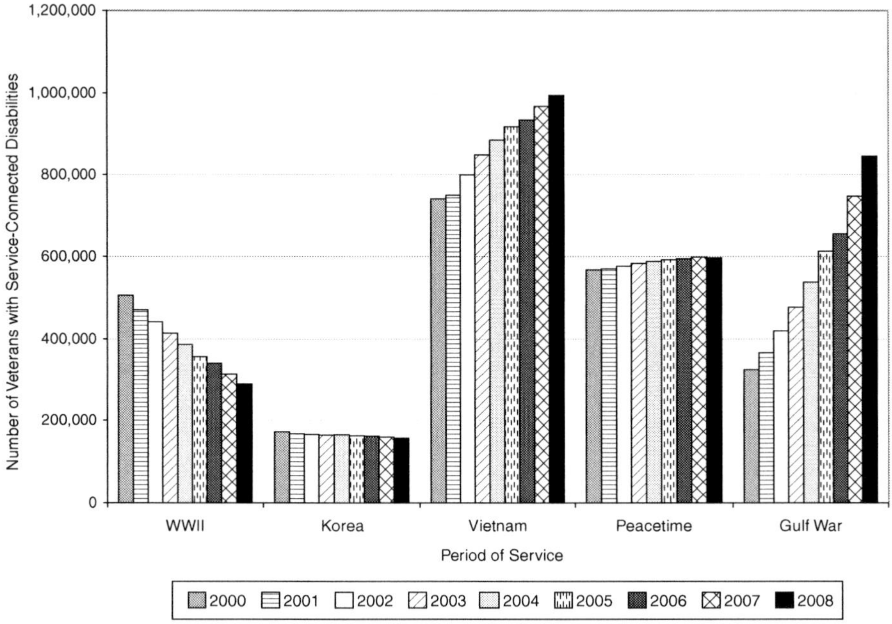

FIGURE 2-3 Number of veterans with service-connected disabilities, by period of service, FY 2000–FY 2008.
NOTE: Gulf War veterans are those who served on or since August 2, 1990, including veterans of OEF/OIF.
SOURCES: VA (2001b, 2002, 2003, 2004a, 2005b, 2006b, 2007a).

ratings. Conditions can be rated 0 percent when they have been determined by VA to be service connected and disabling, but not to the extent that they would affect an average veteran's ability to work.[11] If a veteran has more than one rated condition, VA calculates a combined percentage intended to represent the net impact of the multiple conditions on the veteran. For example, a 40 percent rating and a 20 percent rating result in a combined rating of 50 percent. The combined rating level determines the amount of monthly compensation. (The procedure for combining ratings is described in Chapter 4.)

[11]Technically, as will be explained in Chapter 3, veterans rated 0 percent disabled have minor impairments that are not considered to be disabling on average. For example, the most common impairments rated 0 percent are minor hearing loss, hemorrhoids, and scars. Similarly, someone who has lost both legs but is a successful lawyer or teacher is rated 100 percent for the severity of his or her impairment, rather than 0 percent for lack of disability.

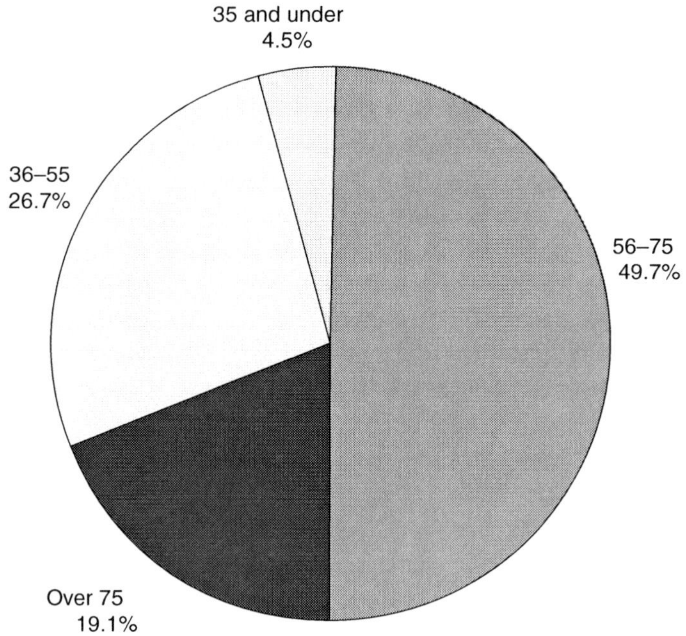

FIGURE 2-4 Veterans receiving disability benefits by age range, FY 2005 (percentages).
SOURCE: VA (2006b).

In FY 2005, veterans with disabilities were being compensated for approximately 7.7 million separate conditions that VA considered disabling, an average of about 3 each. The largest group of the 2.6 million veterans with disabilities had a combined rating of 10 percent (30 percent), followed by those with a 20 percent rating (15 percent). Fewer than 10 percent were rated totally (100 percent) disabled (Figure 2-5).

The distribution of rating levels by individual condition is quite different. Of the total of 7.7 million conditions, the largest number is rated 10 percent, followed by conditions rated at 0 percent. Only 3 percent are rated 100 percent (Figure 2-6).

The Most Prevalent Disabling Conditions

There are two ways to consider prevalence of disabilities, either by the major (i.e., highest-rated) condition of each individual veteran or by the

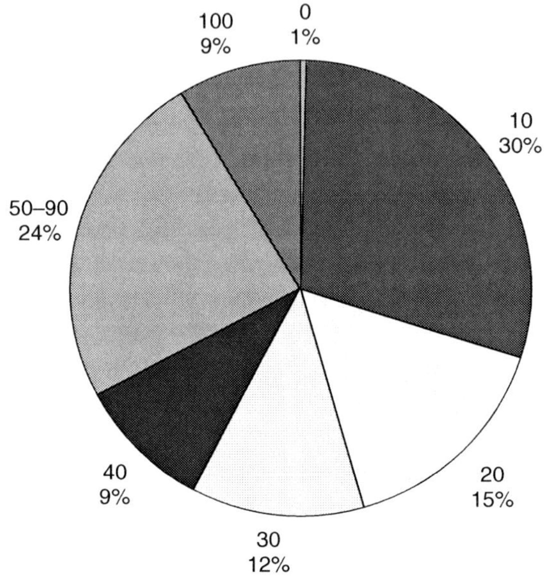

FIGURE 2-5 Veterans by combined rating level, FY 2005 (percentages).
SOURCE: VA (2006b).

7.7 million separate conditions the 2.7 individual veterans have among them. In FY 2005, posttraumatic stress disorder (PTSD) was the major diagnosis for the largest number of veterans, or 203,000, followed by diabetes mellitus and tinnitus, each with 102,000 (left half of Table 2-1).[12] PTSD, diabetes, and tinnitus together were the major diagnosis for 15 percent of service-connected veterans in FY 2005. The three conditions were much less prominent 10 years earlier, however, when they were ranked 9th, 22nd, and 14th, respectively, as major diagnoses, and accounted for less than 5 percent of the veterans with disabilities (VA, 1995). (In FY 1995, the three most prevalent major conditions were impairment of the knee other than ankylosis, generalized anxiety disorder, and lumbosacral strain,

[12]According to the American Tinnitus Association, tinnitus is "the perception of sound in the ears or head where no external source is present." Although often referred to as "ringing in the ears," some people with tinnitus hear hissing, roaring, whistling, chirping, or clicking. Both the volume and the continuity of the perceived sound varies from person to person with tinnitus (ATA, 2007).

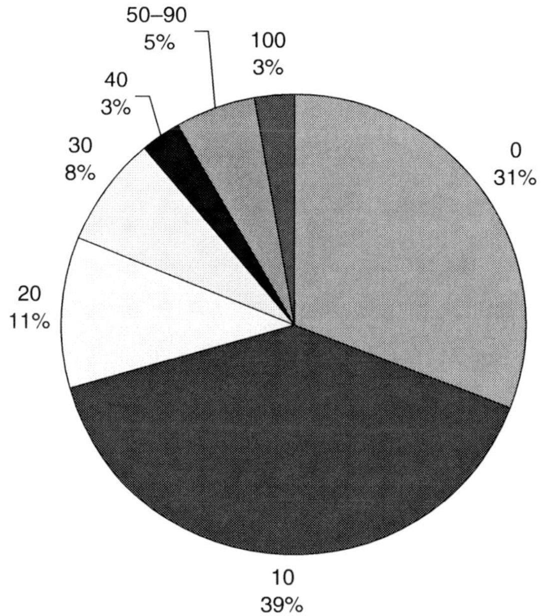

FIGURE 2-6 Disabling conditions by rating level, FY 2005 (percentages).
NOTE: These are the 7.7 million separate conditions for which the 2.7 million service-connected veterans have been rated.
SOURCE: Appendix Table 2-1.

which together accounted for 11 percent of veterans with disabilities at that time.)

The most numerous service-connected conditions in FY 2005 were defective hearing (354,000 ratings), tinnitus (340,000 ratings), and orthopedic conditions for which there was no diagnostic code (300,000 ratings); they were rated using the code for a similar, or "analogous," condition (right half of Table 2-1). These conditions ranked higher because they tend to have lower ratings such as 10 or 0 percent, and while many veterans have these lower ratings, they also have higher ratings for other conditions. For example, 354,000 veterans were rated for impaired hearing, but only 71,000 had it as their highest-rated condition.

Another point of comparison is the prevalence of the same conditions in the general population, although one should bear in mind that some or many veterans may have impairments (e.g., tinnitus, diabetes, PTSD) that are not service connected or for which, if service connected, applications for benefits have not been submitted, making the comparison inexact. The

TABLE 2-1 Number of Veterans and Number of Rated Conditions, by Diagnostic Code, End of FY 2005

	Number of Veterans by Major Condition		Number of Conditions Rated per Diagnostic Code	
Rank	Major Condition (Diagnostic Code)	Number of Veterans	Condition (Diagnostic Code)	Number of Conditions
1	PTSD (9411)	203,378	Defective hearing (6100–6110)	353,897
2	Diabetes mellitus (7913)	101,883	Tinnitus (6260)	339,573
3	Tinnitus (6260)	101,758	Analogous to an orthopedic diagnostic code (5299)	300,098
4	Knee, other impairment of (5257)	98,662	Scars, other (7805)	283,337
5	Arthritis, due to trauma (5010)	98,132	Arthritis, due to trauma (5010)	272,047
6	Intervertebral disc syndrome (5293)	86,469	PTSD (9411)	244,876
7	Analogous to an orthopedic diagnostic code (5299)	75,628	Knee, other impairment of (5257)	235,158
8	Sacroiliac injury and weakness (5295)	74,644	Diabetes mellitus (7913)	220,532
9	Defective hearing (6100–6110)	70,915	Hypertensive vascular disease (7101)	193,055
10	Hypertensive vascular disease (7101)	57,252	Arthritis, degenerative, hypertrophic, or osteoarthritis (5003)	162,004
	All diagnostic codes	2,636,979	All diagnostic codes	7,675,811

SOURCE: VA (2005c).

12-month prevalence of PTSD in U.S. adults ages 18 and older is estimated to be 3.5 percent (Kessler et al., 2005a). The estimated lifetime prevalence of PTSD is 6.8 percent (Kessler et al., 2005b). The baseline analysis of the Millennium Cohort found that the prevalence of PTSD among veterans was 2.4 percent, although it was between 3.5 and 3.8 percent among some subgroups—those without a high school diploma, ages 17–24, or who served

4 years or less (Riddle et al., 2007).[13] Recent studies have found higher rates of PTSD among OEF/OIF veterans, probably because of their younger age and other demographic risk factors, and because of greater exposure to combat and to dead and wounded servicemembers and civilians than the Millenium Cohort (Hoge et al., 2004; Seal et al., 2007).[14] The 245,000 veterans service connected for PTSD in 2005 constituted 1 percent of all veterans at that time (VA, 2006d).

The prevalence of diabetes among U.S. adults ages 20 and older is 9.6 percent (NIDDK, 2005). The 2001 National Survey of Veterans found that 11.2 percent of veterans in the sample were being treated for diabetes with insulin or diet (VA, 2001a:Table 5-16). The number of veterans service connected for diabetes in 2005 was 202,000, or 0.8 percent of all veterans (VA, 2006d).

Between 10 and 15 percent of U.S. adults have prolonged tinnitus requiring medical evaluation (Heller, 2003). In the 1994 National Health Interview Survey, 29 percent of veteran respondents reported having chronic (lasting three months or more) tinnitus, compared with 15 percent of non-veterans (Hoffman and Reed, 2004). The 340,000 veterans service connected for tinnitus constitute 1.4 percent of all veterans (VA, 2006d).

Conditions Rated 100 Percent

Three conditions are the major diagnosis for half the veterans rated 100 percent: PTSD (26 percent), schizophrenia (19 percent), and malignancies of the genitourinary system (e.g., prostate cancer) (5 percent) (Figure 2-7).

The major diagnoses most likely to be associated with combined ratings of 100 percent are relatively rare, except for loss of, or loss of use of, both feet. They include loss of, or loss of use of, two or more limbs; loss of, or blindness in, both eyes; renal diseases; certain cancers; and schizophrenia and other psychoses. All or nearly all veterans with these conditions as their major diagnosis are rated 100 percent.

Conditions by Period of Service

Prevalence and distribution of disabling conditions vary somewhat by service period, reflecting age and other differences, such as attitudes about

---

[13]The Millennium Cohort is a longitudinal study of the health effects of military service. It will follow more than 100,000 servicemembers for 22 years through 2025 using standardized instruments (Ryan et al., 2007).

[14]Hoge et al. surveyed members of four infantry units returning from Iraq and Afghanistan and found that 16–17 and 11 percent, respectively, met screening criteria for major depression, generalized anxiety, or PTSD. Seal et al. found that 25 percent of veterans of OEF/OIF seen at VA health-care facilities between 2001 and 2005 were diagnosed with mental disorders.

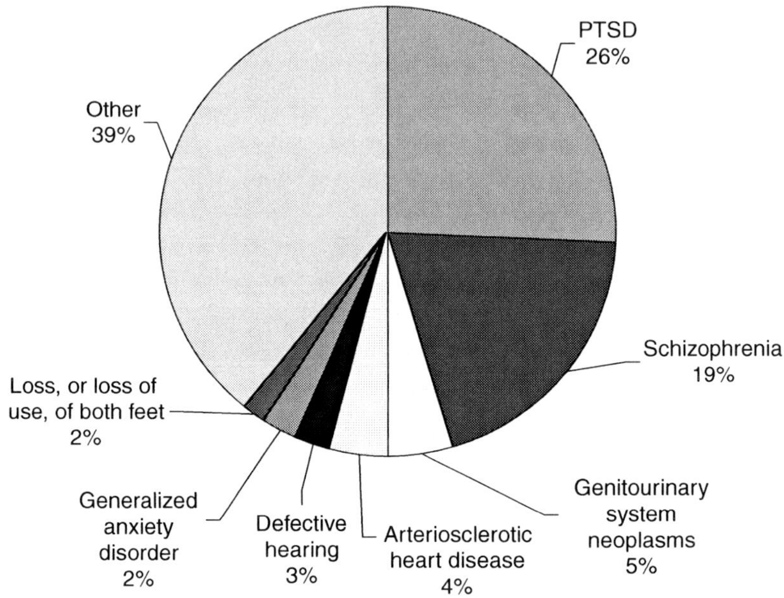

FIGURE 2-7 Service-connected veterans with 100 percent combined rating, by major diagnosis, end of FY 2005 (percentages).
NOTE: Schizophrenia combines codes 9200–9205; defective hearing combines codes 6100–6110; and loss, or loss of use, of both feet combines 5107 and 5710.
SOURCE: VA (2005c).

admitting to having mental illness. Prevalence is also affected by decisions to make certain conditions presumptive for compensation, such as diabetes among veterans who served in Vietnam. Although World War II veterans are age 80 or older, they have the least number of service-connected conditions. The average number of conditions currently being compensated for is 2.0 for World War II, 2.2 for Korea, 3.0 for Vietnam, and 3.7 for Gulf War veterans (i.e., veterans since 1990) (VA, 2006b) (Figure 2-8).[15]

Hearing impairments are very prevalent among veterans of all periods of service. In FY 2005, tinnitus ranked among the top five most prevalent service-connected conditions for all periods of service, and defective hearing ranked among the top five in all periods except the Gulf War (Appendix Table 2-2).

[15]The average was 2.7 for peacetime veterans, meaning those who served between World War II and Korea, between Korea and Vietnam, and between Vietnam and the Gulf War periods.

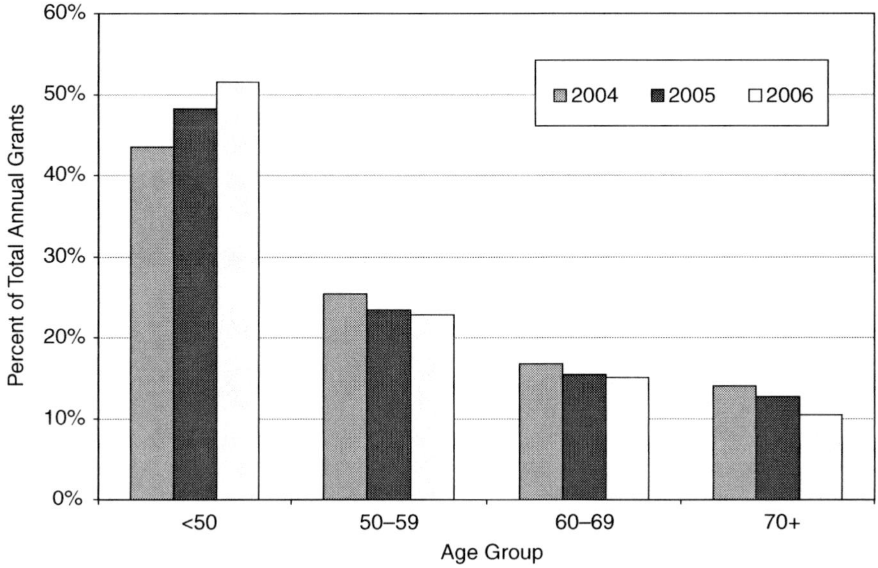

FIGURE 2-8 Percent of conditions granted service connection or higher rating, by age group, calendar year (CY) 2004–CY 2005.
NOTE: The absolute number of grants to veterans younger than age 50 increased by 29 percent (from 315,000 to 406,000) between 2004 and 2006, while the number of grants to older veterans stayed about the same (ages 50–59 and 60–69) or declined (age 70 or older).
SOURCE: IOM (2006).

Other conditions are more prevalent in particular periods of service. Residuals of frozen feet, or immersion foot, were the second and third most common conditions among veterans of World War II and Korea, respectively, but this condition is rare among veterans of other periods. Diabetes and PTSD are the first and second most prevalent disorders among Vietnam veterans, but these conditions are not among even the 10 most prevalent conditions among veterans of other periods. Musculoskeletal conditions are the most prevalent disorders among Gulf War and peacetime veterans, along with hearing impairment.

Women Veterans

Between 1990 and 2000, the population of women veterans increased by one-third, from 1.2 to 1.6 million. There were 1.7 million women veterans at the end of FY 2005, representing approximately 7 percent of the total veteran population. By the year 2015, more than 9 percent of the veteran population is projected to be women (VA, 2004b).

Data on the total number of women receiving VA disability compensation is not reported. For the years 2004 through 2006, however, women veterans were granted compensation for 235,600 conditions, 10 percent of all grants for compensation made during those three years (IOM, 2006). Women were more likely to be younger and be Gulf War veterans than men. Most (84 percent) of the grants to women for disability compensation made during 2004–2006 were to women younger than age 50, and 78 percent were to Gulf War veterans (the comparable figures for men granted disability compensation were 41 and 45 percent, respectively).

Several of the conditions most frequently granted compensation among women between 2004 and 2006 were also the most frequently granted among men. For example, lumbosacral or cervical strain, limitation of flexion of leg, degenerative arthritis of the spine, limited motion of the ankle, and arthritis due to trauma were among the 20 most frequently service-connected conditions for both women and men (Appendix Table 2-3).

Certain disabilities were more prevalent among men, and others among women. Defective hearing and diabetes mellitus were the second and third most frequently granted conditions among men, but these conditions were not among the 20 most frequently service-connected conditions in women. Migraine, major depressive disorder, allergic or vasomotor rhinitis, flatfoot, asthma, and hallux valgus (bunion deformity) were more prevalent in women than in men.

RECENT TRENDS

VA provided the committee with data on disability compensation decisions made during CY 2004, CY 2005, and CY 2006. These data are more detailed than data available before 2004, when Rating Board Automation 2000, the Compensation and Pension (C&P) Service's computerized management information system, became fully operational.

In the three-year period from 2004 through 2006, C&P Service raters decided on compensation for 5.2 million conditions—whether they should be service connected if new, or whether they should be given a higher rating if previously service connected (Table 2-2). They granted (and assigned a rating to) 45 percent of the new conditions claimed and approved a higher rating level for 35 percent of the already service-connected conditions.

The grant rate varied somewhat by the age, sex, and period of service of the veteran claiming the condition. On average, women veterans were slightly more likely to receive a favorable decision. Younger veterans (under age 50) were more likely to have their conditions service connected but not to receive a higher rating of an earlier service-connected condition. Veterans

TABLE 2-2 Disability Compensation Decisions on and Grants of Service Connection and Higher Ratings, CY 2004–CY 2006

Service-Connected Veterans	Service Connection		Higher Rating		Total	
	Decisions	Grants (%)	Decisions	Grants (%)	Decisions	Grants (%)
All	4,313,860	1,947,027 (45%)	926,263	327,543 (35%)	5,240,123	2,274,570 (43%)
Men	3,716,252	1,673,947 (45%)	796,580	283,430 (36%)	4,512,832	1,957,377 (43%)
Women	444,875	207,909 (47%)	69,523	24,740 (40%)	514,398	235,649 (46%)
Unknown	152,733	65,171 (43%)	60,160	19,373 (32%)	212,893	84,544 (40%)
Age <50	1,994,176	997,570 (50%)	260,302	91,163 (35%)	2,254,478	1,088,733 (48%)
50–59	1,092,450	438,987 (40%)	288,699	102,893 (36%)	1,381,149	541,880 (39%)
60–69	694,794	289,455 (42%)	186,171	66,931 (36%)	880,965	356,386 (41%)
70 or older	519,376	215,590 (42%)	186,540	65,372 (35%)	705,916	280,962 (40%)
Unknown	13,064	5,425 (42%)	4,551	1,184 (26%)	17,615	6,609 (38%)
WW II	201,437	88,538 (44%)	72,739	24,551 (34%)	274,176	113,089 (41%)
Korea	110,119	50,890 (46%)	36,627	12,674 (35%)	146,746	63,564 (43%)
Vietnam	1,222,142	540,350 (44%)	333,314	121,448 (36%)	1,555,456	661,798 (43%)
Peacetime	882,988	343,158 (39%)	279,247	97,854 (35%)	1,162,235	441,012 (38%)
Gulf War	1,896,602	924,089 (49%)	200,044	69,236 (35%)	2,096,646	993,325 (47%)
Unknown	571	1 (0%)	4,292	1,780 (42%)	4,863	1,781 (37%)

SOURCE: IOM (2006).

of peacetime periods were less likely to have a new condition service connected than veterans of other periods, while Gulf War veterans were more likely to have a condition service connected. The rate of grants of higher ratings did not vary by age group or service period.

Veterans younger than age 50 not only had the largest number of disability issues granted during the period 2004–2006 (Table 2-2), but their share of grants increased each year relative to the older age groups. The pattern was similar for Gulf War veterans (Figure 2-9).

Claims were evaluated for almost 1 million veterans age 70 or older between 2004 and 2006. This constituted about 13 percent of the total claims filed. Reasons for older veterans applying for VA disability compensation may include increased disability with aging, increased ratings of already service-connected disabilities, and opening of new claims reflective of degenerative problems.

During 2004–2006, the most common disabling conditions considered by raters were defective hearing, tinnitus, PTSD, lumbosacral strain, and diabetes, which accounted for 26 percent of the decisions (left side of Table 2-3). The conditions that were granted service connection or higher rating were the same five, in different order: tinnitus, defective hearing,

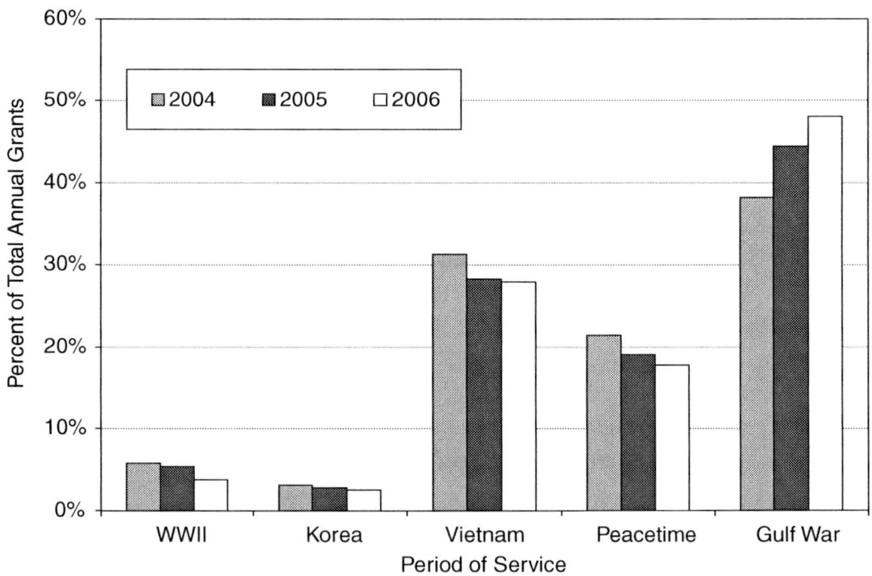

FIGURE 2-9 Percent of conditions granted service connection or higher rating, by period of service, CY 2004–CY 2006.
SOURCE: IOM (2006).

TABLE 2-3 10 Conditions with the Highest Number of Decisions and 10 Most Common Conditions for Which Veterans Were Granted Disability Compensation, CY 2004–CY 2006

	Decisions on Disability Compensation by Diagnosis		Grants of Disability Compensation by Diagnosis	
Rank	Diagnosis (Diagnostic Code)	Number of Decisions	Diagnosis (Diagnostic Code)	Number of Grants
1	Defective hearing (6100)	419,323	Tinnitus (6260)	178,608
2	Tinnitus (6260)	304,773	Defective hearing (6100)	165,476
3	PTSD (9411)	257,191	PTSD (9411)	115,478
4	Lumbosacral or cervical strain (5237)	288,088	Diabetes mellitus (7913)	100,796
5	Diabetes mellitus (7913)	178,126	Lumbosacral or cervical strain (5237)	78,388
6	Hypertensive vascular disease (7101)	162,953	Hypertensive vascular disease (7101)	60,329
7	Limitation of flexion of leg (5260)	112,353	Degenerative arthritis of the spine (5242)	54,036
8	Limited motion of the ankle (5271)	102,141	Limitation of flexion of leg (5260)	49,492
9	Knee impairment other than ankylosis (5257)	101,342	Paralysis of sciatic nerve (8520)	46,402
10	Eczema (7806)	88,558	Limited motion of ankle (5271)	41,923
	All diagnostic codes	5,240,141	All diagnostic codes	2,274,588

SOURCE: IOM (2006).

PTSD, diabetes, and lumbosacral strain (right side of Table 2-3). They accounted for 28 percent of the grants made in that three-year period.

Five conditions accounted for almost half (48 percent) of the 58,000 conditions that were service connected and rated 100 percent during CY 2004–CY 2006: malignant neoplasms of the genitourinary system (prostate cancer), malignancies of the respiratory system (lung cancer), PTSD, arteriosclerotic heart disease, and loss of use of both feet (left side of Table 2-4). Lung and prostate cancer and arteriosclerotic heart disease are related to age, while PTSD and loss of use of both feet are more likely to be related to recent service. Other age-related disabilities in the 20 most numerous condi-

TABLE 2-4 10 Most Common Diagnoses for Which Veterans Were Granted Service Connection and Rated 100 Percent, CY 2004–CY 2006

	All Veterans		Gulf War Veterans	
Rank	Diagnosis (Diagnostic Code)	Number of Veterans	Diagnosis (Diagnostic Code)	Number of Veterans
1	Malignant neoplasms of the genitourinary system (7528)	13,077	PTSD (9411)	624
2	New growths, malignant, any specified part of the respiratory system exclusive of skin growths (6819)	6,410	Loss of use of both feet (5110)	342
3	PTSD (9411)	3,657	Malignant neoplasms of the genitourinary system (7528)	268
4	Arteriosclerotic heart disease (7005)	2,998	Major depressive disorder (9434)	177
5	Loss of use of both feet (5110)	2,051	Rectum and anus, impairment of sphincter control (7332)	166
6	Knee replacement (prosthesis) (5055)	1,989	New growths, malignant, digestive system, exclusive of skin growths (7343)	159
7	Bones, new growths of, malignant (5012)	1,855	Hip replacement (prosthesis) (5054)	158
8	Defective hearing (6100)	1,756	Knee replacement (prosthesis) (5055)	158
9	Non-Hodgkin's lymphoma (7715)	1,732	New growths, malignant, any specified part of the respiratory system exclusive of skin growths (6819)	130
10	Leukemia (7703	1,673	Dementia associated with brain trauma (9304)	130
	All diagnostic codes	58,326	All diagnostic codes	6,185

NOTE: The counts in this table are of diagnoses, not of individual veterans. Grants of higher ratings of already service-connected disabilities are not included in this table.
SOURCE: IOM (2006).

tions rated 100 percent include leukemia, lymphomas, and other cancers; hip and knee replacements; coronary artery bypass surgery; myocardial infarction; and stroke. Some if not many of the cases of renal disorders and dialysis are probably long-term manifestations of diabetes.

The most numerous conditions service connected and rated 100 percent among Gulf War veterans were (in descending order) PTSD, loss of use of both feet, malignant neoplasms of the genitourinary system, major depressive disorder, and impairment of sphincter control (right side of Table 2-4). The 20 most numerous conditions rated 100 percent include more that might be related to recent service in a war zone (e.g., PTSD, loss of use of both feet, major depression, dementia associated with brain trauma, loss of use of both hands, and brain hemorrhage), but they still include a large number of age-related conditions (e.g., prostate and lung cancers, hip and knee replacements, and arteriosclerosis).

VETERANS OF THE WARS IN AND AROUND AFGHANISTAN AND IRAQ

The Department of Defense (DoD) reported that, as of early March 2007, more than 25,000 U.S. servicemembers had been wounded in action in or around Afghanistan or in Iraq.[16] Almost 7,700 servicemembers in OEF/OIF required medical air transport between September 2001 and February 2007 (Embrey, 2007). Of the 25,000 wounded in action in OEF/OIF, the majority (55 percent) were able to return to duty within 72 hours.[17]

Most of the wounded in action in OEF/OIF have been young—30 percent younger than age 22, 25 percent from ages 22 to 24, and 23 percent from ages 25 to 30 (DoD, 2007c). The main source of injury in Iraq has been from explosive devices, such as improvised explosive devices, suicide bombs, and landmines (68 percent of injuries), and from mortar, rocket, or other artillery fire (11 percent of injuries) (DoD, 2007d).[18]

DoD does not provide figures on the number injured or ill in addition to those wounded in action, but reported that in addition to those wounded in action in OEF/OIF, more than 8,000 servicemembers required medical air transport for nonbattle injuries, and 22,600 because of disease or other medical causes (Embrey, 2007).

VA's claims-processing data system cannot separate out veterans who have served in OEF/OIF. They are included within a broader category of

[16]See http://www.defenselink.mil/news/casualty.pdf (accessed March 9, 2007). Iraq figures were as of March 8, 2007; OEF figures were as of March 3, 2007.

[17]See footnote 19.

[18]The percentages are based on the number of wounded for whom the cause was known as of February 10, 2007 (17,500 of the 23,500 wounded).

Gulf War era veterans who have served in the period beginning with the start of the first Gulf War on August 2, 1990. Statistics on this group were presented in the previous section of this chapter.

VA has some information on OEF/OIF veterans obtained by comparing the names of discharged servicemembers who had been deployed to OEF/OIF with the names of claimants for compensation and pension benefits. According to a November 2006 report from VBA's Office of Performance Analysis and Integrity, 1,324,000 servicemembers had been deployed to OEF/OIF from September 11, 2001, through August 31, 2006. Nearly three-quarters were active duty servicemembers; 28 percent were from the reserves.

Of those deployed, 634,000 had been discharged by the end of August 2006. This group of veterans had filed 176,111 claims for compensation and pension benefits. Of the 136,000 claims that had been decided, service connection of one or more disabilities had been granted in 120,000 cases (88 percent). The claims of 16,000 veterans had been denied on all issues. As of the end of August, nearly 40,000 claims were pending adjudication.

Most (55 percent) of the service-connected veterans of OEF/OIF were granted a combined rating of 20 percent or less; 21 percent were rated 50 percent or higher. Compared with all veterans with disabilities, OEF/OIF veterans are rated lower on average (Figure 2-10). They are far more likely to have a combined rating of 0 percent and much less likely to have a rating of 70 to 100 percent. This reflects their age and their recent military service separation. As they become older and their impairments worsen, they will be able to apply for higher ratings.

The most common disabling conditions for OEF/OIF veterans were tinnitus and hearing loss, PTSD, and musculoskeletal conditions (Table 2-5).

VA reported only the 10 most numerous disability conditions at all combined rating degrees; the most numerous conditions rated 100 percent are unknown. The number of seriously wounded veterans, the nature of their disabilities, and how they have fared in the disability claims process is not known, except from scattered reports. VA's Office of Research and Development reported that from the time the OEF/OIF conflicts began through January 2006, almost one-third (more than 600) of servicemembers with battlefield injuries severe enough to warrant evacuation from Iraq to the Walter Reed Army Medical Center had traumatic brain injury, and the majority of these cases were blast-related (VA, 2007b). According to a poster presented by a VA researcher at a conference in November 2006, the four VA polytrauma rehabilitation centers had treated 566 active duty servicemembers during the first four years of OEF/OIF, 188 of whom were injured in OEF/OIF. A little more than half of the OEF/OIF servicemembers had been wounded by blasts, the rest by other means such as gunshots and vehicular crashes. The primary injury in both groups was head trauma,

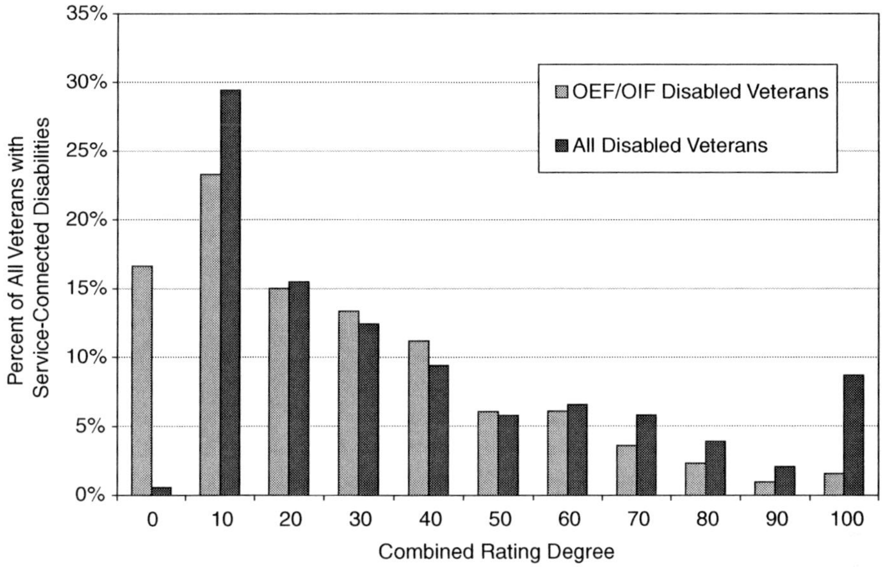

FIGURE 2-10 Distribution of service-connected OEF/OIF veterans and all service-connected veterans by combined rating degree.
NOTE: Figures for OEF/OIF veterans are as of August 30, 2006; figures for all veterans are as of September 30, 2005.
SOURCE: VA (2006a,b).

but soft-tissue wounds and burns, eye, otologic, oral/maxillofacial, and penetrating brain injuries were more common in the group injured by blasts than in the group suffering non-blast injuries. Cognitive impairments, pain, psychiatric symptoms, problems with balance and motor function, and other impairments were prevalent in both groups, but blast-injured servicemembers were more likely to have hearing loss, tinnitus, and PTSD symptoms (Sayer et al., 2006).[19]

According to the head of Disabled American Veterans, as of February 2007, there were 553 amputees from OIF/OEF who had lost one or more arms, legs, hands, and/or feet. Almost a quarter (128) suffered multiple amputations (U.S. Congress, Senate and House of Representatives, Com-

[19]All the differences between the blast-injured and non-blast-injured cited above are statistically significant. Another VA document says, "Through December 2005, the Polytrauma Rehabilitation Centers provided inpatient rehabilitation treatment to 245 OEF and OIF service members with severe traumatic brain injury" (VA, 2007b).

TABLE 2-5 Most Common Conditions of Veterans of the Afghanistan and Iraq Wars, 2001–2006

Diagnostic Code	Condition	Number of Grants
6260	Tinnitus	35,871
5237	Lumbosacral or cervical strain	32,733
6100	Defective hearing	28,907
5299	Conditions analogous to musculoskeletal impairments listed in the VA Rating Schedule	23,892
5271	Limited motion of the ankle	16,454
9411	PTSD	16,131
5260	Limitation of flexion of leg	15,335
5257	Limitation of knee other than ankylosis	12,048
5201	Limitation of motion of arm	11,337
7101	Hypertensive vascular disease	11,303

SOURCE: VA (2006a).

mittees on Veterans' Affairs, 2007a). More than 400 OEF/OIF veterans had suffered major burns by 2006 (Kupersmith, 2006).[20]

According to March 2007 testimony from Blinded Veterans of America, 16 percent of all casualties evacuated from Iraq between March 2003 and April 2005 had eye injuries. Walter Reed Army Medical Center had surgically treated about 690 soldiers for blindness or moderate to severe significant visual injuries. The National Naval Medical Center had surgically treated approximately 450 traumatic eye injuries (U.S. Congress, Senate and House of Representatives, Committees on Veterans' Affairs, 2007b).

Another source of information on the potential disability status of OEF/OIF veterans is the types of conditions for which they seek health care at the Veterans Health Administration (VHA). According to the latest analysis of those data, as of the end of August 2006, 205,097 (32 percent) of the 631,174 OEF/OIF military personnel who had separated from service and become veterans had sought VA health care for a current health problem (VA, 2006c). Most of those who sought care were male, were between the ages of 20 and 29, and had separated from the Army. About equal numbers were former active duty and reserve or National Guard members.

OEF/OIF veterans filed disability claims with VHA for a wide variety of conditions (Appendix Table 2-4). The largest percentage of conditions matched ICD-9 codes that belonged within the category of diseases of the musculoskeletal and connective system (43 percent), followed by mental

[20]Major burns are defined as those covering more than 10 percent of the body.

disorders (36 percent), and symptoms, signs, and ill-defined conditions without an immediately obvious cause or with laboratory abnormalities that cannot be coded elsewhere in the ICD-9 (33 percent).

A total of 73,157, or about one-third of, OEF/OIF veterans received a diagnosis of a possible mental disorder (Appendix Table 2-5). The most common diagnosis was PTSD (33,754), followed by non-dependent abuse of drugs (28,732), and depressive disorders (23,462).[21]

Although these statistics are suggestive, they do not mean that, for example, 36 percent of all OEF/OIF veterans have diagnosable mental disorders. Veterans who seek care at VA are self-selected. If very sick, they are perhaps unemployed or underemployed and lacking health insurance, which they do not need for VA services.

Of OIF soldiers who completed post-deployment health assessments between May 1, 2003, and April 30, 2004, 19 percent reported a mental health concern, compared with 11 percent of soldiers returning from Afghanistan and 9 percent of soldiers returning from other locations. OIF veterans whose post-deployment health was reassessed three to six months after deployment showed even higher rates of mental health concerns; 35 percent reported some kind of mental health concern on at least one general screening question related to PTSD, depression, alcohol use, relationship/interpersonal concerns, or suicidal ideation. Data from the Army's health-care system show that 35 percent of soldiers who returned from Iraq accessed military mental health services at some time during the first year after return, most often within the first two months. Twelve percent of all soldiers who returned from OIF were diagnosed with a mental health problem within the first year after return (U.S. Congress, House of Representatives, Committee on Veterans' Affairs Subcommittee on Health, 2006).

CONCLUSION

Veterans likely to seek disability compensation from VA currently and in the future are a diverse group. Some are veterans of the current wars in Afghanistan and Iraq, and most of them are young. If the wars end soon, and if the same percentage of those deployed as those who were in the first Gulf War leave active service within 10 years (67 percent), and the same percentage of those who have left active service apply for disability compensation as did veterans of the first Gulf War as of September 30, 2001 (about 33 percent), VA can expect to receive about 290,000 claims from veterans of OEF/OIF. The number is likely to be larger, because a higher percentage (28 percent) of the deployed servicemembers have been activated

[21]These three diagnoses alone total more than 73,157, because some veterans had multiple diagnoses of mental disorder.

from the National Guard and reserves than in the first Gulf War. (At this point, 48 percent of those deployed to OEF/OIF have left the service, and 28 percent of them have filed claims for disability compensation.)

If this group continues to have the same impairments as it has had to date, most claims that will be adjudicated will be for hearing problems, musculoskeletal impairments, and mental disorders, especially PTSD. However, the majority of veterans will continue to be from earlier periods of service and, therefore, will be approaching middle or advanced age. They will be filing reopened claims as their service-connected conditions become worse and new conditions appear, either secondary to already service-connected conditions or made presumptive by legislation or regulation. The percentage of reopened claims has declined from 75 percent in 2000, but is still two-thirds of all claims. This means that VA will continue to receive a substantial number of claims for cardiovascular conditions, cancers, diabetes and its complications, deteriorating hearing and vision, joint replacements, and other problems associated with advancing age. Claims for such conditions are likely to continue to increase in number as evaluation tools improve and problems are detected earlier. In addition, there will be a relatively small but important set of mostly younger veterans with multiple impairments, including traumatic brain injuries, which must be adequately evaluated and rated.

REFERENCES

ATA (American Tinnitus Association). 2007. *About tinnitus*. http://www.ata.org/about_tinnitus/ (accessed May 14, 2007).

DoD (Department of Defense). 2007a. *Global war on terrorism [casualties] by reason, October 7, 2001, through February 10, 2007*. http://siadapp.dior.whs.mil/personnel/CASUALTY/ gwot_reason.pdf (accessed March 9, 2007).

DoD. 2007b. *Military casualty information*. http://siadapp.dior.whs.mil/personnel/CASUALTY/castop.htm (accessed March 6, 2007).

DoD. 2007c. *Military casualty information*. http://siadapp.dior.whs.mil/personnel/CASUALTY/OIF-Wounded-After.pdf and http://siadapp.dior.whs.mil/personnel/CASUALTY/OEFWIA.pdf (accessed March 9, 2007).

DoD. 2007d. *Military casualty information*. http://siadapp.dior.whs.mil/personnel/CASUALTY/gwot_reason.pdf (accessed March 9, 2007).

DVBIC (Defense and Veterans Brain Injury Center). 2007. *Blast injury FAQs*. http://www.dvbic.org/blastinjury.html (accessed March 12, 2007).

Embrey, E. P. 2007. *Force health protection*. PowerPoint presentation by the Deputy Assistant Secretary of Defense for Force Health Protection and Readiness. http://www.amsus.org/sm/presentations/Feb07-B.ppt#293,1,Force Health Protection (accessed March 14, 2007).

Heller, A. J. 2003. Classification and epidemiology of tinnitus. *Otolaryngology Clinics of North America* 36(2):239–248.

Hoffman, H. J., and G. W. Reed. 2004. Epidemiology of tinnitus. In *Tinnitus: Theory and management*, edited by J. B. Snow, Jr. Hamilton, Ontario, Canada: B. C. Decker. Pp. 16–41.

Hoge, C. W., C. A. Castro, S. C. Messer, D. McGurk, D. I. Cotting, and R. L. Koffman. 2004. Combat duty in Iraq and Afghanistan, mental health problems, and barriers to care. *New England Journal of Medicine* 351(1):13–22.

IOM (Institute of Medicine). 2006. Staff analyses of claims data provided by VA, December 19, in response to Data Request 07-042, submitted by the Veterans' Disability Benefits Commission.

IOM. 2007. Staff analyses of data from *VetPop2004 Version 1.0 State and National Tables, Table 2L*. http://www.va.gov/vetdata/docs/VP2004B.htm (accessed March 1, 2007).

Kessler, R. C., W. T. Chiu, O. Demler, and E. E. Walters. 2005a. Prevalence, severity, and comorbidity of twelve-month DSM-IV disorders in the National Comorbidity Survey Replication (NCS-R). *Archives of General Psychiatry* 62(6):617–627.

Kessler, R. C., P. A. Berglund, O. Demler, R. Jin, K. R. Merikangas, and E. E. Walters. 2005b. Lifetime prevalence and age-of-onset distributions of DSM-IV disorders in the National Comorbidity Survey Replication (NCS-R). *Archives of General Psychiatry* 62(6):593–602.

Kupersmith, J. 2006. *Global conflicts: Implications for VA research*. PowerPoint presentation by the Chief Research and Development Officer, Veterans Health Administration, VA. http://www.academyhealth.org/2006/kupersmith.pdf (accessed March 9, 2007).

NIDDK (National Institute of Diabetes and Digestive and Kidney Diseases). 2005. *National Diabetes Statistics*. http://diabetes.niddk.nih.gov/dm/pubs/statistics/#7/ (accessed May 18, 2007).

Riddle, J. R., T. C. Smith, B. Smith, T. E. Corbeil, C. C. Engel, T. S. Wells, C. W. Hoge, J. Adkins, M. Zamorski, and D. Blazer. 2007. Millennium Cohort: The 2001–2003 baseline prevalence of mental disorders in the U.S. military. *Journal of Clinical Epidemiology* 60(2):192–201.

Ryan, M. A., T. C. Smith, B. Smith, P. Amoroso, E. J. Boyko, G. C. Gray, G. D. Gackstetter, J. R. Riddle, T. S. Wells, G. Gumbs, T. E. Corbeil, and T. I. Hooper. 2007. Millennium Cohort: Enrollment begins a 21-year contribution to understanding the impact of military service. *Journal of Clinical Epidemiology* 60(2):181–191.

Sayer, N. A., C. Chiros, B. Clothier, H. Lew, T. Pickett, S. Scott, and B. Sigford. 2006. *Predictors of functional improvement during acute inpatient rehabilitation among combat-injured OIF and OEF servicemembers*. Poster presented at 2006 annual meeting of the American Military Surgeons of the United States, San Antonio, TX.

Scott, S. G. 2005. *Polytrauma rehabilitation system of care*. PowerPoint presentation made at February 2005 meeting of the Veterans' Disability Benefits Commission, St. Petersburg, FL. http://www.1888932-2946.ws/vetscommission/e-documentmanager/gallery/Documents/February_2006/DrScottColFryerPresentation.pdf (accessed March 1, 2007).

Seal, K. H., D. Bertenthal, C. R. Miner, S. Sen, and C. Marmar. 2007. Bringing the war back home: Mental health disorders among 103,788 U.S. veterans returning from Iraq and Afghanistan seen at Department of Veterans Affairs facilities. *Archives of Internal Medicine* 167(5):476–482.

U.S. Congress, House of Representatives, Committee on Appropriations. 2007. *Prepared statement of Joel Kupersmith, M.D., Chief Research and Development Officer, VA, before the Subcommittee on Military Construction, Veterans' Affairs and Related Agencies*, 110th Cong., 1st Sess., March 14. https://www.va.gov/OCA/testimony/hac/smqlva/070314JK.asp (accessed May 14, 2007).

U.S. Congress, House of Representatives, Committee on Veterans' Affairs. 2006. *Prepared statement of Colonel Charles W. Hoge, U.S. Army Director of Division of Psychiatry and Neuroscience, Walter Reed Army Institute of Research, before the Subcommittee on Health's hearing on posttraumatic stress disorder and traumatic brain injury*, 109th

Cong., 2nd Sess. September 28. http://veterans.house.gov/hearings/schedule109/sep06/9-28-06/CharlesHoge.html (accessed March 15, 2007).

U.S. Congress, House of Representatives, Committee on Veterans' Affairs. 2007a. *Prepared statement of James R. Nicholson, Secretary of Veterans Affairs, before the Full Committee.* 110th Cong., 1st Sess., February 8. http://veterans.house.gov/hearings/schedule110/feb07/02-08-07/JamesNicholson.html (accessed March 1, 2007).

U.S. Congress, House of Representatives, Committee on Veterans' Affairs. 2007b. *Prepared statement of Steven G. Scott, Medical Director, VA Tampa Polytrauma Rehabilitation Center, before the Subcommittee on Oversight and Investigation.* 110th Cong., 1st Sess., March 8. http://veterans.house.gov/hearings/schedule110/mar07/03-08-07/StevenScott.shtml (accessed March 9, 2007).

U.S. Congress, House of Representatives, Committee on Veterans' Affairs. 2007c. *Prepared statement of Ronald R. Aument, Deputy Under Secretary for Benefits, VA, before the Subcommittee on Disability Assistance and Memorial Affairs.* 110th Cong., 1st Sess., March 13. http://veterans.house.gov/hearings/schedule110/mar07/03-13-07/Aument.pdf (accessed March 9, 2007).

U.S. Congress, Senate, Defense Appropriations Committee. 2007. *Prepared statement of Lt. Gen. (Dr.) James G. Roudebush, Surgeon General of the Air Force, before the Defense Appropriations Subcommittee.* 110th Cong., 1st Sess., March 7. http://appropriations.senate.gov/hearings.cfm (accessed March 9, 2007).

U.S. Congress, Senate and House of Representatives, Committees on Veterans' Affairs. 2007a. *Prepared statement of Bradley S. Barton, National Commander, Disabled American Veterans.* 110th Cong., 1st Sess., February 27. http://veterans.house.gov/hearings/schedule110/feb07/02-27-07/BradleyBarton.shtml (accessed March 9, 2007).

U.S. Congress, Senate and House of Representatives, Committees on Veterans' Affairs. 2007b. *Prepared statement of Larry Belote, National President, Blinded Veterans of America.* 110th Cong., 1st Sess., March 8. http://veterans.senate.gov/index.cfm?FuseAction=Hearings.CurrentHearings&rID=946&hID=256/ (accessed March 16, 2007).

VA (Department of Veterans Affairs). 1995. VA report RCS 20-0227, as of March 31, 1995 (unpublished).

VA. 2001a. *2001 National Survey of Veterans: Final report.* Washington, DC: Department of Veterans Affairs. http://www.va.gov/vetdata/docs/NSV%20Final%20Report.pdf (accessed June 22, 2007).

VA. 2001b. *Veterans Benefits Administration annual benefits report for fiscal year 2000.* Washington, DC: Veterans Benefits Administration. http://www.vba.va.gov/bln/dmo/reports/fy2000_abr_v3.pdf (accessed March 1, 2007).

VA. 2002. *Veterans Administration annual benefits report for fiscal year 2001.* Washington, DC: Veterans Benefits Administration. http://www.vba.va.gov/bln/dmo/reports/FY2001_ABR.pdf (accessed March 1, 2007).

VA. 2003. *Veterans Administration annual benefits report for fiscal year 2002.* Washington, DC: Veterans Benefits Administration. http://www.vba.va.gov/bln/dmo/reports/fy2002/2002_abr_all.pdf (accessed March 1, 2007).

VA. 2004a. *Veterans Administration annual benefits report for fiscal year 2003.* Washington, DC: Veterans Benefits Administration. http://www.vba.va.gov/bln/dmo/reports/fy2003/2003_abr.pdf (accessed March 1, 2007).

VA. 2004b. *VetPop2004 Version 1.0 State and National Tables Table 5L: Veterans 2000–2033 by race/ethnicity, gender, period, age.* http://www.va.gov/vetdata/docs/VP2004B.htm (accessed December 18, 2006).

VA. 2005a. Polytrauma rehabilitation procedures. *VHA handbook 1172.1.* http://www.va.gov/vhapublications/ViewPublication.asp?pub_ID=1317 (accessed March 12, 2007).

VA. 2005b. *Veterans Administration annual benefits report for fiscal year 2004*. Washington, DC: Veterans Benefits Administration. http://www.vba.va.gov/bln/dmo/reports/fy2004/2004_abr.pdf (accessed March 1, 2007).

VA. 2005c. VA report RCS 20-0227, as of September 30, 2005 (unpublished).

VA. 2006a. *Compensation and pension benefit activity among 633,867 veterans deployed to the Global War on Terrorism*. Washington, DC: Office of Performance Analysis and Integrity, Veterans Benefit Administration. Prepared November 8, 2006. Unpublished document provided by VA to the Committee on Medical Evaluation of Veterans for Disability Compensation on March 14, 2007.

VA. 2006b. *Veterans Benefits Administration annual benefits report for fiscal year 2005*. Washington, DC: Veterans Benefit Administration. http://www.vba.va.gov/bln/dmo/reports/fy2005/2005_abr.pdf (accessed March 1, 2007).

VA. 2006c. *Analysis of VA health care utilization among U.S. Southwest Asian war veterans: Operation Iraqi Freedom and Operation Enduring Freedom*. Washington, DC: Office of Public Health and Environmental Hazards, Veterans Health Administration.

VA. 2006d. VA report RCS 20-0227, as of September 30, 2005 (unpublished).

VA. 2007a. *FY2008 budget submission, volume II: National Cemetery Administration, benefits programs, and departmental administration*. Washington, DC: Office of Budget, Department of Veterans Affairs. http://www.vba.va.gov/bln/dmo/reports/FY2001_ABR.pdf (accessed March 1, 2007).

VA. 2007b. *Polytrauma and blast-related injuries*. QUERI (Quality Enhancement Research Initiative) fact sheet. http://www.va.gov/hsrd/publications/internal/polytrauma_factsheet.pdf (accessed March 14, 2007).

VA. 2007c. Unpublished tables of claims data provided by VA Office of Performance Analysis and Integrity to the Committee on Medical Evaluation of Veterans for Disability Compensation.

Warden, D. 2006. *TBI during wartime: The Afghanistan and Iraq experience*. Presentation at 2nd Federal Traumatic Brain Injury Interagency Conference, Bethesda, MD, March 9. http://www.tbi-interagency.org/pdf/dwarden.pdf (accessed March 21, 2007).

APPENDIX TABLE 2-1 Individual Service-Connected Conditions by Rating, FY 1995 and FY 2005

	FY 1995		FY 2005	
Rating	Number of Rated Conditions	Percent of Total	Number of Rated Conditions	Percent of Total
0%	1,775,993	34.9%	2,363,021	31.0%
10%	1,894,441	37.2%	3,052,872	40.0%
20%	476,706	9.4%	813,832	10.6%
30%	433,832	8.5%	593,025	7.7%
40%	145,030	2.9%	212,238	2.8%
50%	91,040	1.8%	166,344	2.2%
60%	88,745	1.7%	142,177	1.8%
70%	27,916	0.5%	97,526	1.3%
80%	9,008	0.2%	10,331	0.1%
90%	2,669	0.1%	3,202	*
100%	140,905	2.8%	221,219	2.9%
Total	5,086,285	100.0%	7,675,787	100.0%

*Less than 0.05 percent.
SOURCE: VA (1995) for 1995 numbers and VA (2006b) for 2005 numbers.

APPENDIX TABLE 2-2 Five Most Common Service-Connected Conditions by Period of Service, All Veterans Receiving Disability Compensation as of FY 2005

Period of Service	Condition	Number of Conditions	Percent of All Conditions
WWII			
	Defective hearing	42,464	5.8%
	Frozen feet, residuals of (immersion foot)	39,169	5.4%
	Tinnitus	32,491	4.5%
	Generalized anxiety disorder	31,367	4.3%
	Scars, other	30,571	4.2%
	PTSD	25,281	3.5%
	Arthritis, due to trauma	24,420	3.3%
	Scars, superficial, tender and painful	15,584	2.1%
	Flatfoot, acquired	15,359	2.1%
	Scars, disfiguring, head, face, or neck	11,718	1.6%
	All	728,911	100.0%
Korea			
	Defective hearing	25,529	7.2%
	Tinnitus	22,100	6.2%
	Frozen feet, residuals of (immersion foot)	19,808	5.6%
	Scars, other	15,476	4.4%
	PTSD	10,994	3.1%
	Arthritis, due to trauma	10,030	2.8%
	Scars, superficial, tender and painful	7,147	2.0%
	Duodenal ulcer	6,825	1.9%
	Scars, disfiguring, head, face, or neck	5,758	1.6%
	Generalized (analogous to) musculoskeletal conditions	5,552	1.6%
	All	355,344	100.0%
Vietnam			
	Diabetes mellitus	190,199	6.9%
	PTSD	179,737	6.5%
	Defective hearing	129,323	4.7%
	Scars, other	121,850	4.4%
	Tinnitus	120,625	4.4%
	Generalized (analogous to) musculoskeletal conditions	78,270	2.9%
	Hypertensive vascular disease	72,169	2.6%
	Arthritis, due to trauma	69,034	2.5%
	Other impairment of knee	62,713	2.3%
	Arthritis, degenerative, hypertrophic, or osteoarthritis	52,920	1.9%
	All	2,745,555	100.0%

continued

APPENDIX TABLE 2-2 Continued

Period of Service	Condition	Number of Conditions	Percent of All Conditions
Gulf War			
	Generalized musculoskeletal conditions	131,092	5.9%
	Tinnitus	104,039	4.7%
	Arthritis due to trauma	100,374	4.5%
	Other impairment of knee	81,677	3.7%
	Hypertensive vascular disease	64,558	2.9%
	Lumbosacral strain	61,658	2.8%
	Scars, other	60,350	2.7%
	Defective hearing	60,023	2.7%
	Arthritis, degenerative, hypertrophic, or osteoarthritis	54,042	2.4%
	Limited motion of ankle	53,002	2.4%
	All	2,233,479	100.0%
Peacetime			
	Generalized musculoskeletal conditions	78,233	4.9%
	Other impairment of knee	77,768	4.9%
	Arthritis due to trauma	68,068	4.2%
	Defective hearing	64,013	4.0%
	Tinnitus	60,278	3.8%
	Scars, other	54,823	3.4%
	Hypertensive vascular disease	50,247	3.1%
	Lumbosacral strain	44,736	2.8%
	Arthritis, degenerative, hypertrophic, or osteoarthritis	39,646	2.5%
	Intervertebral disc syndrome	37,103	2.3%
	All	1,602,697	100.0%

SOURCE: VA (2006b).

APPENDIX TABLE 2-3 20 Most Frequent Service-Connected Conditions Among Women and Men, 2004–2006

Women		Men	
Condition	Number of Grants	Condition	Number of Grants
Lumbosacral or cervical strain	11,113	Tinnitus	161,090
Migraine	10,255	Defective hearing	135,394
Tinnitus	5,901	Diabetes mellitus	85,005
Scars, other	5,807	PTSD	74,491
Limitation of flexion of leg	5,566	Hypertensive vascular disease	51,033
Major depressive disorder	5,378	Lumbosacral or cervical strain	50,136
Tenosynovitis	5,155	Penis, deformity with loss of erectile power	38,719
Degenerative arthritis of the spine	4,997	Paralysis of sciatic nerve	38,356
Scars, superficial, tender, and painful	4,847	Degenerative arthritis of the spine	36,672
Allergic or vasomotor rhinitis	4,687	Limitation of flexion of leg	35,798
Hernia, hiatal	4,671	Scars, other	33,537
Eczema	4,443	Limited motion of the ankle	30,182
Limited motion of the ankle	4,258	Arthritis, due to trauma	29,306
Flatfoot, acquired	3,992	Hernia, hiatal	25,251
Hypertensive vascular disease	3,734	Scars, superficial, tender, and painful	24,924
Asthma, bronchial	3,534	Tenosynovitis	24,806
PTSD	3,313	Eczema	23,666
Hallux valgus	3,303	Paralysis of the median nerve	22,227
Arthritis, due to trauma	3,236	Intervertebral disc syndrome	20,929
Paralysis of the median nerve	2,988	Arteriosclerotic heart disease	19,854

SOURCE: VA (2007c).

APPENDIX TABLE 2-4 Frequency of Diagnoses Among Recent Veterans of Iraq and Afghanistan

Broad ICD-9 Category	Frequency	%
Infectious and parasitic diseases (001–139)	21,362	10.4
Malignant neoplasms (140–208)	1,584	0.8
Benign neoplasms (210–239)	6,571	3.2
Diseases of endocrine/nutritional/metabolic systems (240–279)	36,409	17.8
Diseases of blood and blood-forming organs (280–289)	3,591	1.8
Mental disorders (290–319)	73,157	35.7
Diseases of nervous system/sense organs (320–389)	61,524	30.0
Diseases of circulatory system (390–459)	29,249	14.3
Diseases of respiratory system (460–519)	36,190	17.6
Diseases of digestive system (520–579)	63,002	30.7
Diseases of genitourinary system (580–629)	18,886	9.2
Diseases of skin (680–709)	29,010	14.1
Diseases of musculoskeletal system/connective system (710–739)	87,590	42.7
Symptoms, signs, and ill-defined conditions (780–799)	67,743	33.0
Injury/poisonings (800-999)	35,765	17.4

SOURCE: VA (2006d).

APPENDIX TABLE 2-5 Frequency of Mental Diagnoses Among Recent Veterans of Iraq and Afghanistan

Disease Category (ICD-9CM Code)	Number of OEF/OIF Veterans
PTSD (309.81)	33,754
Nondependent abuse of drugs (305)	28,732
Depressive disorders (311)	23,462
Neurotic disorders (300)	18,294
Affective psychoses (296)	12,386
Alcohol dependence syndrome (303)	5,413
Sexual deviations and disorders (302)	3,239
Special symptoms, not elsewhere classified (307)	3,178
Drug dependence (304)	2,387
Acute reaction to stress (308)	2,273

SOURCE: VA (2006d).

3

Impairment, Disability, and Quality of Life

The primary focus of this study is the extent to which the Department of Veterans Affairs' (VA) Schedule for Rating Disabilities (Rating Schedule) is "an appropriate, valid, and reliable instrument for evaluating medical impairment and determining degree of disability." The statement of work for the committee clarified our assignment to ask how well the Rating Schedule and associated regulations enable VA to determine the proper levels of disability to compensate veterans with injuries and diseases incurred in, or aggravated by, military service for (1) "impact on quality of life" and (2) "impairment in earnings capacity." This chapter begins with a section that provides a model of disability and defines our understanding of quality of life and impairment in earning capacity, as well as other concepts used in the model, including medical impairment and limitations in the activities of daily living.

A MODEL OF DISABILITY AND DEFINITIONS

The most useful model for purposes of this report was developed by an earlier Institute of Medicine (IOM) committee in 1991 (IOM, 1991). It has four domains of disablement: pathology, impairment, functional limitation, and disability (see Figure 3-1). More recent conceptual models, such as the *International Classification of Functioning, Disability and Health* (ICF) (WHO, 2001),[1] are not linear, recognizing, for example, that there is not always a stepwise progression from pathology to impairment to functional

[1]See Figure 1 in WHO (2001).

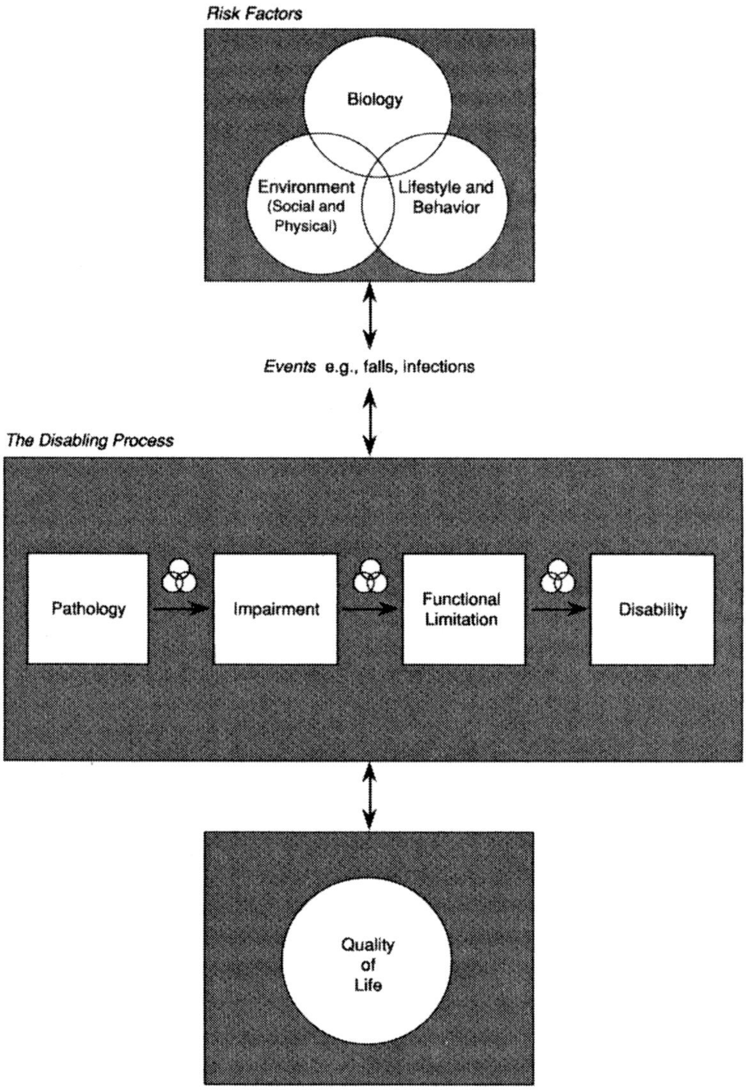

FIGURE 3-1 The four domains of disablement (IOM, 1991:Figure 4).

limitation to disability. A functional limitation may result in yet another impairment, for example, or an impairment may not limit function but be disabling, such as disfigurement.[2]

The 1991 IOM model is practical to use because it not only has the concepts of impairment, functional limitation, and disability and includes mediating factors (e.g., lifestyle and behavioral, biological, and environmental), but also acknowledges the interaction between quality of life and the disablement process. The committee does not find the IOM definition to be inconsistent with the more conceptually sophisticated ICF. (See Box 3-1 for a summary of the disability-related concepts and terms used by the committee in this report.)

Impairment

Impairment is a loss of physiological integrity in a body function or anatomical integrity in a body structure (WHO, 2001). Impairment is caused by disease, injury, or congenital defect. It may be a secondary consequence of yet another impairment, as when a person has a shorter leg from an injury and later develops arthritis in the hip because the abnormal gait resulting from the short leg causes trauma in the joint. Disability compensation systems, such as VA's or workers' compensation programs, generally determine the amount of compensation by rating the severity of the permanent impairment—the sequelae or residuals of a disease or injury. Impairments can be defined in relation to a physiological or anatomical structure or functional limitations.

The next chapter will assess the extent to which the Rating Schedule bases compensation on degree of impairment alone, but below are some examples of ratings of disability based on severity of impairment:

- Ribs, removal of (diagnostic code 5297):

More than six	50 percent
Five or six	40 percent
Three or four	30 percent
Two	20 percent
One or resection of two or more ribs without regeneration	0 percent

- Paralysis of fifth (trigeminal) cranial nerve (8205):

Complete	50 percent
Incomplete, severe	30 percent
Incomplete, moderate	10 percent

[2]This complexity was recognized in the text of IOM (1991: 8–10).

BOX 3-1
Basic Concepts and Definitions of Terms Used

activities of daily living/instrumental activities of daily living—functional limitations at the person level; measures of the net impact of an impairment or impairments on an individual's ability to engage in life situations.

disability—a broad term that includes work disability and quality of life.

disabling process—a product of the interaction of the person and the environment, thereby influencing one's quality of life.

domains—aspects of an individual's activities, such as the physical, psychological, and social.

functional assessment—measure of the degree to which an individual can perform chosen roles (as well as duties and responsibilities) without physical, social, psychological, or cognitive limitation.

health-related quality of life—measures what an individual values and whether there is much satisfaction in one's life; components can include signs or symptoms, treatment side effects, or physical, cognitive, emotional, and social functioning.

impairment—loss of physiological integrity in a body function or anatomical integrity in a body structure; caused by disease, injury, or congenital defect (WHO, 2001).

IOM model of disablement domains—the model's four domains are (1) pathology, (2) impairment, (3) functional limitation, and (4) disability. The model encompasses the concepts of impairment, functional limitation, and disability, and includes mediating factors—lifestyle and behavioral, biological, and environmental—and acknowledges the interaction between quality of life and the disablement process (IOM, 1991).

loss in quality of life—the consequences of an injury or disease other than work disability.

quality of life—includes the cultural, psychological, physical, interpersonal, spiritual, financial, political, temporal, and philosophical dimensions of a person's life; reflects changes in people and the environment over time across many of its domains (Tate et al., 1996); the perception of physical and mental health over time (CDC, 2007).

work disability—(1) actual loss of earnings resulting from the injury or disease and (2) presumed loss of earning capacity [or *impairments of earning capacity*] resulting from the injury or disease.

Note: Dependent upon relative degree of sensory manifestation or motor loss.

Some kinds of impairments are rated according to the degree of functional limitation of the body structure or process. These include range of motion of limbs and decreased capacity of an organ (loss of breathing capacity of the lung has already been described above):

- Thigh, limitation of flexion of (5252):

Flexion limited to 10°	40 percent
Flexion limited to 20°	30 percent
Flexion limited to 30°	20 percent
Flexion limited to 45°	0 percent

- Arteriosclerotic heart disease (coronary artery disease) (7005):

  100 percent—Chronic congestive heart failure; or workload of 3 metabolic equivalents of task (METs)[3] or less results in dyspnea, fatigue, angina, dizziness, or syncope; or left ventricular dysfunction with an ejection fraction of less than 30 percent

  60 percent—More than one episode of acute congestive heart failure in the past year; or workload of greater than 3 METs but not greater than 5 METs results in dyspnea, fatigue, angina, dizziness, or syncope; or left ventricular dysfunction with an ejection fraction of 30 to 50 percent

  30 percent—Workload of greater than 5 METs but not greater than 7 METs results in dyspnea, fatigue, angina, dizziness, or syncope; or evidence of cardiac hypertrophy or dilatation on electrocardiogram, echocardiogram, or X-ray

  10 percent—Workload of greater than 7 METs but not greater than 10 METs results in dyspnea, fatigue, angina, dizziness, or syncope; or continuous medication required

[3]One MET is equivalent to a metabolic rate that consumes 3.5 milliliters of oxygen per kilogram of body weight per minute (roughly the oxygen uptake of someone sitting quietly). http:// prevention.sph.sc.edu/tools/compendium.htm (accessed May 1, 2007).

Limitations in the Activities of Daily Living

It is common to differentiate functional limitations at the physiologic or anatomic level, as in the examples above, from functional limitations at the person level, which are measured by scales of activities of daily living (ADLs) and instrumental activities of daily living (IADLs) (Box 3-2). ADLs and IADLs are considered to be measures of the net impact of an impairment or impairments on an individual's ability to engage in life situations. The distinction is useful because physicians are trained to evaluate impairment but rarely are taught to evaluate the capacity of individuals to function in daily life. Evaluation of impairment is based on an examination of a patient and his or her test results, medical history, and symptoms, while evaluating the functional capacity of an individual is based on performance measures (e.g., ambulation, lifting specified loads).

The Veterans Health Administration (VHA) uses ADL and IADL assessments, for example, in deciding whether a post-stroke patient needs inpatient rehabilitation, the level of inpatient care needed, and readiness for discharge (VA, 2007). The Veterans Benefits Administration (VBA) does not use ADLs, IADLs, or other whole-person functional assessments to evaluate service-connected injuries and diseases, except for mental disorders. For mental disorders, the Rating Schedule has criteria to assess the degree of occupational and social impairment on a six-point scale from 0 to total.

BOX 3-2
ADLs and IADLs

Activities of daily living (ADLs) scales were developed beginning in the 1960s to assess ability to perform self-care activities such as dressing, bathing, grooming, toileting, transferring (getting into or out of bed or a chair), and eating. The original purpose was to assess the disability of individuals in inpatient rehabilitation settings and nursing homes to determine what kind of help they need and to monitor their progress (Katz et al., 1963; Mahoney and Barthel, 1965). ADL scales have been adapted to clinical settings.

Instrumental activities of daily living (IADLs) were developed to assess the ability of elderly and disabled individuals to live independently in the community (Lawton and Brody, 1969). These activities include managing money, using a telephone, preparing meals, performing light or heavy housework, walking across the room, climbing up stairs, going outside, shopping, and getting around in the community.

Neither ADLs nor IADLs directly measure capacity to work.

The Australian Department of Veterans' Affairs uses ADLs to determine impairment ratings of conditions for which criteria either do not exist in the body system tables or are inadequate or inappropriate. The intent of using ADLs is to assess conditions that result in a veteran being housebound or nearly housebound, chairbound, or bedridden (e.g., effects of severe strokes, Parkinson's disease, heart failure, respiratory disease, or liver or kidney failure) or to assess non-specific indicators of disease or injury (e.g., pain, lethargy, or poor prognosis of life expectancy). An ADL-based rating of a single condition can be combined with body system-based ratings of other conditions, or the ADLs can be used to rate all conditions. The evaluator grades six ADLs—movement in bed, transfers, locomotion, dressing, personal hygiene, and feeding—on a scale from 0 to 8. The total of the six scores is converted using a table to an impairment rating ranging from 0 to 70. The evaluator also uses a second set of criteria based on effects of symptoms such as pain or lethargy and decreased life expectancy to derive an impairment rating from 0 to 35. The higher of the two ratings is used to determine the amount of compensation (Australian DVA, 2005).

Disability

This chapter uses *disability* as a broad term that includes work disability and quality of life in order to be responsive to the tasks assigned to the committee. Work disability refers to the loss of earning capacity (or impairment in earning capacity) or the actual loss of earnings resulting from an injury or disease. Loss in quality of life refers to the consequences of an injury or disease other than work disability. These definitions are refined in the rest of this chapter.

Impairments of Earning Capacity (Work Disability)

Work disability has two meanings. Actual loss of earnings is the extent of actual loss of earnings resulting from the injury or disease. Loss of earning capacity (which is the same as impairments of earning capacity) is the presumed loss of earning capacity resulting from the injury or disease. Loss of earning capacity is more a legal or economic concept than a medical concept. It is used in the legal system as a basis for determining damages in personal injury cases. It was carried over into workers' compensation programs, which were established in the early 20th century to replace the tort system in dealing with accidents at work. When disability benefits for veterans were established by an amendment of the War Risk Insurance Program in 1917, the concept of a rating schedule to compensate for diminished earning capacity was borrowed from state workers' compensation programs.[4]

Conceptually, loss of earning capacity is not the same as loss of actual earnings because, for various reasons, some people earn less than they could earn, or they earn more than expected given the seriousness of their injuries. In legal proceedings, there must be a reasonable basis for determining earning capacity. Vocational specialists often have a key role in determining what jobs a person might be able to perform given his or her age, education, occupation, skills, knowledge, and experience, and what such jobs usually pay. In practice, past earnings are usually the basis for tort awards, because there is little evidence of earning capacity except actual preinjury earnings (Horner and Slesnick, 1999).

Quality of Life

Despite the limitations of our current models for measuring disability, researchers have pointed out the importance of including more global measures of health status and health-related quality of life (HRQOL) when measuring outcomes (IOM, 1997). It is also important to emphasize that these measures are not meant to replace traditional measures of impairment, limitations in ADLs, or work disability. The current role of these broader measures of outcomes such as HRQOL is to expand the scope of evaluation research and the scope of policy making. More research is needed to better understand how HRQOL relates to work disability, including loss of earning capacity. According to the IOM model of disability (1997), the disabling process is a product of the interaction of the person and the environment, thereby influencing one's quality of life.

Defining Quality of Life

The concept of quality of life (QOL) can be traced back to the ancient Western philosopher Aristotle, who described it as "happiness," a "certain kind of virtuous activity of the soul" (Zhan, 1992). Attempts to define QOL in the United States at the societal level were initiated by President Eisenhower's Commission on National Goals (Weisgerber, 1991). Later during the 1970s the concept began being used in reference to the individual (Wolfensberger, 1994). Historically, the United States has measured the success of its efforts to improve the health of its citizens on the basis of mortality statistics. Gains in human longevity no doubt have been accompanied by

[4]The 1917 amendments authorized "monetary payments, for disability incurred or aggravated in armed service, based largely upon the practices of state employees compensation laws, and called 'disability compensation' instead of 'pensions'" (Griffith, 1945).

increases in the incidence and prevalence of morbidity and accompanying disabilities (IOM, 1997). Within the last few decades, the emphasis on such measurement has changed from the quantity to the quality of life.

Both the economic and human costs of disability are enormous. Approximately one-third of people with physical, mental, or sensorial disabilities have disabilities so severe that they are unable to carry out the major activities of their age group, such as attending school, working, parenting, or providing self-care (IOM, 1997). As a result, attention must be focused not only on preventing disease and injury but on treatment and rehabilitation.

By definition, the concept of QOL covers many dimensions of one's life: cultural, psychological, physical, interpersonal, spiritual, financial, political, temporal, and philosophical. Furthermore, QOL is dynamic because it reflects changes in people and the environment over time across many of its domains (Tate et al., 1996).

Shumaker et al. (1990) define QOL on three levels varying from global to specific. The global dimension or overall assessment is "an individual's overall satisfaction with life, and one's general sense of well-being." The middle level includes the four domains of physical, psychological, social, and economic aspects of QOL, and the lowest level includes all aspects of each domain that are specifically assessed by different QOL measures. Psychological well-being, therefore, might be determined by a combination of factors such as the absence of negative states such as depression, anxiety, or posttraumatic stress disorder, and by the presence of positive states such as effective coping skills and a healthy self-esteem.

Different approaches have been used to evaluate the QOL of individuals with disease and injury. Highlighting its importance to successful rehabilitation, the concept has been studied in a variety of conditions including cardiovascular disease, cancer, renal disease, spinal cord injury, traumatic brain injury, stroke, and lung disease, to mention a few. QOL is viewed as an important indicator of a patient's overall health across time. HRQOL components can include signs or symptoms, treatment side effects, or physical, cognitive, emotional, and social functioning. During the progression of chronic disease or disability, HRQOL components can interact with other QOL dimensions (e.g., financial, workplace, and environmental accessibility factors) in a number of situations. These dimensions also may affect a person's ability to cope with injury or disease and successfully respond to interventions.

The concept of QOL is thus critical to the enabling-disabling process as outlined in *Enabling America*, which assessed the state of rehabilitation science and engineering (IOM, 1997). This report illustrated how biological, environmental (physical and social), and lifestyle/behavioral factors are involved in reversing the disabling process. The availability of more comprehensive health services is particularly important and timely because of the growing needs of veterans with disabilities and the demand for rehabilitation services that extend beyond the physical realm. New developments in rehabilitation science and engineering are essential to restore human functional capacity and to improve a person's quality of life and interactions with the surrounding environment.

QOL Assessments

There are many approaches to assessing the health of a person. Most include measurements in several domains. The term *domain* is used to describe the physical, psychological, and social aspects of an individual's activities. For example, measures of physical impairments, which might include anatomical or physiological abnormalities, are thought to contribute to overall function and quality of life. In addition, measures of limitations of function, such as gait velocity or prehension, are done because they provide an accurate and quantitative picture of what an individual is able to perform. Measures of disability are also acknowledged as being useful because they place the abnormalities within the context of an individual's daily routines.

In 1948, the World Health Organization (WHO) prompted a major departure from the disease-driven orientation previously adopted to define the concept of health and to assess outcomes. WHO stated that "physical, mental, and social well-being and not merely absence of disease" defines health. The definition helped set the conceptual framework for what constitutes treatment goals, thereby acknowledging the importance of using multidimensional outcome measures that would include the domains of physical, mental, and social health, and measures of function and disability. Toward this end, WHO devised the *International Classification of Functioning, Disability and Health* (ICF) to reflect advances in science and to acknowledge the individual's values and goals within the context of his or her unique social and physical environment. The ICF comprises four domains:

1. measures of body function;
2. measures of body structures;
3. measures of activity and participation at the level of the person; and
4. environmental support (physical and social).

There has been considerable interest in the multi-domain approach to assessment for several reasons:

- The information age has educated individuals about what is possible
- The public has higher expectations about what can be achieved by an individual following illness and injury
- The Americans with Disabilities Act has identified regulations about the need to remove environmental barriers and increase opportunities for people with disabilities
- Medical practice and health services have advanced such that amelioration of disability and restoration of function is feasible with greater frequency

In general, the health-care establishment is committed to helping reduce the burden of disease, but has become increasingly aware of patient priorities, which include the desire to be independent, to maintain valued activity, and to have a sense of well-being in all aspects of daily life—in short, to achieve a good quality of life. The Centers for Disease Control and Prevention (CDC) defines QOL as the perception of physical and mental health over time (CDC, 2007). When it is referred to as HRQOL, QOL is frequently linked with function and/or health status.

Function is not the same as QOL. Functional assessment is designed to measure *what* individuals are doing. It is a measure of the degree to which an individual can perform chosen roles (as well as duties and responsibilities) without physical, social, psychological, or cognitive limitation. What distinguishes the functional assessment from the QOL or the HRQOL instrument is the component of measuring patient satisfaction. HRQOL is designed to measure what an individual values and whether there is much satisfaction in one's life. Many instruments have been developed. Some have been designed to rate specific activities based on their importance to an individual and others to assess the impact of these activities on the individual's feelings of satisfaction and competence.

QOL measures address the value of the activity to the individual. Functional measures and QOL indicators are measures of different but complementary phenomena, and a substantial body of data show that physical findings and disease severity do not always correlate with patient self-reported QOL.

Controversy exists about whether such measures are more about life than health and whether health care should consider QOL measures as relevant given that the social, financial, and spiritual components of life usually most influence quality. Nevertheless, as individuals become more knowledgeable about health-care options, and as data are provided about the risks and benefits of these options, individuals are (and should be) participating more in decision making. As a result, an increasing number of studies include HRQOL measurements as outcomes, and investigators suggest they provide meaningful information that informs clinical practice.

Programs That Compensate for Loss of QOL

There are several concepts of QOL at the Department of Defense (DoD) and VA. First, while in the service, veterans benefit from what DoD calls quality-of-life programs and services. Military QOL programs provide services that improve the life circumstances of servicemembers and/or their families. For example, the annual Military Construction, Military Quality of Life, and Veterans Affairs Appropriations Act funds family housing and recreational facilities. QOL programs also include the range of services to take care of families while members are deployed or when they return injured.

At VHA, QOL usually refers to the concept described earlier. VHA has developed an HRQOL instrument, the Veterans SF-36 (SF-36V), to assess veterans in outpatient settings. The SF-36V has been shown to be valid and reliable in the population served by VHA (Perlin et al., 2000), and use of the SF-36V in outcomes research is widespread in VHA medical research studies (Kazis, 2000). At VBA, however, *quality of life* refers to impacts of service-connected injuries and diseases that are not likely to affect a veteran's employment prospects. These include scars, minor hearing loss, and loss of a procreative organ.

The Canadian veterans disability compensation program and some provincial workers' compensation programs compensate for loss of QOL. Veterans Affairs Canada, for example, measures degree of interference with ability to

- carry out usual and customary ADLs;
- maintain appropriate and customary personal relationships; and
- participate in recreational and community activities.

The standard for comparison is, as much as possible, the usual or accustomed activities that the veteran was engaged in before becoming disabled. A QOL level determination table sets out criteria for three levels of QOL, ranging from mild limitations or reductions of ability to carry out the three kinds of activities listed above (level 1) to moderate interference or limitations (level 2) to extreme inability to carry them out (level 3).

The next step is to use a QOL conversion table to determine the percentage ranging from 1 to 20 percent that should be added to the "medical impairment rating." The higher the medical impairment rating, the larger the QOL percentages given in the table. For example, those rated 11–20 percent impaired can receive up to 5 additional percentage points for loss of QOL, while those rated rated 71–80 percent may receive up to 20 additional percentage points for loss of QOL.[5] The resulting total of the medical impairment rating and the QOL rating is called the "disability assessment." This is done for each condition, and the results are combined to determine the overall rating, which forms the basis for the amount of compensation.[6] The Canadian method of compensating for loss of QOL is administratively feasible but far from a full assessment of QOL.

Most Canadian provinces compensate workers for non-economic loss in addition to or, in some cases, when compensation for non-economic loss would be higher, in place of compensating for loss of earning capacity. Non-economic loss is usually based on degree of impairment, measured by the American Medical Association's (AMA's) *Guides to the Evaluation of Permanent Impairment* or similar impairment schedule. Although intended to compensate for losses suffered despite ability to work, Sinclair and Burton's study of the Ontario workers' compensation program found that impairment ratings based on the AMA *Guides* did not well predict loss of quality of life (Sinclair and Burton, 1995).

The Australian Department of Veterans' Affairs (DVA) compensates veterans for "permanent impairment, pain and suffering and the lifestyle restrictions which are a result of the accepted [i.e., service-connected] injury or disease" (Australian DVA, 2006). First, DVA determines an impairment rating between 5 and 100 percent using a *Guide to Determining Impairment and Compensation* (Australian DVA, 2005). Second, DVA determines a lifestyle rating based on the extent an individual is limited in fulfilling roles normal for a veteran without a service-connected injury or disease. The lifestyle rating is an average of ratings on four scales—personal relationships, mobility, recreational and community activities, and employment and domestic activities (Australian DVA, 2005).[7] The impairment rating and lifestyle rating are then combined using a table, and the resulting compensation factor (expressed as a percentage between 0 and 1) is multiplied by the maximum permanent impairment pay amount to produce the monthly amount of compensation (Australian DVA, 2005). The lifestyle factor accounts for 15 percent of the compensation factor for impairment ratings up to 50, a lesser amount for impairment ratings between 50 and 80, and 0 percent of the compensation factor for impairment ratings 80 and higher (because the compensation factor for impairment ratings of 80 and higher is 1, the maximum that can be awarded).

---

[5]The maximum rating for impairment plus loss of QOL is 100 percent.

[6]The rating manual is available at http://www.vac-acc.gc.ca/clients/sub.cfm?source=dispen/2006tod/ch_02_2006/ (accessed March 19, 2007).

[7]There are two scales for the last domain, one for domestic activities and one for employment activities. The higher of the two ratings is used.

THE RELATIONSHIPS AMONG THE CONCEPTS IN THE DISABILITY MODEL

The preceding section provided a model of disability and definitions and discussions of the salient concepts embedded in that model, including impairment, limitations in ADLs, work disability (including impairments in earning capacity), and QOL. One crucial point is that a distinction must be made between the purpose of a disability compensation program (a topic considered in the next section) and the operational basis for the benefits (a topic considered in this section, in the next chapter, and in Appendix C).

Use of Proxies for Wage Loss in Workers' Compensation

State workers' compensation programs differ with respect to whom they cover, which injuries and diseases are covered, benefit levels, and administrative rules. All states provide benefits for temporary disabilities (that is, benefits between the date of injury and the date of "maximum medical improvement," when the healing period is completed). During the temporary disability period, workers' compensation benefits are only paid if the worker has an actual loss of earnings.

After the date of maximum medical improvement, states differ in their approaches to permanent disability benefits. Almost all state workers' compensation statutes have a schedule, or list, of body parts that are covered and an indication of how loss of each body part, such as a finger, hand, leg, eye, or hearing, is compensated for workers with permanent partial disability, which constitutes the vast majority of cases with permanent consequences. Scheduled permanent partial disability benefits are based on an assessment of the degree of permanent impairment, where the permanent impairment is used as a proxy for the expected losses of earnings. Spine injuries, head injuries, organ damage, and occupational diseases, however, are usually not on the schedule. Nonscheduled permanent partial disability cases are paid on the basis of three approaches. The most common approach is to pay for the degree of permanent impairment without regard to future earnings losses, usually based on use of the AMA *Guides*, where the permanent impairment is used as a proxy for actual losses of earnings. The second approach pays permanent partial disability benefits after a determination of the worker's loss of earning capacity, based on the extent of permanent impairment and other factors, such as his or her age and previous work experience. A few states pay permanent partial disability benefits based on the worker's actual wage losses, which is much more complicated to administer. Some states use a combination of two or even all three approaches, depending on the type and severity of the worker's injury (Barth, 2003/2004; Burton, 2005).

Use of Proxies for Wage Loss in the Veterans Disability Compensation Program

Although the official name of the VA Rating Schedule is the Veterans Administration Schedule for Rating Disabilities, it mostly uses proxy measures of assessing the extent of work disability. Proxy measures include

- degree of anatomic loss (e.g., 70 percent for amputation or loss of use of a dominant hand);[8] and
- extent of functional loss of an organ (e.g., 10, 30, 60, or 100 percent for diminished lung capacity because of asthma, bronchitis, emphysema, or chronic obstructive pulmonary disease).[9]

The Rating Schedule considers social and economic impacts only in rating mental disorders. For example, 30 percent is given for

> occupational and social impairment with occasional decrease in work efficiency and intermittent periods of inability to perform occupational tasks (although generally functioning satisfactorily, with routine behavior, self-care, and conversation normal [sic]), due to such symptoms as: depressed mood, anxiety, suspiciousness, panic attacks (weekly or less often), chronic sleep impairment, mild memory loss (such as forgetting names, directions, recent events).[10]

Although the veterans disability compensation program borrowed the ideas of a schedule of monthly benefits for particular impairments and loss of earning capacity from workers' compensation, some significant changes were made. In the state programs, the schedule normally lists a duration of benefits that depends on the severity of the permanent impairment, which is paid out weekly at a fraction of the worker's preinjury wages (typically two-thirds) until the total is reached. In the veterans compensation program, the monthly amount is paid for life. The VA approach assumes the impairment is permanent, an assumption at odds with current thinking on rehabilitation. The schedule also included all injuries and diseases, not just specific body parts. The loss of earning capacity rather than actual wage loss probably seemed more appropriate because many veterans do not have a civilian job before entering the service. Implicitly, the policy

---

[8]Diagnostic codes 5124 (amputation) and 5125 (loss of use) in the Rating Schedule (loss, or loss of use, of the non-dominant hand is rated 60 percent).

[9]As measured by a FEV_1 (forced expiratory volume in one second) test. An FEV_1 result of less than 40 percent of predicted value equals a rating of 100 percent, 40–55 percent equals 60 percent, 56–70 percent equals 30 percent, and a 71–80 percent equals 10 percent (diagnostic codes 6600 and 6602–6604 in the Rating Schedule).

[10]These are the criteria for all of the mental disorders except eating disorders (diagnostic codes 9201–9440 in the Rating Schedule).

acknowledged the difference between impairment and disability by (1) recognizing that individuals with the same severity of impairment will have a range of earnings and (2) allowing veterans with impairments to earn as much as they want without affecting the amount of their compensation. In 1933, VA officially recognized that some individuals are not able to earn as much as others with the same degree of impairment, by establishing the individual employability (IU) benefit and, further, allowing individuals who do not meet the minimum schedular rating degree to quality for IU to appeal to the administrator for total disability benefits.

Perhaps because earning capacity is not the same as actual earnings, successive VA Rating Schedules, including the current one, have not been based on empirical comparisons of the actual earnings of veterans at the various rating levels with veterans who are not rated for disability. In 1945, for example, VA's Disability Policy Board, mostly made up of physicians and some lawyers, set the criteria for rating the conditions in the Rating Schedule:

> According to a former Director of VA's Compensation and Pension Service, VA's Department of Medicine and Surgery, now the Veterans Health Administration, provided the Board with a medical monograph—a detailed description of etiology and manifestations—for each of the conditions included in the schedule at that time. The Board used these monographs to estimate the relative effects different levels of severity of a condition have on the average veteran's ability to compete for employment in the job market . . . [and] set the ratings on this basis (GAO, 1997).

According to VA, the 1945 Rating Schedule was "more detailed than the 1933 schedule." It "reflected society's reduced reliance on manual labor and had a greater appreciation of the effect of mental disability." "The 1945 scheme remains in effect with changes made as the need arose and with the assistance from Veterans Health Administration" (Pamperin, 2006). The Disability Policy Board of eight physicians and lawyers was responsible for revising the Rating Schedule until it was abolished in 1969 (GAO, 1989).

In 1956, the President's Commission on Veterans' Pensions, chaired by retired Army general Omar Bradley, commissioned surveys of representative samples of veterans and of veterans receiving disability compensation and compared the median earnings of each group, for example, veterans without disabilities, veterans rated 10 percent, veterans rated 20 percent, and so on, up to veterans rated 100 percent. The results showed veterans had lower earnings as rating levels increased, with an especially sharp drop off at 100 percent (President's Commission, 1956). When the amount of monthly compensation was added in, however, veterans with disabilities had about the same income as veterans without disabilities except at the

100 percent rating level. On average, veterans rated 100 percent earned about 10 percent less than veterans without disabilities. Probably as a result of this finding, Congress raised the benefit amount for 100 percent in 1957 relative to the rest of the rating levels, a difference that has widened over the years (Economic Systems, 2004a). When the Bradley Commission looked at the average income of veterans with mental and neurological diseases and those with general medical and surgical conditions separately, it found that the former group had 10–20 percent less income than the latter at most rating levels (President's Commission, 1956).

In 1971, VA conducted an "economic validation" of the Rating Schedule, with a sample size large enough to compare 1967 earnings of veterans at one or more rating levels of most of the diagnostic categories with those of veterans without disabilities with similar demographic characteristics. Known as the ECVARS study, for *Ec*onomic *Va*lidation of the *R*ating *S*chedule, it found that the difference between the earnings plus compensation of veterans with disabilities at a given rating level and the earnings of veterans without disabilities varied by condition, in some cases giving veterans with disabilities higher rating percentages than percentages of actual earnings losses, in other cases giving them lower rating percentages than actual earnings losses.[11] Like the Bradley Commission, ECVARS found that the drop-off in earnings was especially severe for those rated 100 percent, and that those with mental conditions consistently had substantially lower earnings. In all, ECVARS found that for about 330 of the 700 conditions studied, the rating criteria overestimated average loss in earnings, and for about 75, the rating criteria underestimated the average loss in earnings (GAO, 1997). VA submitted a Rating Schedule with criteria adjusted according to the ECVARS findings, but Congress declined to act on it (U.S. Congress, Senate, Committee on Veterans' Affairs, 1973).

In conclusion, average impairments in earnings is an abstract concept that cannot be measured directly. Its origins are legal, not medical. As used by VA, it is based on judgment, and it is not linked to observed average losses of actual earnings by veterans at each rating level or with particular conditions.

PURPOSE OF SERVICE-CONNECTED DISABILITY COMPENSATION

Compensation for average loss of earning capacity is the official statutory purpose of the veterans disability compensation program. The concept of average loss dates from the War Risk Insurance program amendments of 1917:

---

[11]The ECVARS is also discussed in Chapter 4 and in Appendix C.

> A schedule of ratings of reductions in earning capacity from specific injuries or combinations of the injuries of a permanent nature shall be adopted and applied by the Bureau. The ratings shall be based as far as is practicable upon the average impairments of earning capacity resulting from such injuries in civil occupations, and not upon the impairment in each individual case, so that there shall be no reduction in the rate of compensation for individual success in overcoming the handicap of a permanent injury (Douglas, 1918:473).[12]

Several widely accepted conceptual models of disability exist and, although they differ in details, all in some way distinguish among medical impairment, functional capacity, and disability (WHO, 2001; IOM, 1991, 1997; NCMRR, 1993; Nagi, 1976). Rather than assuming that the level of impairment is highly correlated with the extent of disability, they conceive of disability as the result of the interaction between an individual's functional limitations and his or her environment, unlike the anatomical approach of the Rating Schedule. This approach accounts for the fact that individuals with similar impairments have different degrees of disability.

These models of disability also conceive of disability as broader than inability to work. Disability also includes the inability to engage in any of the range of activities that most people enjoy, such as going to school, interacting socially, having a family, traveling, and managing one's legal and economic affairs. The ability to participate in this range of activities represents a person's QOL. *Disability in America* included QOL as a factor in disability. The report called for improved QOL measurement to use in assessments of health and disability because QOL corresponds to overall well-being with both physical and psychosocial dimensions and is more than the absence of disease or injury (IOM, 1991).

The Rating Schedule is a tool or instrument used by VA to rate disability on a scale ranging from 0 to 100 percent in intervals of at least 10 percent. As a tool, the Rating Schedule is a means to an end or a method of achieving a purpose. Therefore, to evaluate the performance of the Rating Schedule and to make recommendations for improving it, the purpose of the compensation program should be as clear as possible. If there are multiple purposes, each should be clear, and the appropriate desired trade-offs should be specified.

There are differences in views about what is or should be the purpose or the intent of compensating veterans. The statutory purpose is clearly economic: To compensate veterans for "the average impairments of earning capacity resulting from such injuries in civil occupations." The intent may not have been to compensate for each individual's actual loss

---

[12]The Bureau referred to in the law is the Bureau of War Risk Insurance, a predecessor agency of today's VA.

of earnings, but the fundamental reason for the program was to provide economic assistance to servicemembers and their families.[13] At the time it was established, the program was clearly seen as a form of social insurance to protect veterans and their families from economic hardship (Douglas, 1918). A recent study of veterans disability compensation legislation cites a number of indications of congressional intent to provide economic security (Economic Systems, 2004b).

Another view of the purpose of the disability compensation program is that it is in part an indemnification against enduring losses, such as blindness, amputation, or PTSD, and other permanent effects, such as pain, and it includes losses that do not seem likely to affect a veteran's earning capacity or ability to work. Proponents of the latter opinion point out features of the program, many mandated by Congress, that imply compensation for losses other than earning capacity, such as disfigurement, loss of a limb or an organ, pain and suffering, social maladjustment, and diminished QOL. The same legislative history cited above for references to the economic intent of disability compensation also found instances of intent to compensate for loss of QOL (Economic Systems, 2004b). VA itself acknowledges a broader purpose in its 2006–2011 strategic plan. Strategic goal one is "Restore the capability of veterans with disabilities to the greatest extent possible, and improve the quality of their lives and that of their families." Objective two under this goal is "Provide timely and accurate decisions on disability compensation claims to improve the economic status and quality of life of service-disabled veterans" (VA, 2006:36).[14]

In addition, using the degree of anatomic and functional loss of body structures and processes (i.e., impairment) as the basis for amount of compensation, rather than evaluating the veteran's ability to function in daily life and earn a living (i.e., disability), makes the compensation in part an indemnification or recognition of permanent damage or loss.

FINDINGS AND RECOMMENDATIONS

The conceptualization of disability and disability rating has evolved since the Rating Schedule was developed. For the most part, the statutory and regulatory provisions of the VA disability compensation program are based on impairments used as a proxy for work disability. There are, however, policies within the disability compensation system that do not strictly follow the view that the sole purpose of benefits is to compensate for work

[13]Other sections of the act as amended in 1917 provided for allowances for families with a member serving in the military and for life insurance for servicemembers.

[14]Objective one is provision of specialized health care to maximize the functioning of disabled veterans.

disability. The Rating Schedule seems intended to evaluate impairments as proxies for a diverse set of objectives (indemnification against limitations in the ADLs, work disability, and losses in QOL) without making clear the relationships among these constructs.

This inconsistency in the VA system in part reflects the evolving concepts and approaches to assessing disability. Today, disability is seen to be more than impairment of earning capacity. Over the years, VA and Congress have implicitly recognized the extent of impact that service-connected injuries and diseases can have on veterans by including conditions in the Rating Schedule that have little if any effect on ability to work. These expansions of the conditions covered by the Rating Schedule have been ad hoc, however, and may not address the full range or extent of nonwork impacts of injuries and diseases suffered while in military service.

A clear legislative statement of the purpose or purposes of the veterans disability compensation program would be tremendously helpful in evaluating and updating the Rating Schedule and the procedures for its application, which would include the appropriateness of the rating criteria, which tests and examinations should be used, and determination of the appropriate types and amounts of expertise needed for implementation, such as using medical rather than vocational experts.

A conceptual model—the ICF—links impairment and limitations in ADLs to work disability as well as nonwork disability (e.g., pain and suffering, distress, and poor personal relationships). The ICF, and similar models such as Nagi's and the IOM's (Nagi, 1976; IOM, 1991, 1997),[15] reflect the way we think about disability today. These more modern conceptual models of disability require broader thinking about impairments, functional limitations, and their relationship to disability (both work and nonwork). It calls for more complex assessments from disability determination systems. It requires more data to make the determinations, and it also requires more empirical evidence about the relationships among the components of the model. Empirical evidence measuring the relationships among impairment, functioning of the individual, work disability, and quality of life is key to a valid and fair system of disability determination. In the absence of empirical evidence, the relationships should be based on up-to-date expert opinion.

The VA disability assessment process also provides a key opportunity to assess the rehabilitation needs of veterans with impairments, and then to ameliorate them and restore function, when possible. It also provides for an opportunity to prevent disability. A system of services for veterans transitioning to civilian life, including health, vocational rehabilitation,

[15]An appendix to the 1991 IOM report contains perhaps the most complete explication of Nagi's conceptual framework.

employment, and education services, calls for multidimensional qualitative and quantitative measures to assess disability.

> **Recommendation 3-1. The purpose of the current veterans disability compensation program as stated in statute currently is to compensate for average impairment in earning capacity, that is, work disability. This is an unduly restrictive rationale for the program and is inconsistent with current models of disability. The veterans disability compensation program should compensate for three consequences of service-connected injuries and diseases: work disability, loss of ability to engage in usual life activities other than work, and loss in quality of life. (Specific recommendations on approaches to evaluating each consequence of service-connected injuries and diseases are in Chapter 4.)**

The committee is aware that adopting Recommendation 3-1 would be difficult and costly. Legislative endorsement would be very helpful, if not required, to ensure its adoption and implementation. If the recommendation is adopted, the Rating Schedule and the procedures needed to implement it will need to be revised to reflect the expanded purposes for disability benefits endorsed by the committee. This can be done in phases after appropriate research and analysis and pilot projects to study the feasibility of changes have been effected. This issue is addressed in Chapters 4 and 5.

Expanding the bases for veterans disability compensation also has cost implications. There will be start-up costs incurred in developing the instruments for evaluating degree of functional limitation and loss of QOL, transitional costs, probably higher administrative costs, and possibly greater compensation costs (if the current Rating Schedule does not adequately compensate for loss of function and QOL). Although the committee was not asked to consider costs in recommending improvements in medical evaluation of veterans for disability benefits, the issue is addressed at the end of Chapter 4.

In addition, if disability compensation is considered in the larger context of veterans benefits and is taken in conjunction with today's views on the rights of individuals with disabilities to live as full a life as possible, it is possible to justify a more comprehensive evaluation of a veteran's needs—medical, educational, vocational, and compensation. Currently, the assessment process is piecemeal and fragmented. Either the veteran must receive a rating to access related services, such as health care and vocational rehabilitation and employment services, or the other service is separate, such as with education. This issue is addressed in Chapter 6.

REFERENCES

Australian DVA (Department of Veterans' Affairs). 2005. *Guide to determining impairment and compensation*. Instrument No. M9 of 2005. Military Rehabilitation and Compensation Commission, Australian Government. http://www.comlaw.gov.au/ComLaw/Legislation/LegislativeInstrument1.nsf/0/18CD3003DD8A7A1DCA25700E0019A473?OpenDocument/ (accessed May 22, 2007).

Australian DVA. 2006. *Permanent impairment compensation payments*. Fact Sheet MRC 07. Department of Veterans' Affairs, Australian Government, October 31. www.dva.gov.au/factsheets/default.htm (accessed May 22, 2007).

Barth, P. S. 2003/2004. Compensating workers for permanent partial disabilities. *Social Security Bulletin* 65(4):16–23. http://www.ssa.gov/policy/docs/ssb/v65n4/v65n4p16.pdf (accessed March 19, 2007).

Burton, J. F., Jr. 2005. Permanent partial disability benefits. In *Workplace injuries and diseases: Prevention and compensation*, edited by K. Roberts, J. F. Burton, Jr., and M. M. Bodah. Kalamazoo, MI: W. E. Upjohn Institute for Employment Research. Chapter 4.

CDC (Centers for Disease Control and Prevention). 2007. *Health-related quality of life*. http://www.cdc.gov/hrqol/ (accessed March 23, 2007).

Douglas, P. H. 1918. The War Risk Insurance Act. *Journal of Political Economy* 26(5):461–483.

Economic Systems, Inc. 2004a. *VA disability compensation program: Literature review*. Washington, DC: Department of Veterans Affairs. http://www.va.gov/op3/docs/Final_Report-LiteratureReview.pdf (accessed March 19, 2007).

Economic Systems, Inc. 2004b. *VA disability compensation program: Legislative history*. Washington, DC: VA. http://www.va.gov/op3/docs/Disability_Comp_Legislative_Histor_Lit_Review.pdf (accessed March 19, 2007).

GAO (Government Accountability Office). 1989. *Veterans' benefits: Need to update medical criteria used in VA's disability rating schedule*. GAO/HRD-89-28. Washington, DC: GAO. http://www.gao.gov/archive.gao.gov/d17t6/137639.pdf (accessed March 19, 2007).

GAO. 1997. *VA disability compensation: Disability ratings may not reflect veterans' economic losses*. GAO/HEHS-97-9. Washington, DC: GAO. http://www.gao.gov/archive/1997/he97009.pdf (accessed March 19, 2007).

Griffith, C. M. 1945. The Veterans Administration. In *Doctors at war*, edited by M. Fishbein. New York: E. P. Dutton & Company. Chapter XIV.

Horner, S. M., and F. Slesnick. 1999. The valuation of earning capacity definition, measurement and evidence. *Journal of Forensic Economics* 12(1):13–32.

IOM (Institute of Medicine). 1991. *Disability in America: Toward a national agenda for prevention*, edited by A. M. Pope and A. R. Tarlov. Washington, DC: National Academy Press.

IOM. 1997. *Enabling America: Assessing the role of rehabilitation science and engineering*, edited by E. Brandt and A. M. Pope. Washington, DC: National Academy Press.

Katz, S., A. B. Ford, R. W. Moskowitz, B. A. Jackson, and M. W. Jaffe. 1963. Studies of illness in the aged. The Index of ADL: A standardized measure of biological and psychosocial function. *Journal of the American Medical Association* 185(12):914–919.

Kazis, L. E. 2000. The Veterans SF-36 health status questionnaire: Development and application in the Veterans Health Administration. *Medical Outcomes Trust Monitor* 5:1–2.

Lawton, M. P., and E. M. Brody. 1969. Assessment of older people: Self-maintaining and instrumental activities of daily living. *The Gerontologist* 9(3):179–186.

Mahoney, F. I., and D. W. Barthel. 1965. Functional evaluation: The Barthel Index. *Maryland State Medical Journal* 14:61–65.

Nagi, S. Z. 1976. An epidemiology of disability among adults in the United States. *Milbank Memorial Fund Quarterly* 54:439–467.

NCMRR (National Center for Medical Rehabilitation Research). 1993. *Research plan for the National Center for Medical Rehabilitation Research*. NIH Publication No. 93-3509. Bethesda, MD: NCMRR. http://www.nichd.nih.gov/publications/pubs/upload/plan.pdf (accessed February 20, 2007).

Pamperin, T. 2006. *Overview of the department and the schedule for rating disabilities*. Presentation to the IOM Committee on Medical Evaluation of Veterans for Disability Compensation, Washington, DC, May 25.

Perlin, J., L. Kazis, K. Skinner, et al. 2000. *Health status and outcomes of veterans: Physical and mental component summary scores, Veterans SF-36, 1999 large health survey of veteran enrollees*. Washington, DC: Office of Quality and Performance, Veterans Health Administration, VA.

President's Commission (The President's [Bradley] Commission on Veterans' Pensions). 1956. *A Report to the President: Veterans' benefits in the United States, Volume I, Parts I and II: Findings and recommendations*. 84th Cong., 2nd Sess. House Committee Print No. 236. Washington, DC: U.S. Government Printing Office.

Shumaker, S. A., R. T. Anderson, and S. M. Czajkowski. 1990. Psychological tests and scales. In *Quality of Life Assessments in Clinical Trials*, edited by B. Spilker. New York: Raven Press. Pp. 95–114.

Sinclair, S., and J. F. Burton, Jr. 1995. Development of a schedule for compensation of non-economic loss: Quality-of-life values vs. clinical impairment ratings. In *Research in Canadian Workers' Compensation*, edited by T. Thomason and R. P. Chaykowski. Kingston, Ontario: IRC Press.

Tate, D. G., M. Dijkers, and L. Johnson-Greene. 1996. Outcome measures in quality of life. *Topics in Stroke Rehabilitation* 2(4):1–17.

U.S. Congress, Senate, Committee on Veterans' Affairs. 1973. *Veterans Administration proposed revision of Schedule for Rating Disabilities*. 93rd Cong., 1st Sess. February 12. Senate Committee Print No. 3. Washington, DC: U.S. Government Printing Office.

VA (Department of Veterans Affairs). 2006. *Department of Veterans Affairs strategic plan, FY 2006-2011*. http://www1.va.gov/op3/docs/VA_2006_2011_Strategic_Plan.pdf (accessed November 15, 2006).

VA. 2007. *Stroke rehabilitation VA/DoD clinical practice guidelines*. http://www.oqp.med.va.gov/cpg/STR/STR_base.htm (accessed June 21, 2007).

Weisgerber, R. A. 1991. *Quality of life for persons with disabilities: Skill development and transitions across life stages*. Rockville, MD: Aspen.

WHO (World Health Organization). 1980. *International classification of impairments, disabilities and handicaps*. Geneva, Switzerland: WHO.

WHO. 2001. *International classification of functioning, disability and health: Short version*. Geneva, Switzerland: WHO.

Wolfensberger, W. 1994. Let's hang up "quality of life" as a hopeless term. In *The Quality of life for persons with disabilities. Disabilities: International perspectives and issues*, edited by D. A. Goode. Cambridge, MA: Brookline Books.

Zhan, L. 1992. Quality of life: Conceptual and measurement issues. *Journal of Advanced Nursing* 17:795–800.

4

The Rating Schedule

This chapter reviews the Department of Veterans Affairs' (VA's) Schedule for Rating Disabilities (Rating Schedule) and makes recommendations for improving its effectiveness as the basis for compensating for service-connected disabilities. It is judged specifically for its ability to compensate for impairments in earning capacity and impacts on quality of life, as well as disability more generally. The processes for applying the Rating Schedule are addressed in Chapter 5. This chapter describes how the Rating Schedule came about and its substantive medical content, as well as how it is managed organizationally, including how revisions are made to it. The committee also reviews the currency of medical knowledge represented in the Rating Schedule and makes recommendations for improving the medical basis of the Rating Schedule and keeping it up to date.

The first part of this chapter describes the long and complex history and development of the Rating Schedule into the current century. It should be noted that, although the practice of providing pensions for veterans with disabilities began in the English colonies in North America, the first national pension law in the United States was adopted by the Continental Congress on August 26, 1776. A number of amendments, consolidations, and veterans acts followed, leading up to the current Rating Schedule used in the determination of eligibility for disability compensation.

The second part of this chapter delves into a detailed description of the Rating Schedule as it currently exists and discusses the numerous aspects of its maintenance and updating to serve the expanded purposes of veterans disability compensation recommended in Chapter 3.

HISTORY

> *There has never been any question but that it is the Government's duty and responsibility to provide, and to provide generously, for those who, while or as a result of serving their country in time of war, suffered disease or injury which resulted in their being unable to support themselves—in other words, those with service-connected disability. It has been accepted that the Government should compensate them in accordance with their disability. . . . Criticism of Government's actions in this area of veterans' benefits has been as much that the compensation paid these beneficiaries has been too small as that it has been too large* (President's Commission, 1956b:65).

The English set a precedent for providing benefits to men disabled in the military service (President's Commission, 1956b:5). Another precedent was set in 1636, when the Plymouth Colony enacted the first law in the English colonies in North America, which provided money to veterans who acquired disabilities as a result of battles with Pequot Indians (VA, 2007a). Other colonies followed this example. The Continental Congress passed the new country's first pension law in 1776 to encourage enlistments and curtail desertions (VA, 2007a,b). Compensation for service-connected disability at "half pay for life or during disability" was provided "to every officer, soldier, or sailor losing a limb in any engagement or being so disabled in the service of the United States as to render him incapable of earning a livelihood," and those partially disabled from getting a livelihood were promised proportionate relief (President's Commission, 1956b:5). Because the Continental Congress lacked the authority or the money to make the pension payment, it was left to the individual states to make the payments. At most, only 3,000 Revolutionary War veterans drew any pension because the obligation was met differently by the individual states (VA, 2007a). The impact of the Revolutionary War was important because awarding the pensions to these veterans set a precedent for later wars. Another key development was the recognition of the political importance of the veterans, although no formal organization among veterans for political purposes would come about until later. The most important development "was the establishment of the idea that the Government owed it to the veterans to protect them against indigency in their old age and also owed a debt of gratitude to all veterans which should be paid in the form of pensions" (President's Commission, 1956b:9).

Basic benefits for veterans remained unchanged for 35 years following the end of the Revolutionary War (President's Commission, 1956b:7). The U.S. Constitution was ratified and the first federal pension legislation was passed in1789. The payment of benefits to veterans was assumed by the first Congress, and the Continental Congress pension law was continued. In 1802, the Secretary of War requested the U.S. Attorney General to interpret military pension law:

> . . . the connexion [sic] between the inflicting agent and consequent disability need not always be so direct and instantaneous. It will be enough if it be derivative, and the disability be plainly, though remotely, the incident and the result of the military profession . . . such are the changes and uncertainties of the military life . . . that the seeds of disease, which finally prostrate the constitution, may have been hidden as they were sown, and thus be in danger of not being recognized as first causes of disability in a meritorious claim.[1]

By 1808, the Bureau of Pensions under the Secretary of War administered all veterans programs. In 1811, the federal government authorized the first domiciliary and medical facility for veterans (VA, 2007a,b). The War of 1812 and the Mexican War, which intervened between the Revolutionary and the Civil Wars, did not reflect significant developments regarding the nature or scope of veterans benefits; compensation for service-connected disability was provided for veterans of these wars at their onset (President's Commission, 1956b:10).Veterans and dependents of the War of 1812 were included through subsequent laws, and benefits to dependents and survivors were extended as well. By 1816, there were 2,200 pensioners, and in that year Congress raised allowances for all veterans with disabilities and granted half-pay pensions for five years (and later for a longer time period) to widows and orphans of soldiers of the War of 1812 to acknowledge the growing cost of living and a Treasury surplus (VA, 2007a,b).[2]

As a result of the surplus, President Monroe suggested in December 1817 that provision be made for the surviving Revolutionary War veterans; he anticipated that the cost would be minimal because there were so few of them remaining. Impassioned arguments urging this expression of gratitude of the country for these veterans prevailed although there was a lack of unanimity expressed by a minority in both houses of Congress as to the proper approach that should be taken to compensating them. For example, Senator William Smith, South Carolina, condemned the measure because he felt it was based on good feelings and sentiment, which he did not believe to be appropriate guides to a legislator. He pointed out that veterans of the War of 1812 would be the next to have as good a claim to such pensions, and

---

[1]Opinion of Richard Rush (U.S. Attorney General), April 15, 1815. See 1 Op. Att'y Gen. 181 (1815).

[2]The compensation for a private was raised from $5 to $8 a month, and for officers of the lower ranks by $2 or $3 a month (3 Stat. L., 296). In 1816, 1,757 disabled officers and men of the Revolutionary War were receiving compensation (President's Commission, 1956a:7).

predicted that this measure's precedent would be regretted later (President's Commission, 1956b:7-8).[3]

The Revolutionary War Pension Act of 1818 (3 Stat. L., 410) transferred administration of pensions to the Secretary of War (under the War Department), replacing the service pension programs run by a few states. Veterans who had served at least nine months in the Continental Army and who were also "in reduced circumstances" received lifetime pensions at half-pay of the rank held during the Revolutionary War. It was anticipated that the program would be "brief" and "inexpensive," an expression of gratitude and an act of charity for the benefit of indigent veterans who would otherwise be put in the humiliating position of having to search for evidence or produce surgeons' certificates. According to this legislation, every person who had served in the war and was in need of assistance would receive a fixed pension for life, at a rate of $20 a month for officers and $8 a month for enlisted men. Prior to this time, pensions were granted only to veterans with disabilities (VA, 2007a). There was an immediate rush of applications and efforts to prove need where none existed, perhaps indicating a sense of entitlement regardless of need (President's Commission, 1956b:8). From 1816 to 1820, the number of pensioners increased from 2,200 to 17,730 and the cost of pensions rose from $120,000 to $1.4 million (VA, 2007a).

The act was amended in 1820 because the original program was found to be "long, costly, and divisive." The program was converted to a hybrid of pension and poor-law provisions, and all recipients were suspended from the rolls pending proof of poverty. Claimants ages 65 and older were allowed the maximum rate only for senility.

There were about 80,000 war veterans at the time of the 1861 Civil War. By the end of the war in 1865, 1.9 million Union forces veterans were added to the rolls.[4] Disability payments based on rank and degree of disability were provided by the General Pension Act of 1862 (12 Stat. L., 566) (the General Law), and it "applied to the Civil War and to any or all future wars in which the United Sates might be engaged" (President's Commission, 1956b:13). Some changes in detail were made, and more liberal benefit provisions for widows, children, and dependent relatives came about, but it continued the same provisions and philosophy:

> The claimant must show that his disability was the result of his military service, or, if it did not arise until after his separation from service, he must show that it arose from causes which could be directly traced to injuries

---

[3]For debates on the measure, see *Annals of Congress*, 15th Cong., 1st Sess., 1, pp. 130–159.

[4]Congress pardoned Confederate service members and extended benefits for the first time in 1958, to the single remaining Confederate survivor.

> received or diseases contracted while in the military service (President's Commission, 1956b:14).

With this act, included for the first time, was compensation for diseases (e.g., tuberculosis) incurred while in service (VA, 2007a).

The rise in importance of veterans groups developed during the Civil War:

> The Civil War was fought under conditions well calculated to impress upon veterans their political power and importance as a group. During the war there was continuous jockeying for political power. Each time an important election was held large numbers of soldiers were furloughed to come home and vote. Particularly was this true in the election of 1864. The importance placed upon the soldier vote in this election was impressed upon the Army and helped lay the groundwork for the later emergence of the Grand Army of the Republic as a potent political force. Since the Republicans were in power, their party became the one which made efforts to save the Union by defeating the rebels; the Democrats, because they were the opposition party, became largely identified with the Copperheads. Service in the Armed Forces also became extremely important politically for candidates for national office for many years after the war (President's Commission, 1956b:11).

After the Civil War, veterans groups (e.g., the Grand Army of the Republic representing Union Veterans of the Civil War) organized to seek increased benefits (VA, 2007a):

> . . . the post-Civil War period was the first one when veterans had been organized for the purpose of exerting political pressure in favor of higher benefits for veterans. . . . The Civil War group was the forerunner of a whole series of veterans' organizations which have been formed along similar lines for the purpose of representing veterans with an organized voice (President's Commission, 1956b:12).

In 1866, to address the needs of the large number of veterans with disabilities, Congress authorized the National Asylum for Disabled Volunteer Soldiers, which in 1873 was called the National Home for Disabled Volunteer Soldiers. The 1873 Consolidation Act revised pension legislation, basing payment on the degree of disability rather than on service rank (VA, 2007a). The act came about because the laws had become so complex and conflicting, leading to the need for codification (President's Commission, 1956b:21).

The Arrears Act was passed in 1879, and it applied to claims filed prior to 1880. Its expense was unanticipated, and it generated an influx of applications. It was precipitated by the 1873 consolidation; payment of arrears of compensation to veterans or dependents of veterans who had not applied for compensation until after the five years specified by the law had elapsed was at issue:

> For the individual who had applied within 5 years, the compensation commenced at the death or discharge of the person on whose account the compensation was granted; for anyone who did not apply within 5 years, the compensation commenced with the filing of the last evidence necessary to complete the claim. It was contended that this discriminated unfairly against the person who tried to get along without compensation and on that account delayed the filing of his application (President's Commission, 1956b:21).

Until 1890, Civil War pensions were granted only to servicemen discharged because of illness or disability as a result of military service. However, that year the scope of eligibility was substantially broadened, and pensions were provided to veterans incapable of manual labor. By 1893, the number of veterans receiving pensions increased from 489,000 to 996,000, while the expenditures for the program doubled. There were no new pension laws after the Spanish-American War (1898)[5] or after the Philippine Insurrection (1899 to 1901) (VA, 2007a).

With the passage of the Sherwood Act of 1912, all veterans were awarded pensions, whereas in the 19th century, recipients had been limited by a similar law to veterans of the Revolutionary War. Under the Sherwood Act, veterans from the Mexican War and Union veterans of the Civil War could receive pensions automatically at age 62 even if they were not sick or disabled. The record shows that of the 429,354 Civil War veterans on pension rolls in 1914, 52,572 qualified on the basis of disability (VA, 2007a).

Military factors clearly led to developments in pension policies prior to World War I; however, the poor medical care and service received by soldiers in all wars prior to World War I may have been a more significant factor:

> Disease became a part of the disability picture, killing more men and probably disabling more men than did the bullets of the enemy. These disabilities due to disease, however, were very difficult to establish service connection for, and brought about much of the demand for pensions, particularly following the Civil War and the Spanish-American War. Confused and incomplete records of all kinds gave rise to much difficulty in establishing the facts of service and the facts of medical records on the basis of which to establish service connection of disabilities.
>
> During this entire period there were no general social welfare programs of any kind in existence for either the entire population or for special groups within the general population. The ruling thought pattern seems to have been that the individual should be responsible for providing for his own

[5]The military conditions were significant, however, in that pension demands increased.

> welfare without aid from the Government or from any other organization. Aid given to individuals was provided by private charity. There was no protection against such hazards as losing one's job because of disability, because of old age, or for any other reason. Veterans' pensions, especially those for Civil War Veterans, provided a comprehensive plan of security for eligible veterans against the hazards resulting in loss of income or in death (President's Commission, 1956b:24).

Prior to World War I, the War Risk Insurance Act of 1914 (40 Stat., 398–411) was passed to insure American ships and their cargoes. In 1917, after the war began, benefits legislation reflected readjustment and rehabilitation. It is estimated that 4.7 million Americans fought in this war, which left 116,000 dead and 204,000 wounded. The War Risk Insurance Act Amendments of 1917 were enacted to provide insurance against loss of life, personal injury, or capture by the enemy of personnel on board American merchant ships (VA, 2007b). Government-subsidized life insurance for veterans with an option for dependent death or disability coverage was provided. Under the act, a dependent's pension in case of death or disability was approved, as well as a $60 discharge allowance at war's end in recognition of service rendered.

Other provisions included the authority to establish courses for rehabilitation and vocational training for veterans with dismemberment, sight, hearing, and other permanent disabilities, with eligibility established retroactively to April 6, 1917, when the United States entered World War I. Veterans injured in service were retrained for new jobs.

An average earnings impairment disability rating schedule was introduced and, for the first time, service-connected "aggravation" of preexisting conditions applied (Gosoroski, 1997). Section 302 of the War Risk Insurance Act of October 6, 1917, provided the following:

> A schedule of ratings of reductions in earning capacity from specific injuries or combinations of injuries of a permanent nature shall be adopted and applied by the bureau. Ratings may be as high as one hundred per centum. The ratings shall be based, as far as practicable, upon the average impairments of earning capacity resulting from such injuries in civil occupations and not upon the impairment in earning capacity in each individual case, so that there shall be no reduction in the rate of compensation for individual success in overcoming the handicap of permanent injury. The bureau shall from time to time readjust this schedule of ratings in accordance with actual experience (cited by Paul Ising, retired VA executive, in a written communication provided to the committee).

The Act of June 25, 1918, further amended the War Risk Insurance Act of 1914 (Ch. 104, part 10, 40 Stat. 609, 611). It stated that in determining disability entitlement individuals having active service in the military "shall be held and taken to have been in sound condition when examined, accepted, and enrolled in service."

The Vocational Rehabilitation Act of 1918 authorized the establishment of the Federal Board for Vocational Education, an independent agency. Any honorably discharged veteran of World War I was made eligible for vocational rehabilitation training; those unable to undertake gainful occupation were also eligible for a special maintenance allowance (VA, 2007b).

In 1921, during the administration of President Harding, a committee investigating the administration of the laws pertaining to veterans recommended that

> . . . there should be created a Veterans' Service Administration, an independent agency to which should be transferred the Bureau of War Risk Insurance, the Rehabilitation Division of the Federal Board for Vocational Education, and such part of the Public Health Service as was necessary in dealing with the beneficiaries of the Bureau of War Risk Insurance and the Rehabilitation Division (Secretary of the Treasury, 1921).

Further, the committee recommended that the Secretary of the Treasury be empowered to consolidate veterans benefits under the Bureau of War Risk Insurance except for hospital and medical care. These recommendations led to the passage of P.L. No. 47 (67th Cong.) in 1921, under which the administration of all laws pertaining to World War I veterans was concentrated (President's Commission, 1956b:30). The Veterans Bureau was established and the first codified Schedule for Rating Disabilities was drafted that same year. In debate on July 20, 1921, Senator Walsh argued:

> It is very apparent to me that this wave of tuberculosis and nervous and mental disease that has taken such a deadly hold and grip of late upon our ex-service men must have been contracted in the service. I feel, therefore, that we ought not continue this requirement of endless affidavits, necessarily involving long delay, in demonstrating the fact that their illness is of service origin. The delays resulting from this affidavit requirement have often resulted in men dying before they ever got their compensation.

The 1921 Rating Schedule amended the presumption of soundness to exclude defects, disorders, or infirmities recorded at the inception of active service. It also provided for presumption of service connection for tuberculosis and neuropsychiatric conditions,[6] and for creation of local rating boards around the country instead of a single rating board in Washington, D.C. (VBA, 2005).

---

[6]These are the first presumptions and were made on a floor amendment to a bill for the then Bureau of Pensions, the precursor organization to the Veterans Administration.

The World War Veterans' Act of 1924 required a new Rating Schedule, which was created and placed into operation January 1, 1926. Known as the 1925 Rating Schedule, it had evaluation percentages in increments of 1 percent. On the positive side, unlike the 1945 Rating Schedule presently in effect, it did not require an increase of 10 percent for each upward adjustment. On the negative side, the scale required arbitrary discrimination to determine the difference between one or two percentage points. This schedule provided a disability rating based on assumptions about the skills and functions needed for specific occupations. For example, a veteran with a disability resulting from an ocular disorder would receive a higher disability evaluation if the individual worked as an accountant as opposed to a laborer with the same disability. Put differently, good eyesight was considered to be more important to a veteran who worked with written materials and numbers than to a veteran who performed manual tasks. This kind of determination provided the original rationale for including an occupational specialist on the rating board.

This act consolidated, codified, and liberalized the regulations and made significant changes in benefits; however, it was not definitive. It extended the presumption of service connection for tuberculosis and neuropsychiatric diseases to January 1, 1925, and added paralysis agitans, encephalitis lethargica, and amoebic dysentery to the presumptive list, which if they appeared before January 1, 1925, were presumed to be service connected (President's Commission, 1956b:33).

The next major liberalization occurred in 1926, with the establishment of a statutory tuberculosis award of not less than $50 a month for any ex-service person shown to have had a tuberculous disease of a compensable degree who had reached complete arrest of the disease; 43,719 veterans were receiving this benefit by June 30, 1932 (President's Commission, 1956b:33). In 1930, P.L. No. 522 (71st Cong.) was passed to grant aid in the form of a pension to needy, disabled World War I veterans with other than service-connected disabilities, with payments ranging from $12 to $40 a month depending on the degree of disability; within a little over two years, 440,954 veterans were receiving pensions. This law was passed when the United States was going into the Depression and no Treasury surplus was available to pay for it (President's Commission, 1956b:33–34).

The Economy Act of March 30, 1933 (P.L. No. 2, 73rd Cong.), which eliminated payments to all veterans without service-connected disabilities except those who were totally disabled and could meet an income test (President's Commission, 1956b:39), authorized the next version of the Rating Schedule. The 1933 Rating Schedule eliminated evaluations in increments of 1 percent and substituted multiples of 10 percent. It also eliminated the difference between temporary and permanent evaluations.[7] Additionally, it provided for the bilateral anatomical loss (e.g., two eyes, two feet, two hands, or any combination thereof) factor as it is used today. Further, the 1933 Rating Schedule eliminated the occupational variance and substituted the concept of average impairment in civilian occupational earnings capacity resulting from certain diseases and injuries. Historically, the War Risk Insurance Act of 1917 had called for implementing a Rating Schedule to be based on "the average impairment in earning capacity" caused by a disability. *Average impairment* was to be based on average loss of earnings for all occupations performing manual labor. Legislation in 1924 provided that the Rating Schedule should still be based on the concept of average impairment with the recognition of the effects of the disability on the preservice occupation of the veteran. However, this 1933 legislation led to reverting back to "average impairment of earnings capacity" (Economic Systems Inc., 2004b).

The advent of the Economy Act brought Executive orders into the system of veterans benefits:

> The Economy Act of 1933 cancelled all previously established benefits for veterans of wars since 1898 and substituted instead a system of veterans' benefits established by Executive order. The new system drastically curtailed all benefits, reduced pension payments to those with total disability, sharply reduced the payments going to those with service-connected disabilities, removed many cases for the rolls altogether, and cut down sharply on the benefits. Some liberalizations were made in the Executive orders during the following 2-year period, and by the end of 2 years, former laws, with the exception of that one granting disability pensions to veterans with non-service-connected disabilities, were substantially reenacted. Pensions continued to be limited to those suffering from total disability (President's Commission, 1956b:45).

The 1945 Rating Schedule became effective April 1, 1946, and formed the basis for the current schedule. This schedule raised the percentages of disability for some impairments and lowered them for others. It also provided for a review of all ratings under the 1925 and 1933 Rating Schedules. Under the 1945 Rating Schedule, a higher evaluation was assigned when possible, but "protection" of a higher rating under the prior Rating Schedule was not provided. (Protection in this context means that a disability rating would not be reduced solely on the basis of the application of the new Rating Schedule. However, a rating could be reduced if

[7]Legislation in 1919 established temporary and permanent disability compensation rates, payable based on the degree of reduction in earning capacity resulting from the disability (Economic Systems Inc., 2004a).

medical evidence establishes that the disability being evaluated has actually improved.) In the 1925 and 1933 Rating Schedules, if the application of the new schedule resulted in a reduction in the rating, the disability rating under the prior Rating Schedule was retained in a protected status. Thus, the assigned rating could only increase. Under the 1945 Rating Schedule, however, the assigned rating could decrease.

According to a July 1954 General Accounting Office (GAO) report:

> The disability ratings provided in the rating schedules are not based on an actual determination of the effect of the various disabilities on the average earning capacity of individuals in civil occupations. The Chairman of the VA Rating Schedule Board, in a statement dated January 21, 1952, regarding various aspects of the disability rating problems . . . indicated that the 1945 schedule is an outgrowth of other rating schedules which had been in use at various times from 1921 to April 1, 1946. He stated that the disability ratings provided in the 1921 schedule were not calculated on statistical or economic data regarding the average reduction in earning capacities from any disability because such data were not available, and that they undoubtedly represented the opinions of the physicians who had developed the schedules as to the effect of the various disabilities upon the earning capacity of the average man. He also stated that the disability percentage ratings provided in the 1945 schedule are based on very little calculations but that they represent the consensus of informed opinion of experienced rating personnel, for the most part physicians, and reflect many compromises of their views (as cited in President's Commission, 1956a:33).

Currently, VA uses the 1945 Rating Schedule and its medical criteria with some revisions to evaluate veterans for disability compensation.

THE CURRENT RATING SCHEDULE

Body Systems and Rating Disability

The current Rating Schedule assigns a percentage of disability, called a *rating*, based mostly on the severity of the veteran's medical impairment or diagnosis. The underlying assumption of this system of rating is that degree of disability is the equivalent or reasonably similar to percentage of impairment. The differences between impairment and disability, and the need to broaden the rating system to take account of dimensions of disability beyond impairment, were discussed in Chapter 3.

As discussed in Chapter 3, although the purpose of the current Rating Schedule is to determine the extent to which impairment reduces earning capacity (*work disability*), the operational basis for these ratings is an evaluation of the severity of impairments resulting from the service-connected injury or disease. Impairments or diagnoses in 14 body systems are delineated, as follows:

1. musculoskeletal
2. organs of special sense (vision and hearing)
3. infectious diseases, immune disorders, and nutritional deficiencies
4. respiratory
5. cardiovascular
6. digestive
7. genitourinary
8. gynecological conditions and disorders of the breast
9. hemic and lymphatic
10. skin
11. endocrine
12. neurological conditions and convulsive disorders
13. mental disorders
14. dental and oral conditions

The assigned percentages are in increments of 10 in a scale of 0 to 100. (Many service-connected conditions have relatively minor consequences and are rated zero.) When the disability is judged to be service connected and a compensable evaluation (at least 10 percent) is assigned, the veteran is entitled to receive monthly monetary benefits. Currently, the benefits range from $115 a month for a 10 percent rating to $2,471 a month for 100 percent or total disability rating for a single veteran. (Depending on the rating level, a veteran may be eligible for additional benefits, which are discussed in Chapter 6.)

The Rating Schedule contains about 700 diagnostic codes. If the veteran has a condition that is not listed in the Rating Schedule, the rater uses an analogous condition listed in the Rating Schedule to evaluate it.

The medical evidence must support both the diagnosis and the percentage assigned for the condition. Following the spirit of the law as reflected in the grateful nation principle, when the rater assigns a disability rating higher than one evaluation, but not sufficiently high to qualify for the next higher evaluation, the higher evaluation must be assigned as a matter of policy, backed by regulation.

The Rating Schedule also includes regulations and provides guidance pertaining to such topics as the

- essentials of evaluative rating (assigning evaluation percentages);
- interpretation of examination reports;
- resolution of reasonable doubt;
- evaluation of evidence;

- analogous ratings;
- attitude of rating officers;
- use of diagnostic code numbers; and
- assignment of a zero-percent rating.

Status of Rating Schedule Updates

> *The rating schedule was originated and designed hopefully on a scientific basis; and was to be revised and readjusted in accordance with actual experience. This "experience" has materialized, and the schedule of ratings has undergone several revisions, but the question or questions still remain—Whose actual experience? What kind of actual experience? When should this actual experience dictate a revision? Who was to designate the time of revisions, after actual experience dictated? Or, does actual experience dictate any revision of the veterans schedule for rating disabilities? . . . What are the criticisms of the current schedule? Is it outmoded? Is it in accord with the accepted medical principles and standard nomenclature? Are the ratings for the various disabilities equitable* (President's Commission, 1956c:155)?

The Rating Schedule has been updated unevenly over the years since this 1956 observation made by the Bradley Commission, which was published 11 years after the last revision had been made and after the addition of nine amendments by extensions. At that time, medical specialists were asked to review the Rating Schedule and respond to the following questions:

- (K) Are the disability ratings in accord with present-day accepted medical principles?
- (L) Is the disease nomenclature in accord with present-day medical standards?
- (M) Do the medical criteria reflect accurately the residuals of the injury or disease for different percentage ratings?
- (N) Is it medically feasible to assign graduations (sic) within an accuracy of 10 percent, when determining the percentage of bodily and mental impairment? If not, what scale of graduations do you regard as feasible?
- (O) In your opinion, do the ratings fairly represent the average impairment of earning capacity resulting from the various degrees of severity of physical impairment?
- (P) Do the disabilities at 10 percent and 20 percent constitute a material impairment of earning capacity?
- (Q) Do you know of any medical data which can be used to set

percentage ratings to represent the average impairment in earning capacity resulting from various diseases or injuries and their residual conditions for civil occupations (President's Commission, 1956c:156)?

Concerns expressed in response to the above questions, which are useful to the reader and illustrative of some of the same issues discussed in this report regarding the current Rating Schedule, are summarized in the Bradley Commission report:

- (K—accepted medical principles) ". . . a considerable number of respondents, who were of the majority [favorable] opinion, agreed with the minority that numerous disability ratings and items in the schedule need revision in the light of changes in modern treatment, both surgical and medical, as disability ratings are changed when residuals of injuries and diseases are improved by operations, prostheses, and other mechanical aids, and particularly in the light of the new dug and surgical treatment of pulmonary tuberculosis. A large number of disability ratings do not properly take into account recent advances in medical rehabilitation, improved prostheses, reconstructive orthopedic surgery, and improved plastic surgery procedures" (p. 161).
- (L—nomenclature) ". . . some of the majority took exception to the outmoded terminology in the psychiatric section of the schedule. This viewpoint was taken by all of the respondents practicing psychiatry. Standard nomenclature of diseases should be required for the physical disability processing and evaluation of the serviceman while in the service and after he becomes a veteran beneficiary. There is confusion of disease nomenclature between the agencies which have to use the schedule for rating disabilities in their physical disability processing and evaluation" (p. 165).
- (M—residuals of the injury or disease) ". . . it appears that the majority opinions are that medical criteria accurately reflect the residuals of the injury or disease . . . with exceptions. . . . The minority opinion maintained . . . that the criteria did not . . . the majority and minority did agree that a revision of the criteria was required and that the medical criteria should be modernized and more clearly correlated to percentages, disability, and average impairment in earning capacity. The criteria for tuberculosis were singled out, as an example, as requiring revision" (p. 171).
- (N—medical basis and percentages) "Although there was a slight majority of the respondents who believed that it is not medically feasible to assign gradations within an accuracy of 10 percent when determining the percentage of bodily and mental impairment, this majority were divided in their recommendations as to what scale of gradations they regarded as feasible. Still, a sizable minority were definite and clear in their opinion, that it is medically feasible. . . . Both the majority and the minority recognized

the fact that any scale adopted was an arbitrary scale. It is not medically feasible . . . in any patient with tuberculosis—according to the 8 medical respondents practicing this medical specialty. One tuberculosis specialist suggested the scale of 'slight, moderate, severe, and total disability'" (p. 176).

- (O—average impairment in earning capacity) "Some respondents believe, and others do not, that the ratings do or do not represent the average impairment of earning capacity resulting from the various degrees of severity of physical impairment. Lower ratings do not fairly represent the average impairment in earning capacity . . . particularly those ratings below 30 percent" (p. 180).
- (P—disabilities rated at 10 percent and 20 percent) "Most of the medical specialists who responded to the question, two-thirds, said that the disabilities rated 10 and 20 percent did not constitute a material impairment of earning capacity" (p. 184).
- (Q—known medical data) "Two-thirds of the respondents commented that they did not know of any medical data which could be used to set percentage ratings to represent the average impairment in earning capacity resulting from various disease or injuries and their residual conditions for civil occupations . . . of the group of respondents who state they knew of medical data . . . some made reference to certain medical publications; some made references to commercial insurance companies; State industrial commissions; and other State compensation commissions; other respondents in this group referred to miscellaneous sources" (p. 189).

The most recent revisions for body systems or sections within body systems went into effect between 1994 and 2002. In addition, one revision has been pending since 1999, one is under review, and two were withdrawn in 2004 (see Tables 4-1 and 4-2). Although the codes within a single body system classification may appear to have been revised as a whole by the issuance of an overarching *Federal Register* item, some of the contents of the sections (e.g., descriptive material, guidance) or specific diagnostic codes have been updated at different times over the years, while others have not been revised since the 1940s or 1950s (e.g., musculoskeletal body system). (See Appendix Table 4-1 for more detailed information about the changes that have occurred, including those in the descriptive text that accompany the diagnostic codes, which revise the criteria for assigning rating levels.) The orthopedic components of the musculoskeletal system and the neurological system have undergone the fewest revisions (see Table 4-1). This is yet another obstacle to providing a valid disability rating for veterans.

TABLE 4-1 Revisions of Diagnostic Codes, by Body System, Since 1945

Body System	Number of Current Codes[a]	Number and Percent of Codes Not Revised Since 1945[b]	Number and Percent of Codes Revised, 1945 Through 1989	Number and Percent of Codes Revised Since 1990
Musculoskeletal: *Orthopedic*	162	105 (64.8%)	54 (33.3%)	3 (1.9%)
Musculoskeletal: *Muscle injuries*	29	0 (0.0%)	0 (0.0%)	29 (100.0%)
Organs of Special Sense: *Vision*	60	29 (48.3%)	31 (51.7%)	0 (0.0%)
Organs of Special Sense: *Hearing*	26	1 (3.8%)	1 (3.8%)	24 (92.3%)
Infectious Diseases, Immune Disorders, and Nutritional Deficiencies	22	0 (0.0%)	0 (0.0%)	22 (100.0%)
Respiratory	82	0 (0.0%)	9 (11.0%)	73 (89.0%)
Cardiovascular	36	0 (0.0%)	0 (0.0%)	36 (100.0%)
Digestive	52	20 (38.5%)	24 (46.2%)	8 (15.4%)
Genitourinary	42	12 (28.6%)	3 (7.1%)	27 (64.3%)
Gynecological Conditions and Disorders of the Breast	19	0 (0.0%)	0 (0.0%)	19 (100.0%)
Hemic and Lymphatic	16	0 (0.0%)	0 (0.0%)	16 (100.0%)
Skin	31	1 (3.2%)	0 (0.0%)	30 (96.8%)
Endocrine	19	0 (0.0%)	0 (0.0%)	19 (100.0%)
Neurological Conditions and Convulsive Disorders	119	105 (88.2%)	13 (10.9%)	1 (0.8%)
Mental Disorders	67	0 (0.0%)	8 (11.9%)	59 (88.1%)
Dental and Oral	16	8 (50.0%)	1 (6.3%)	7 (43.8%)
Total	798	281 (35.2%)	144 (18.0%)	373 (46.7%)

[a]This table does not include the number of diagnostic codes that have been dropped, or added and subsequently dropped, since 1945, although this number would provide additional information on how much each body system has been revised since the Schedule for Rating Disabilities was issued in 1945. It also does not include analogous codes, although substantial increase in use of an analogous code in a body system might indicate a new code is needed.

[b]In other words, these codes were in the original 1945 Schedule for Rating Disabilities.

TABLE 4-2 Dates of Rating Schedule Changes in the 14 Body Systems

Body System	Proposed	Final	Effective Date
Genitourinary	12/02/91	01/18/94	02/17/94
Dental and oral conditions	01/19/93	01/18/94	02/17/94
Gynecological conditions and disorders of the breast	03/26/92	04/21/95	05/22/95
Hemic and lymphatic	04/30/93	09/22/95	10/23/95
Endocrine	01/22/93	05/07/96	06/06/96
Infectious diseases, immune disorders, and nutritional deficiencies	04/30/93	07/31/96	08/30/96
Respiratory	01/19/93	09/05/96	10/07/96
Mental disorders	10/26/95	10/08/96	11/07/96
Musculoskeletal: *Muscles*	06/16/93	06/03/97	07/03/97
Cardiovascular	01/19/93	12/11/97	01/12/98
Organs of special sense: *Hearing*	04/12/94	05/11/99	06/10/99
Skin	01/19/93	07/31/02	08/30/02
Digestive: *Gastrointestinal*	08/07/00	(withdrawn in 2004)	
Musculoskeletal: *Orthopedic*	02/11/03	(withdrawn in 2004)	
Organs of special sense: *Vision*	05/11/99		
Neurological conditions and convulsive disorders	(under review)		
Digestive	(under review)		

Updating Process

In 2002, the General Accounting Office (now known as the Government Accountability Office) pointed out that the procedures for revising the Rating Schedule contributed to the obsolete medical knowledge found in significant portions of the schedule. Currently, all proposed changes must be reviewed by VA's legal counsel, the Veterans Health Administration (VHA), the VA Office of Congressional and Legislative Affairs, the VA Office of Inspector General, and the Office of Management and Budget. Further, the number of staff assigned to coordinate the updates and train the raters is not sufficient for the complex task: one staff person is assigned less than half-time to coordinate such efforts. GAO found that "VA does not have a well-defined plan to conduct the next round of medical updates" (GAO, 2002).

In 1989, to address some of the existing shortcomings with the rating system, VA hired a contractor to convene practicing physicians, organized by teams according to specific body systems, to review and update criteria for several of the body systems. The physicians were asked to propose changes in the Rating System that were consistent with modern medical practice and phrased in language that rating personnel could easily interpret. VA in-house staff reviewed the teams' results, made necessary adjustments, and forwarded that information to various VA offices for review. The proposed changes were published in the *Federal Register* for comments and final rules were issued. As of March 2002, VA had finalized the criteria for 11 of 14 body systems (GAO, 2002).

In general, VA publishes an Advance Notice of Proposed Rulemaking (ANPRM) in the *Federal Register* prior to issuance of a Notice of Proposed Rulemaking (NPRM) for each body system revision, or for revision of a specific diagnostic code or explanatory note in a body system, to allow the public preliminary commentary on revisions VA is planning to propose. There are comment periods for both the ANPRM and the NPRM (generally 30 or 60 days). These notices explain in detail the reasons why revisions are deemed necessary and the specific revisions being proposed. The public comments and other pertinent information received are recorded and considered in light of their medical and regulatory appropriateness. The NPRM item contains agency responses indicating whether or not and why in each case the comments made in response to the ANPRM were used as part of the revisions. The new rules go into effect shortly after the Final Rule is published in the *Federal Register*. The Final Rule document contains the agency's responses to commentators' suggestions regarding the NPRM.

Revising the Rating Schedule has not been based on systematic studies of the reliability or validity of the rating criteria for the various conditions. Few such studies have been done. In 1983, VA had the regional offices (then numbering 56) rate 16 sample claims with 26 claimed disabilities.

The evaluation concluded that it was possible for raters to assign different ratings to the same condition because of the lack of precision of some rating criteria, inadequate medical records and reports, and reluctance of raters to ask for additional or clarifying information because of time pressures (VA, 2005). In 2005, the Veterans Benefits Administration (VBA) initiated a study of the consistency of decisions on three conditions: hearing loss, post-traumatic stress disorder, and knee conditions. VBA had 10 subject matter experts review 1,750 regional office decisions and planned to follow up with additional studies of particular conditions and review areas identified with consistency problems every two to three years (FY05 PAR:221). The results were briefed to VA leaders but not made public. Also in 2005, VA contracted with the Institute of Defense Analyses to determine the major factors contributing to state and regional variation in disability compensation claims, ratings, and payments. VA expects the results to help in identifying corrective actions to increase consistency (IDA, 2007).

Evaluation of the Medical Knowledge in the Current Rating Schedule

The Rating Schedule contains a number of obsolete diagnostic categories, terms, tests, and procedures, and does not recognize many currently accepted diagnostic categories. Some examples of these are provided below. In other cases, the diagnostic categories are current but do not specify appropriate procedures to measure disability for the conditions.

Examples of Conditions in Need of Updating

Craniocerebral Trauma As an example of a condition that needs to be based on more current medical knowledge, the criteria for rating severity of craniocerebral trauma are not adequate because the description is out of date and does not provide guidance for the rating of multiple neurological disorders associated with craniocerebral trauma. The chronic effects of craniocerebral trauma include cerebrospinal fistula, pneumocephalus, carotid-cavernous fistula, vascular injury with thrombosis (although hemiplegia, seizures, and cranial nerve paralyses can be coded), infections, chronic headache, new onset migraine headaches, visual disorders, sleep disturbances, and (rarely) movement disorders. These criteria should be differentiated conceptually; they need to be updated to coincide with current knowledge and medical practice and should include not only more specific problems, such as acute and chronic sequelae, but also focal abnormalities from brain injury and symptomatic response to medication.

Neurodegenerative and Neurological Disorders As another example, the criteria for rating severity of neurodegenerative disorders are inadequate, principally because most of the disorders currently considered to be neurodegenerative have not been included. Moreover, among the four that are listed in the Rating Schedule, only one (amyotrophic lateral sclerosis) is currently considered to be neurodegenerative. Among the three others, both multiple sclerosis and myasthenia gravis are now classified as autoimmune, and syringomyelia is usually a developmental abnormality, often associated with the Chiari type I or type II malformation. In present practice, the neurodegenerative diseases are defined as disorders characterized by the progressive loss of neurons in focal, multifocal, or more widespread parts of the nervous system. The diseases commonly considered neurodegenerative include Alzheimer's disease, Parkinson's disease, dementia with Lewy bodies, multiple system atrophy, frontotemporal dementia, corticobasal degeneration, progressive supranuclear palsy, and amyotrophic lateral sclerosis. Similar concerns exist regarding neurological conditions such as spinal cord injury (SCI). There are no clear criteria by which to evaluate neurological impairment and functional limitations related to SCI in the current Rating Schedule. Information used is based on cranial nerve impairments and very outdated, suggesting the need for adopting a more widely known classification system such as the one used by the American Spinal Injury Association (known as the ASIA Classification System for Neurological Disorders).

Posttraumatic Arthritis An additional example of inappropriate medical knowledge used in the current Rating Schedule is that of posttraumatic arthritis. The existing criteria for determining disability in posttraumatic arthritis depend on anatomical findings and the assessment of *working movement*, a term that is both archaic and imprecise. Specifically included are X-ray evidence of past trauma and loss of range of motion. This does not use the most commonly used imaging techniques, such as computed tomography (CT) and magnetic resonance imaging (MRI), which provide significantly more anatomical specificity than X-ray films and are most frequently used in clinical settings in which trauma is assessed. Using imaging techniques to assess disability assumes a strong correlation between anatomy or range of motion loss and functional ability. This relationship is often not linear. Hence, these measures are inadequate in determining disability. However, the musculoskeletal guidelines provide detailed information on the range of factors that need to be considered. They include an opportunity to record pain or fatigue during repetitive motion, which are needed in this type of assessment.

Mental Disorders Since the ratings for mental disorders were last revised in 1996, VA has used a single rating formula to evaluate all mental conditions. Each rating level is based on a mix of symptoms that is not appropriately applicable to any particular mental disorder but reflects psychopathology more broadly. When evaluating claims for mental disorders, raters (or the Board of Veterans Appeals) may request a Global Assessment of Functioning (GAF) score.

The GAF is used to assess *functioning* on Axis V of the multiaxial assessment system within the *Diagnostic and Statistical Manual of Mental Disorders* (DSM-IV) (APA, 1994). The GAF, derived from the Global Assessment Scale (Endicott et al., 1976), assesses *psychological functioning* (i.e., severity of symptomatology) and *social and occupational functioning* together on a single 100-point scale. This combined assessment approach was criticized for producing confusing and sometimes uninterpretable ratings by the multiaxial workgroup that design this portion of the DSM-IV (Goldman et al., 1992). The authors proposed separating the GAF into two separate scales (Goldman et al., 1992), and the resulting Social and Occupational Assessment Scale (SOFAS) was introduced in the appendix to DSM-IV (APA, 1994).

In addition to these limitations, GAF scores have not been shown to be reliable without systematic training of evaluating psychiatrists or psychologists: "Evidence suggests that without training, some raters may base their ratings on average symptom occurrence or functionality over time, while others will rate the most recent episode or lowest level of these two components. In disorders such as posttraumatic stress disorder (PTSD), where symptom severity and functionality can fluctuate, these two approaches will yield very different GAF scores" (VA, 2002). There are also different interpretations of *mild*, *moderate*, and *severe* in assigning levels of severity. The GAF also measures both functional impairment and disability (APA, 2002). Therefore, "two patients with severe delusions may function at completely different levels but will still receive the same GAF score of 20 because of the symptoms" (APA, 2002:212). Because of such problems with validity and reliability, the American Psychiatric Association might drop or greatly revise the GAF in DSM-V (Narrow, 2006).

Since the Social Security Administration (SSA) revised its mental impairment standards in the early 1980s, a single rating scale has been used to assess work-related functional limitations. The Psychiatric Review Technique Form (PRTF) assesses functional limitations on four dimensions (activities of daily living; social interaction; concentration, persistence, and pace; and adaptive functioning or decompensation) using an ordinal scale (none, mild, moderate, marked, and extreme) or a frequency count. The PRTF has been assessed and found to be reliable and also to measure functional loss related to work disability (Pincus et al., 1991).

Other Examples The classification of epilepsy is totally out of date and should be replaced with the current international classification of the epilepsies. The distinction between *neuritis* and *neuralgia* is no longer in keeping with current practice or knowledge of neuropathological changes in peripheral nerves. Examiners cannot reasonably be expected to provide information needed to apply the criteria, as the criteria are conceptually inadequate, out of date, and incomplete.

FINDINGS AND RECOMMENDATIONS

The first order of business should be to ensure that the Rating Schedule is up to date medically. Up to date medically means that

- the diagnostic categories reflect the classification of injuries and diseases currently used in health care, so that the appropriate condition in the Rating Schedule can be more easily identified and confirmed using the medical evidence;
- the criteria for successively higher rating levels reflect increasing degrees of anatomic and functional loss of body structures and systems (i.e., impairment), so that the greater the extent of loss, the greater the amount of compensation; and
- current standards of practice in assessment of impairment are followed and appropriate severity scales or staging protocols are used in evaluating the veteran and applying the rating criteria.

Making the Rating Schedule medically current and keeping it up to date is addressed in the first recommendation, below.

The second order of business should be to see if and how measures of a veteran's ability to function in everyday life could be integrated with or be used to adjust the impairment criteria. The third area that needs addressing is the assessment of disability and rehabilitation needs. It should be possible to establish a more effective process for coordinating VA benefits for veterans to maximize their capacity to function by developing and implementing an initial assessment process for all VBA programs. Would it be possible to base compensation partly on this assessment of disability, if it is more severe than the degree of impairment? Fourth, an effort should be made to determine if it would be possible to measure health-related quality of life and develop a way to compensate for its loss, if it turns out that the criteria in the Rating Schedule do not predict loss of quality of life. These issues are addressed in the recommendations below, along with the need to collect information on the economic aspects of disability and compensation.

Updating the Medical Aspects of the Rating Schedule

The Rating Schedule mostly assesses the medical severity of service-related injuries or diseases rather than the impact of the injuries or diseases on the veteran's life and work, although there is an assumption that degree of impairment and its social and economic consequences are roughly related, on average. Given the importance of impairment rating in the veterans disability compensation program, it is critical that the categories and criteria in the Rating Schedule are based on current medical knowledge and practice.

We began the study with a careful review of a number of the medical conditions included in the current Rating Schedule and were very concerned by what we found. In many cases, the medical knowledge used in the Rating Schedule is inadequate, often because the information is obsolete or there has been inadequate integration of current and accepted diagnostic procedures. In some instances, the nomenclature used for some of the ratings is obsolete, many modern diagnoses are not included, and even when symptoms (e.g., pain, fatigue) are mentioned, they are not included in a systematic fashion as possible contributors to the rating. In some instances, the percentages recommended do not reflect the level of severity of specific conditions the committee reviewed. For example, the assignment of 10 percent disability for symptoms of dizziness and shortness of breath associated with exercise of more than 7 and less than 10 metabolic equivalents of task (equivalent to jogging 3 miles in 30 minutes, something most Americans cannot do) is a reasonable assessment of disability. It may be an underestimate of the functional impact of the cardiac condition for certain specific vocational activities. For example, any dizziness would ground a pilot or a courier on bicycle, and they would be more than 10 percent disabled. This creates a situation in which the Rating Schedule may correctly rate the condition, and it is medically agreed that it has properly scaled the impairment, but the rating has not properly reflected the disability.

In exceptional cases, when the Rating Schedule does not adequately evaluate the condition in the opinion of the rater, the case can be referred to the director of the Compensation and Pension (C&P) Service for special consideration of a higher percentage, but this is not a frequent occurrence.

The Rating Schedule should be revised to remove ambiguous criteria and obsolete conditions and language, reflect current medical practice, and include medical advances in diagnosis and classification of new conditions. For a number of reasons, however, as indicated above, updates have been made slowly and relatively randomly, and the Rating Schedule remains outdated in both its organization and the current body system content, thereby hindering raters from providing accurate assessments of veterans' disabilities.

The body system structure of the Rating Schedule is not necessarily based on current knowledge of relationships among conditions and comorbidities (e.g., autoimmune disorders, neurodegenerative diseases). Some related conditions are scattered throughout the body systems, such as diabetes, a multisystem disease, and malignancies, should they become metastatic. We now understand that a common process underlies them wherever they occur.

The committee considers it important for VA to be as up to date as possible in current medical approaches to diagnosis and terminology as pertains to the Rating Schedule in order to serve veterans with disabilities more effectively and help them integrate or reintegrate into a productive and meaningful civilian life. VA should undertake a comprehensive revision of the Rating Schedule now and make it a formal process to revise the schedule every 10 years thereafter. One possible approach would involve the revision of several body systems each year on a staggered basis.

> **Recommendation 4-1. VA should immediately update the current Rating Schedule, beginning with those body systems that have gone the longest without a comprehensive update, and devise a system for keeping it up to date. VA should reestablish a disability advisory committee to advise on changes in the Rating Schedule.**

The disability advisory committee should be appointed by and report to the head of VBA, although it might be staffed by the C&P Service. Its members should be experts in medical care, disability evaluation, functional and vocational assessment, and rehabilitation, and include representatives of the health policy, disability law, and veteran communities. The committee would meet several times a year to review developments in medicine and rehabilitation and consider the implications for the Rating Schedule. The committee could also advise on research needs and plans related to measurement of veterans' disability and quality of life.

To make Recommendation 4-1 feasible, VA will also need to increase its staff capacity to update and revise the Rating Schedule. As an example, SSA's disability program has an Office of Medical Policy with six doctors, representing a range of fields, and several times that number of analysts for the revision process. SSA is guided by the same Administrative Procedures Act in revising regulations, including the publication of ANPRMs, NPRMs, and Final Rules in the *Federal Register*. In the SSA process, however, health-care professionals are more systematically and extensively involved by serving as in-house medical experts. SSA also gathers feedback on relevant medical issues from state officials who help the agency make disability decisions. In addition, SSA uses its in-house expertise to keep current with advances in medicine and identify aspects of the criteria that need to be revised (GAO, 2002). In its informal notice and comment period, after the issuance of an ANPRM, SSA hosts at least one outreach conference, which includes invited medical experts, advocates, and patients. SSA staff review the input from the outreach conferences and uses this input to inform the development of the NPRM. In contrast, VBA has one physician who works with staff in a unit responsible for all C&P regulations.

The Uses of the Rating Schedule

The Rating Schedule should be based on the best current medical evidence, which was the topic examined in the previous portions of this chapter. The Rating Schedule should also be designed to serve the purposes of the veterans disability compensation program, which is the topic examined in the balance of the chapter. Those purposes were identified in Chapter 3, namely to provide compensation for the impact of service-connected injuries and diseases on (1) work disability (loss of earning capacity), (2) the degree of nonwork disability incurred (loss of ability to engage in usual life activities other than work), and (3) loss in the quality of life (QOL).

The discussion of how the Rating Schedule serves the purposes of the veterans disability compensation program is based in part on the paper in Appendix C of this report, "The Relationship Between Impairments and Earnings Losses in Multicondition Studies" (Relationship Study). The Relationship Study examines the relationship of ratings to earned income in the workers' compensation programs in Wisconsin and California and the *Economic Validation of the Rating Schedule* Study.

One of the important contributions of the Relationship Study is the distinction between the *purposes* of the disability benefits and the *operational basis* for the benefits. That distinction can be illustrated by the entries in Figure 4-1.[8]

The concepts in Figure 4-1 correspond to the operational measures actually or potentially used to determine the amount of cash benefits provided by the workers' compensation and veterans disability programs, as well as the outcome measures used in research on disability and health-care programs. (The terms are defined in greater detail in Appendix C.)

IA. *Medical impairment: anatomical loss* refers to impairment ratings that are based on anatomical loss, such as amputation of the leg.

IB. *Medical impairment: functional loss* refers to impairment ratings that are based on the extent of functional loss, such as loss of motion of the wrist.

II. *Limitations in the activities of daily living* refers to limitations on the veteran's ability to engage in the activities of daily living, such as bending, kneeling, or stooping, resulting from the impairment, and to participate in usual life activities, such as socializing and maintaining family relationships.

---

[8]Figure 4-1 corresponds to Figure A2 in the Relationship Study.

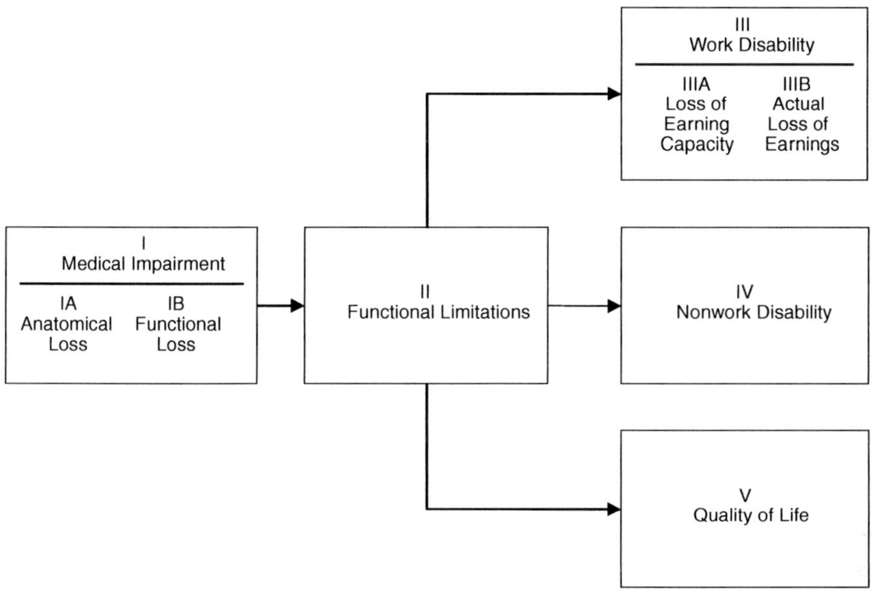

FIGURE 4-1 The consequences of an injury or disease.

IIIA. *Work disability: loss of earning capacity* refers to the presumed loss of earning capacity resulting from the impairment and limitations in the activities of daily living.

IIIB. *Work disability: actual loss of earnings* refers to the actual loss of earnings resulting from the impairment and limitations in the activities of daily living.

IV. *Nonwork disability* refers to limitations on the veteran's ability to engage in usual life activities other than work. This includes ability to engage in activities of daily living, such as bending, kneeling, or stooping, resulting from the impairment, and to participate in usual life activities, such as reading, learning, socializing, engaging in recreation, and maintaining family relationships.

V. *Loss of quality of life* refers to the loss of physical, psychological, social, and economic well-being in one's life.

The essential point of the distinction between the purposes of the disability benefits and the operational basis for the benefits is this: While the *purpose* of the workers' compensation benefits and the current veterans disability compensation program is to compensate for work disability, the *operational basis* for the benefits is almost invariably one of the other concepts shown in Figure 4-1, such as ratings based on an assessment of the extent of anatomical loss (IA) or functional loss (IB). In essence, the ratings of impairment are being used as predictors or proxies for the work disability that is assumed to follow from the impairments. Whatever the merits of the assumption, the use of proxies from the left side of Figure 4-1 as the operational basis for benefits that are provided for a purpose on the right side of the figure is ubiquitous in disability programs. Whether that assumption is warranted is one of the issues examined in Appendix C and in the balance of this chapter.

The Rating Schedule and Work Disability

One of the purposes of the veterans disability compensation program endorsed in Chapter 3 is to provide compensation for work disability resulting from service-connected injuries and diseases. For the Rating Schedule to support this purpose, several questions need to be resolved.

Question One: What Is the Measure of Work Disability That the Rating Schedule Is Supposed to Compensate?

The current Rating Schedule states that "the percentage ratings represent . . . the average impairment in earning capacity . . . in civil occupations."[9] This corresponds to the loss of earning capacity concept (IIIA) in Figure 4-1. However, there is no meaningful test of the accuracy of the current Rating Schedule if a comparison is made between (1) the *ratings* produced by application of the criteria for evaluating medical conditions contained in the Rating Schedule and (2) the *average reduction in earning capacity* because in practice they are the same thing. The meaningful test is whether the ratings produced by the Rating Schedule (which are the estimates of loss of earning capacity) correspond to the actual average loss of earnings among veterans with the same rating degree (IIIB) in Figure 4-1. This is the test that has been consistently used by researchers in the disability field, and corresponds to the test used in the Relationship Study for the workers' compensation programs in Wisconsin and California and VA's veterans disability compensation program.

The methodology used to calculate the actual loss of earnings resulting from a work-related or service-related injury or disease is explicated in the Relationship Study. A comparison is made between persons with disabilities

[9]The full text of § 4.1 of the *Code of Federal Regulations* is provided in Section A.4.b of Appendix C.

and persons without disabilities who have similar age, education, and other factors that affect earnings.

Question Two: How Should the Rating Schedule Be Evaluated?

The Rating Schedule should be evaluated by the ability of the ratings produced by the schedule to accurately predict the extent of actual losses of earnings for veterans with disabilities. The Relationship Study in Appendix C provides such evaluations for the Wisconsin and California workers' compensation programs and for the veterans disability compensation program as of 1967. We are not suggesting that the results from these three programs should be used to evaluate the current Rating Schedule for the veterans program, in large part because we are aware that a study of the current schedule is being conducted by the Center for Naval Analysis. Rather, we are suggesting that the criteria that should be used to evaluate the accuracy of the current Rating Schedule for the veterans disability compensation program are the extent of horizontal and vertical equity in the relationship between the ratings and the actual loss of earnings for veterans with disabilities.

There is a long-standing tradition of the use of the equity criterion to evaluate programs for persons with disabilities. An example is the *Report of the National Commission on State Workmen's Compensation Laws* (National Commission on State Workmen's Compensation Laws, 1972), which defined equitable as

> Delivering benefits and services fairly as judged by the program's consistency in providing equal benefits or services to workers in identical circumstances and its rationality in providing benefits and services in proportion to the impairment or disability for those with different degrees of loss.

One variant of the equity test—*intra-injury horizontal equity for ratings*—requires that the actual wage losses for workers or veterans with the same disability ratings and the same type of injury should be the same or similar. In the case of the Rating Schedule, this test is whether all veterans with the same rating for a given condition have approximately the same earnings. For example, say veterans rated 70 percent for loss of a hand average 50 percent less earnings than veterans without service-connected conditions. One would not want to see a substantial number of veterans earning significantly less than the average. The evidence from the Wisconsin workers' compensation program suggests this equity test is very difficult to satisfy (see Figure C-5 in Appendix C).

Another variant of the equity test—*inter-injury horizontal equity for ratings*—requires that the actual wage losses for workers with the same disability ratings, but different types of injuries, should be the same or similar. Regarding the Rating Schedule, the test is whether veterans rated at the same degree for different conditions experience approximately the same loss of earning capacity. For example, are the average earnings of veterans rated 50 percent for depression and the average earnings of veterans rated 50 percent for a bad knee or loss of all fingers about the same? To put it another way, the Rating Schedule is not fulfilling the statutory intent if veterans at any given rating degree for impairments in one body system average substantially lower earnings than those with the same rating degree in another body system.

The evidence indicates that the Rating Schedule in use in 1967, as well as the two workers' compensation programs, had serious deficiencies meeting this test. Each of the programs systematically treated some injuries or medical conditions differently than other injuries in terms of the extent of earnings losses associated with similar disability ratings (see Figures C-6, C-11 and C-12, and C-14 and C-15 in Appendix C for results from the Wisconsin workers' compensation, California workers' compensation, and VA disability compensation programs circa 1967, respectively).

A third variant of the equity test—*vertical equity*—requires that actual wage losses increase in proportion to increases in disability ratings. To meet this test, the Rating Schedule would consistently assign higher ratings to veterans with a given disabling condition who have lower average earnings. For example, veterans rated 30 percent for arteriosclerotic or coronary heart disease should earn less, on average, than those rated 10 percent, while those rated 60 percent should earn, on average, less than those rated 30 percent, and so on. At the aggregate level (the entire sample of workers or veterans), the evidence indicates that the Wisconsin rating system did an excellent job, the California rating system did a moderately good job, and the VA Rating Schedule in use in 1967 did a fairly poor job meeting the vertical equity criterion (see Figures C-4, C-13, and C-16 in Appendix C, respectively).

The answers to the first two questions in this section are the basis for our next recommendation.

> **Recommendation 4-2. VA should regularly conduct research on the ability of the Rating Schedule to predict actual loss in earnings. The accuracy of the Rating Schedule to predict such losses should be evaluated using the criteria of horizontal and vertical equity.**

Question Three: What Factors Should Be Included in the Rating Schedule in Order to Improve the Accuracy of the Predictions of Actual Loss in Earnings?

The current Rating Schedule largely relies on assessments of medical impairment (concepts 1A and 1B in Figure 4-1) to determine the disability ratings. Would the inclusion of other permanent consequences of an injury or disease in the rating formula improve the accuracy of the predictions of actual loss of earnings?

One threshold issue is whether to base the disability ratings on direct measures of the actual loss of earnings for each veteran since that is the purpose of the benefits. There are two reasons why disability systems have generally avoided this approach. First, the earnings of a particular person are affected by a myriad of factors, and the workers' compensation programs that have used the actual wage loss approach have generally abandoned it because it was found to be unworkable.[10] Second, as discussed in Appendix C, the direct link between disability ratings (and the accompanying disability benefits) and the actual loss of earnings can create incentive problems for active participation in the labor force.[11]

The more relevant issue is whether the predictions of actual loss of earnings (IIIB in Figure 4-1) would be improved by adding more information about the veteran, such as age, education, or work experience, which typically are used to predict loss of earning capacity. However, the examination in Appendix C of the two workers' compensation programs and VA's disability compensation program as of 1967 provided some evidence that the accuracy of the predictions of actual wage loss was worse in terms of horizontal and vertical equity. We are not endorsing this finding as typical or necessary but rather as a warning that an attractive assumption—including data from more factors in the disability process is worthwhile—needs to be tested empirically, which leads to our next recommendation.

Recommendation 4-3. VA should conduct research to determine if inclusion of factors in addition to medical impairment, such as age, education, and work experience, improves the ability of the Rating Schedule to predict actual losses in earnings.

---

[10]The difficulties that the Florida workers' compensation program had with the wage-loss approach for permanent partial disability benefits adopted in 1979 are described by Berkowitz and Burton (1987:283–312). The Florida program subsequently largely abandoned the wage-loss approach.

[11]The possible inducement to reduce earnings in order to increase the cash benefits provided by the veterans disability compensation program is discussed by Greenberg and Rosenheck (2007).

Question Four: How Can the Ability of the Rating Schedule to Predict Actual Losses of Earnings Be Improved?

The evidence from the research produced by Recommendations 4-2 and 4-3 can be used to improve the accuracy of the predictions of earnings losses made by the Rating Schedule. The study in Appendix C provides examples of how certain medical conditions may consistently have more (or less) earnings losses than predicted by the disability rating systems used in the workers' compensation programs and VA's disability compensation program as of 1967. A current study of the disability compensation program is likely to produce similar findings. Likewise, research can determine whether the inclusion of additional factors (such as measures of the limitations in activities of daily living) produces more accurate estimates of the actual losses of earnings.

These research results can be used in at least two ways to improve the accuracy of the Rating Schedule. First, the disability ratings assigned to a particular medical condition can be increased (or decreased) to incorporate the research results. Second, the value of the ratings in the Rating Schedule can be maintained, but a series of modifiers can be used to translate the "standard rating" from the Rating Schedule into an "adjusted rating" that will serve as the basis for calculating benefits. This second approach may be preferable because the expertise and knowledge needed by the people conducting the disability ratings will not have to be updated each time that research indicates changes are needed to improve the accuracy of the predictions of losses of earnings.

Recommendation 4-4. VA should regularly use the results from research on the ability of the Rating Schedule to predict actual losses in earnings to revise the rating system, either by changing the rating criteria in the Rating Schedule or by adjusting the amounts of compensation associated with each rating degree.

The Rating Schedule and Nonwork Disability

Several issues need to be resolved if the veterans disability compensation program is to compensate for nonwork disability resulting from service-connected injuries and diseases, as recommended in Chapter 3.

Issue 1: Definition of Nonwork Disability

Disability is a broad concept. Individuals may have disabilities affecting multiple aspects of their lives. According to the *International Classification of Functioning, Disability and Health* (ICF), disability is a person's functional limitations in various health and health-related domains. Health domains include seeing, hearing, walking, learning, and remembering, whereas health-related domains include transportation, education, employment, and social interactions (WHO, 2001). Theoretically, then, nonwork disability covers all domains of disability except employment.

The basis for this distinction is that a veteran may be working but unable to participate in other usual life activities. For example, a veteran may be employed in a good job but suffer from the symptoms of post-traumatic stress disorder (PTSD). A veteran with severe mobility restrictions might be able to use a computer linked to the Internet to earn a good living from home, especially if there are adequate social supports (e.g., friends or family to help with food shopping). There are many ways in which the lives of veterans with service-connected injuries and diseases can be changed by the effects of injuries or diseases.

Issue 2: Measures of Nonwork Disability

The next issue is the feasibility of measuring the degree or extent of nonwork disability in a way that would be valid and practical as a basis for compensation. One approach is to perform functional assessments using such established scales as activities of daily living (ADLs) and instrumental activities of daily living (IADLs) and develop a method for converting the scores into benefit amounts. Or VA could use condition-specific functional scales, although achieving parity across conditions might be a challenge. Validated functional assessment instruments have been developed for most conditions, such as the Extended Glasgow Outcome Scale and Community Integration Questionnaire for brain injury; the National Institutes of Health's Stroke Scale; the Functional Independence Measure and Spinal Cord Independence Measure; St. George's Respiratory Questionnaire; Guyatt's Chronic Respiratory Questionnaire; the University of California at San Diego's Shortness of Breath Questionnaire for chronic obstructive pulmonary disease; and the Diabetes Health Profile.

Some veterans disability benefits programs assess and compensate for functional limitations under certain circumstances. The Veterans Affairs Canada system for augmenting impairment ratings with a quality-of-life rating of ability to participate in activities of independent living, take part in recreational and community activities, and initiate and take part in personal relationships was described in Chapter 3. The Australian Department of Veterans' Affairs has a scale for grading six activities of daily living (movement in and out of bed, transferring [e.g., from bed to chair], locomotion, dressing, personal hygiene, and eating and drinking). There is also a scale for nonspecific indicators of disease such as pain, lethargy, and poor prognosis. These scales are used to assess veterans who are bedridden or unable to leave the house because of such conditions as severe stroke, Parkinson's disease, heart failure, respiratory disease, liver failure, severe kidney failure, and some dementias. The higher score of the two scales is taken and compared with the appropriate body system-specific impairment rating. If it is higher, it is used to determine the amount of compensation instead of the impairment rating.

Recommendation 4-5. VA should compensate for nonwork disability, defined as functional limitations on usual life activities, to the extent that the Rating Schedule does not, either by modifying the Rating Schedule criteria to take account of the degree of functional limitation or by developing a separate mechanism.

It is possible that the Rating Schedule, when updated, will provide accurate ratings for both work disability and nonwork disability, even though its primary purpose is to compensate for loss of earning capacity. This is an empirical question that VA should address by developing a functional limitation scale (or adapting an existing scale) to a sample of veterans with and without disabilities and determining if it would lead to ratings different from those given by the Rating Schedule. Given the variance in the correlation of impairment measures and disability across conditions, it is possible that ratings based on impairment and ratings based on functional measures will differ more or more consistently in some body systems than others.

If the result is that functional measures capture disability where the Rating Schedule does not, VA should decide how to compensate for it. The Canadian approach of adding points to the impairment rating, while perhaps arbitrary, is administratively simple. The Australian approach of computing an impairment rating and a functional limitation rating and compensating on the basis of the higher rating is another possibility to be considered.

The Rating Schedule and Losses in the Quality of Life

One of the purposes for the veterans disability compensation program endorsed in Chapter 3 is to provide compensation for loss in QOL resulting from service-connected injuries and diseases. For the Rating Schedule to support this purpose, several questions need to be resolved.

Question One: What Is the Measure of Quality of Life the Rating Schedule Is Supposed to Compensate?

Although the measurement of QOL has no precedent in the veterans disability compensation program, the impact of injury or disease on QOL has been studied in a number of other areas where monetary valuations for a loss is the ultimate outcome. As noted by Sinclair and Burton (1995):

> Quality of life is frequently measured by ascertaining the preferences of individuals or groups for particular health states or treatment outcomes. Determining the opinions or preferences of relevant populations for alternative health states is a measurement technique that has been used extensively in the quality-of-life measures in health-care, economic, and social sciences research over the past 20 years.

An example of QOL research is the noneconomic loss survey of approximately 12,000 injured workers who received benefits from the Ontario, Canada, workers' compensation program, plus 300 individuals from the general population of Ontario who served as a control group. Seventy-eight medical conditions covering a wide range of impairments were selected as subjects for videos. Each video portrayed the limitations and adaptations to lifestyle required of the workers with a given condition. The workers discussed their condition with a therapist and demonstrated their capacity to perform various tasks of daily living. The procedure used to ascertain the quality-of-life ratings was described by Sinclair and Burton (1995):

> Each survey respondent spent 30 minutes viewing four or six of the videos, randomly assigned, excluding videos depicting his or her condition. Respondents were asked to rate, on an "opinion meter" scale, the loss of enjoyment of life they believed they would suffer if they had the condition portrayed. These ratings were on a scale of 0 to 100, with 0 representing normal health and 100 representing death.

A similar methodology can be used to develop a QOL rating system for veterans with disabilities. The ratings can be customized to recognize the special needs and interests of veterans.

> **Recommendation 4-6. VA should determine the feasibility of compensating for loss of quality of life by developing a tool for measuring quality of life validly and reliably in the veteran population, conducting research on the extent to which the Rating Schedule already accounts for loss in quality of life, and if it does not, developing a procedure for evaluating and rating loss of quality of life of veterans with disabilities.**

The purpose of the current Rating Schedule is to compensate for work disability, not losses in QOL, and so it is likely that the relationship between ratings under the current schedule and the measures of QOL are not particularly close. Nonetheless, the relationship is worth examining empirically. The research could be similar to the study by Sinclair and Burton (1995) of the relationship between the permanent impairment ratings produced by the American Medical Association *Guides to the Evaluation of Permanent Impairment* (AMA *Guides*) and QOL values for injured workers in Ontario, Canada. The findings indicated that the permanent ratings systematically underpredicted the loss of QOL that workers associated with the various permanent impairments. The results also indicated a "body-system effect," with different body systems having greater losses in QOL for a given rating than other body systems.[12]

VA should compare the results of the Rating Schedule and evaluations of loss of QOL to see where and how they differ. These research results can be used in at least two possible ways to improve the accuracy of the Rating Schedule. First, the disability ratings assigned to a particular medical condition can be increased (or decreased) to incorporate the research results. Second, the value of the ratings in the Rating Schedule can be maintained, but a series of modifiers can be used to translate the standard rating from the Rating Schedule into an adjusted rating that will serve as the basis for calculating benefits. This second approach may be preferable because the expertise and knowledge needed by the persons conducting the disability ratings will not have to be updated every time that research indicates changes are needed to improve the accuracy of the predictions of loss of earnings.

If research shows a disparity between the Rating Schedule and loss of QOL measures, VA should develop a way to compensate for loss of QOL that the Rating Schedule does not. This could be done by adapting the Rating Schedule to be used for both work disability and loss in QOL, or there could be separate Rating Schedules for these two consequences of service-related injuries and diseases. The committee recommended in Chapter 3 that the current purpose of the Rating Schedule—to compensate for work disability—should be expanded to provide compensation for both work disability and losses in QOL. Whether this means there should be one or two rating schedules will have to be decided by VA. Among the factors to be considered are

- Will there be a single cash benefit to serve the two purposes (compensating work disability and compensating loss in quality of life) or will there be separate cash benefit programs to serve the two purposes? If there are separate cash benefit programs, then separate rating schedules for each of the two programs may make more sense.

---

[12]For example, a 10 percent permanent impairment rating of the musculoskeletal system and a 10 percent permanent impairment of the nervous system received very different loss-of-enjoyment-of-life values, 32 and 62 percent, respectively (Sinclair and Burton, 1995).

- Are the factors that produce accurate predictions of the extent of actual loss of earnings similar or different from the factors that produce accurate predictions of the extent of loss of quality of life? If the explanatory factors are different, then separate rating schedules for each of the two benefit programs may make more sense.

IMPLEMENTATION AND COST ISSUES

This section suggests a phased approach to implementing the recommendations made in this chapter that VA compensate for the impact of military service on veterans, including impairment, loss of ability to function and participate in usual activities of everyday life, and loss in quality of life. The development of practical measures of functional capacity and loss of QOL involve research and development, experimentation, and pilot testing before full implementation.

Expanding the bases for veterans disability compensation also has cost implications. These include start-up costs incurred in developing and testing the instruments for evaluating degree of functional limitation and loss of QOL, transitional costs such as training, probably higher operating costs because of additional time and skills needed to evaluate losses of function and QOL, and possibly greater compensation costs, if functional and/or QOL deficits are greater on average than accounted for in the current impairment ratings. Although the committee was not asked to consider costs in recommending improvements in medical evaluation of veterans for disability benefits, it was cognizant of the magnitude of the changes recommended and aware that its recommendations for updating and improving the system for evaluating veterans for disability benefits would entail additional short- and long-term administrative costs and probably benefit costs.

Phase 1

Recommendation 4-1 calls for updating the Rating Schedule immediately. The updating should begin with the body systems that have gone the longest without a comprehensive update, namely, the orthopedic part of the musculoskeletal system, neurological conditions, and the digestive system. The revised rating criteria should rely to the extent possible on validated severity ratings and disease-staging systems, which are condition specific. Revisions of the remaining systems could be done on a rolling basis, several a year, possibly taking them in the order in which they were updated during the 1990s.

These revisions of the Rating Schedule will entail the establishment of a staff of medical experts and experienced raters, who would work in conjunction with experts in VHA and the reestablished medical advisory committee.

The medical advisory committee might be renamed the disability advisory committee, in recognition of the broadened basis for compensation.

Phase 2

The next step would be to investigate the relationship between the ratings and average earnings to see the extent to which the Rating Schedule as revised is meeting vertical and horizontal equity criteria (Recommendation 4-2). This would build on the analyses being conducted by the CNA Corporation, but use samples large enough to study the most prevalent conditions being rated. In fiscal years 2004–2006, for example, 38 conditions were the basis for at least 10,000 claims a year, including defective hearing, tinnitus, PTSD, lumbosacral or cervical strain, diabetes mellitus, hypertension, impairments of the leg, limitation of flexion of leg, limitation of motion of the ankle, and impairment of knee (other than ankylosis, degenerative arthritis of the spine, migraine, and arteriosclerotic heart disease). These 38 conditions accounted for 66 percent of the compensation rating decisions during 2004–2006. Conditions that are most often rated at 100 percent, if not already included on the basis of overall prevalence, also might be included, such as brain trauma.

Based on the results of the analysis of the relationship between the ratings and average earnings, VA could adjust the criteria to increase vertical and horizontal equity (Recommendation 4-4).

Phase 3

Next, to implement Recommendation 4-5, VA should develop a set of functional measures (e.g., ADLs, IADLs) and specific performance measures, such as time to ambulate a certain distance, or ability to do specific work-related tasks in both physical domains (e.g., climbing stairs or gripping) and cognitive domains (e.g., communicating or coordinating with other people). After the measures are validated in the disability compensation population, VA would conduct a study of functional capacity among applicants to see how well the revised Rating Schedule compensates for loss of functional capacity. There may be a correlation between the rating levels based on impairment and degree of functional limitations (i.e., the higher the rating, the more functional capacity is limited).

If the correlation is not high or does not exist, VA should develop a mechanism to compensate for loss of function that exceeds degree of impairment. Functional criteria could be included in the Rating Schedule or it could be rated separately with compensation based on the higher of the two ratings (see Appendix E for a diagram of a possible process for assessing impairment and functional disability). The use of such a mechanism should be thoroughly tested for reliability and validity in pilot studies and experiments.

A side benefit of functional assessment, if performed by interdisciplinary teams whose members are trained to assess function (e.g., physical, occupational, and other therapists; rehabilitation physicians and nurses; and vocational rehabilitation [VR] counselors), is that it would provide a basis for determining a veteran's needs for ancillary services (discussed in Chapter 6). In addition, VA could use the results of disability evaluations in making decisions on individual unemployability, particularly if a VR counselor or other vocational specialist is involved in the multidisciplinary assessment (see Chapter 7).

Phase 4

Quality-of-life assessment is relatively new and still at a formative stage, which makes implementation of Recommendation 4-6 more long-term and experimental. Health-related quality-of-life (HRQOL) instruments are the most developed and validated. VHA already uses a psychometric HRQOL instrument, the SF-36, to assess the effectiveness of medical interventions, and it has been adapted and validated for the population of veterans receiving care in an ambulatory setting (SF-36V). Preference-based HRQOL instruments are less well developed but have the potential to be more useful in a compensation system, because the results can be quantified and located on an interval scale (the SF-36V does not, for example, provide a summary score).

VA should begin a program of empirical research and development to determine the QOL effects of service-connected injuries and diseases. The goal would be to find out whether a global HRQOL instrument could reliably and validly measure the QOL of disabled veterans and be the basis for compensating its loss. A preference-based HRQOL measure would also have to place values on losses about which veterans and the remainder of the community agree, so that compensation based on HRQOL losses would be acceptable to both groups. While it is not clear, based on the current status of the science, that it is possible to measure HRQOL with a significant degree of accuracy, the committee believes there is a good chance this goal can be achieved and, because of its importance, should be attempted.[13]

---

[13]VA should be cognizant of the Patient-Reported Outcomes Measurement Information System (PROMIS), an effort by the National Institutes of Health (NIH) "to develop ways to measure patient-reported symptoms, such as pain and fatigue, and aspects of health-related quality of life across a wide variety of chronic diseases and conditions." The aim is to produce well-validated measures of HRQOL that will increase the quality and comparability of clinical research results (NIH, 2007).

If a reliable quality-of-life instrument can be validated, VA should ascertain the degree to which the Rating Schedule, as revised in phases 1-3 (above) accounts for loss of QOL (i.e., the higher the rating, the greater the loss in QOL). If the Rating Schedule does not do a good job of compensating for severe loss in QOL, VA should develop a mechanism for doing so.

REFERENCES

APA (American Psychiatric Association). 1994. *Diagnostic and statistical manual of mental disorders*, 4th ed. Washington, DC: APA.

APA. 2002. *A research agenda for DSM-V*, edited by D. J. Kupfer, M. B. First, and D. A. Regier. Washington, DC: APA. http://www.appi.org/pdf/kupfer_2292.pdf (accessed April 27, 2007).

Berkowitz, M., and J. F. Burton, Jr. 1987. *Permanent disability benefits in workers' compensation*. Kalamazoo, MI: W. E. Upjohn Institute for Employment Research.

Economic Systems Inc. 2004a. *VA Disability Compensation Program: Legislative history*. Washington, DC: VA Office of Policy, Planning, and Preparedness. http://www.va.gov/op3/docs/Disability_Comp_Legislative_Histor_Lit_Review.pdf (accessed December 28, 2006).

Economic Systems Inc. 2004b. *VA Disability Compensation Program: Literature review*. Washington, DC: VA Office of Policy, Planning, and Preparedness. http://www1.va.gov/op3/docs/Final_Report-LiteratureReview.pdf (accessed December 28, 2006).

Endicott, J., R. Spitzer, J. L. Fleiss, and J. Cohen. 1976. The global assessment scale. *Archives of General Psychiatry* 33:766–771.

GAO (General Accounting Office). 2002. *SSA and VA disability programs: Re-examination of disability criteria needed to help ensure program integrity*. Report GAO-02-597. Washington, DC: GAO.

Goldman, H. H., A. E. Skodol, and T. R. Lave. 1992. Revising axis V for DSM-IV: A review of measures of social functioning. *American Journal of Psychiatry* 149:1148–1156.

Gosoroski, D. M. 1997. Brotherhood of the damned: Doughboys return from the world war. *VFW Magazine*. http://www.worldwar1.com/dbc/vetsorg.htm (accessed April 26, 2007).

Greenberg, G. A., and R. A. Rosenheck. 2007. Compensation of veterans with psychiatric or substance abuse disorders and employment and earnings. *Military Medicine* 172:162–168.

IDA (Institute for Defense Analyses). 2007. *Support to the Department of Veterans Affairs*. http://www.ida.org/researchareas/resourceandsupportanalyses/acquisition%20planning%20and%20resource%20management.php (accessed May 22, 2007).

Narrow, W. E. 2006. Presentation to the IOM Committee on Medical Evaluation of Veterans for Disability Compensation, Washington, DC, September 21.

National Commission on State Workmen's Compensation Laws. 1972. *Report of the National Commission on State Workmen's Compensation Laws*. Washington, DC: Author. http://www.workerscompresources.com/National_Commission_Report/national_commission_report.htm (accessed February 28, 2007).

NIH (National Institutes of Health). 2007. *What is PROMIS? Overview*. http://www.nihpromis.org/what_is_promise/default.asp (accessed May 29, 2007).

Pincus, H. A., C. Kennedy, S. J. Simmens, H. H. Goldman, P. Sirovatka, and S. S. Sharfstein. 1991. Determining disability due to mental impairment: APA's evaluation of Social Security Administration guidelines. *American Journal of Psychiatry* 148(8):1037–1043.

President's Commission (The President's [Bradley] Commission on Veterans' Pensions). 1956a. *The administration of veterans' benefits: A study of the interrelationship of organization and policy.* Staff Report No. V1, June 19. House Committee Print No. 244, 84th Cong., 2nd Sess. Washington, DC: Government Printing Office.

President's Commission. 1956b. *The historical development of veterans' benefits in the United States.* Staff Report No. 1, May 9. House Committee Print No. 244, 84th Cong., 2nd Sess. Washington, DC: Government Printing Office.

President's Commission. 1956c. *The Veterans' Administration disability rating schedule: Historical development and medical appraisal.* Staff Report No. 8, Part B, July 18. House Committee Print No. 244, 84th Cong., 2nd Sess. Washington, DC: Government Printing Office.

Secretary of the Treasury. 1921. *Annual report*, Pp. 96–100, as cited in The President's Commission on Veterans' Pensions (1956).

Sinclair, S., and J. F. Burton, Jr. 1995. Development of a schedule for compensation of noneconomic loss: Quality-of-life values vs. clinical impairment ratings. In *Research in Canadian Workers' Compensation*, edited by T. Thomason and R. P. Chaykowski. Kingston, ON: IRC Press of Queen's University.

VA (Department of Veterans Affairs). 2002. *Best practice manual for posttraumatic stress disorder (PTSD) compensation and pension examinations.* Washington, DC: VA. http://www.avapl.org/pub/PTSD%20Manual%20final%206.pdf (accessed June 22, 2007).

VA. 2005. *Review of state variances in VA disability compensation payments.* Report No. 05-00765-137. Washington, DC: Office of Inspector General, VA. http://www.va.gov/oig/52/reports/2005/VAOIG-05-00765-137.pdf (accessed May 22, 2007).

VA. 2007a. *History of the Department of Veterans Affairs.* Part 1. http://www.va.gov/opa/feature/history/history1.asp (accessed March 9, 2007).

VA. 2007b. *History – VA history.* http://www.va.gov/about_va/vahistory.asp (accessed March 9, 2007).

VBA (Veterans Benefits Administration). 2004. *Trainee workbook for basic ratings—Prerequisite training.* VBA Training & Performance and Support System (accessed March 2006 from VA Intranet).

VBA. 2005. *General policy in rating: Student guide.* Washington, DC: VA (accessed March 2006 from VA Intranet).

VBA. 2006. *Claims recognition: Student guide.* Washington, DC: VA (accessed March 2006 from VA Intranet).

WHO (World Health Organization). 2001. *International classification of functioning, disability and health: ICF.* Geneva: WHO.

APPENDIX TABLE 4-1 Summary of Key Revisions to Diagnostic Codes Since 1945

Body System	Revisions
Musculoskeletal	• E91 was published as proposed 68 FR 6998, Feb. 11, 2003. This proposed rule was withdrawn at 69 FR 22757, Apr. 27, 2004. It would have been the first comprehensive revision since 1945. Nonetheless, some codes have been revised. • The diagnostic code for atrophic rheumatoid arthritis (5002) was revised at 70 FR 75399, Dec. 20, 2005. • The diagnostic code for degenerative hypertrophic arthritis or osteoarthritis (5003) was revised at 68 FR 51454, Aug. 27, 2003. • The diagnostic codes for prosthetic implants (5051, 5052, 5053, 5054, 5055, and 5056) were revised at 43 FR 45348, Oct. 2, 1978. • The diagnostic code for fibromyalgia (5025) was revised at 64 FR 32410, June 17, 1999. • Four codes for anatomical losses were revoked at 41 FR 11291, Mar. 18, 1976, while two codes for loss of use of hands and feet (5104 and 5105) were revised. • Terminology was updated for a number of multiple finger amputations diagnostic codes (5127, 5128, 5130, 5131, 5132, 5135, 5136, 5138, 5139, 5141, 5143, 5146, 5149, and 5150) at 67 FR 48784, July 26, 2002. A substantive revision was made to the diagnostic code for the amputation of two digits (the ring and little fingers) of one hand (5151). • Terminology was updated for a single finger amputation code (5154) at 67 FR 48784, July 26, 2002. • At 43 FR 45348, Oct. 2, 1978, one diagnostic code for amputation of lower extremity (5166) was revised, while another (5174) was revoked. • For the elbow and forearm diagnostic codes, impairment of ulna (5211) and impairment of radius (5212) were revised at 43 FR 45348, Oct. 2, 1978. • The diagnostic code for ankylosis of the wrist (5214) was revised at 43 FR 45348, Oct. 2, 1978. • The ankylosis section was revised at 67 FR 48784, July 26, 2002, affecting multiple digits: unfavorable ankylosis (5216–5219), multiple digits; favorable ankylosis (5220–5223); ankylosis of individual digits (5224–5227); and limitation of motion of individual digits (5228–5230). • The spine section underwent a major revision at 68 FR 51454, Aug. 27, 2003, with the creation of a number of new diagnostic codes under which previous codes were subsumed. Diagnostic codes 5285–5295 were therefore deleted. • The section on shortening of the lower extremity (5275) was revised at 43 FR 45348, Oct. 2, 1978. • The muscle injuries section underwent a major revision at 62 FR 30235, June 3, 1997, affecting diagnostic codes 5301–5329.

APPENDIX TABLE 4-1 Continued

Body System	Revisions
Organs of Special Sense	• NPRM 64 FR 25246, May 11, 1999, which would be a body system revision, is anticipated to become a final rule in October 2006. Some revisions have been made since the 1970s. • The diagnostic code for unilateral or bilateral ptosis (6019) was revised at 43 FR 45348, Oct. 2, 1978. • The diagnostic code for aphakia (6029) was revised at 43 FR 45348, Oct. 2, 1978. • Table V: Ratings of Central Visual Acuity Impairment was revised at 53 FR 50955, Dec. 19, 1988. Diagnostic codes in this section were revised: anatomical loss of both eyes (6061) at 41 FR 11291, Mar. 18, 1976; and 6063–6079 for defective visual acuity at 43 FR 45348, Oct. 2, 1978. • Impairment of field vision (6080) was revised at 43 FR 45348, Oct. 2, 1978, while pathological, unilateral scotoma (6081) was revised at 41 FR 11291, Mar. 18. 1976. • Diplopia (6090) was revised at 53 FR 30261, Aug. 11, 1988. • The section on diseases of the ear was revised at 64 FR 25202, May 11, 1999, including changes in all diagnostic codes except otosclerosis (6202), which was revised at 59 FR 17295, Apr. 12, 1994, when the code for otitis interna (6203) was deleted. Recurrent tinnitus (6260) was revised at 68 FR 25822, May 14, 2003. • In the section for other sense organs, the diagnostic codes for sense of smell (6275) and sense of taste (6276) were revised at 64 FR 25202, May 11, 1999. Diagnostic codes 6277–6297 had been removed at 52 FR 44117, Nov. 18, 1987.
Infectious Diseases, Immune Disorders, and Nutritional Deficiencies (formerly Systemic Diseases)	• The entire body system was revised at 61 FR 39873, July 31, 1996. • Prior to that, the diagnostic codes for AIDS-related complex (6352) and HIV antibody positive (6353) were removed at 57 FR 10134, Mar. 24, 1992, and it was indicated that they would be rated under the diagnostic code for HIV-related illness (6351). • The diagnostic code for HIV-related illness (6351) was further revised at 61 FR 39873, July 31, 1996.
Respiratory	• The entire body system was revised at 61 FR 46720, Sept. 5, 1996. • Diagnostic codes 6707–6710 and 6725–6728 under diseases of the lung and pleura—tuberculosis was removed. • Diagnostic codes 6800–6809 (bacterial infections of the lung) and 6810–6818 (restrictive lung diseases) were removed and replaced by new diagnostic codes 6822–6824 and 6840–6847, respectively. • 71 FR 52457, Sept. 6, 2006, made substantive revisions to the "Guidelines for the Application of Evaluation Criteria for Certain Respiratory and Cardiovascular Conditions; Evaluation of Hypertension with Heart Disease."

continued

APPENDIX TABLE 4-1 Continued

Body System	Revisions
Cardiovascular	• The entire body system was revised at 62 FR 65207, Dec. 11, 1997. • Diagnostic codes 7010–7014 were removed, and the conditions moved to codes 7010 or 7011 for evaluation purposes. The diagnostic code for arteriosclerosis (7100) was also removed, and the condition's manifestations were indicated to be rated under the body system they affect. • Section 4.104 was amended at 63 FR 37778, July 14, 1998, by revising the diagnostic code for cold injury residuals (7122). • 71 FR 52457, Sept. 6, 2006, made substantive revisions to the "Guidelines for the Application of Evaluation Criteria for Certain Respiratory and Cardiovascular Conditions; Evaluation of Hypertension with Heart Disease."
Digestive	• Some revisions have been made since the 1970s. • The diagnostic code for ventral postoperative hernia (7339) was revised and the code for wounds (7341) was removed at 41 FR 11291, Mar. 18, 1976. The code for vagotomy (7348) was addressed, but no specific revision was made. • Section 4.112 was revised at 66 FR 29486, May 31, 2001, addressing weight. • The diagnostic codes for residuals of injury to the liver (7311) and cirrhosis of the liver (7312) were revised at 66 FR 29486, May 31, 2001, and residuals of abscess of the liver (7313) was removed because the condition is now considered treatable. • Diagnostic codes 7343–7345, 7351, and 7354 were revised at 66 FR 29486, May 31, 2001.
Genitourinary	• The entire body system was revised at 59 FR 2523, Jan. 18, 1994. • New diagnostic codes 7532–7542 were added. • The diagnostic code for pyelitis (7503) was removed because the term is no longer used and the condition is included under diagnostic code 7504. • The diagnostic code for cystitis, interstitial (Hunner), submucous or elusive ulcer (7513) was removed, and included under diagnostic code 7512. • The diagnostic code for tuberculosis of the bladder (7514) was removed because it is now uncommon and ratings for nonpulmonary tuberculosis are prescribed by sections 4.88b and 4.89. • The diagnostic code for resection or removal of the prostate gland (7526) was removed, included under code 7527, and residuals are evaluated according to the severity of the individual disability. • Section 4.115b, nephritis, was revised at both 59 FR 14566, Mar. 29, 1994, and 59 FR 46338, Sept. 8, 1994. • Raters were instructed to review the diagnostic codes for deformity of the penis with loss of erectile power (7522), complete testis atrophy (7523), and testis removal (7524) for entitlement to special monthly compensation at 59 FR 46338, Sept. 8, 1994.

APPENDIX TABLE 4-1 Continued

Body System	Revisions
Gynecological Conditions and Disorders of the Breast	• The entire body system was revised at 60 FR 19851, Apr. 21, 1995. • New diagnostic codes for benign neoplasms of the gynecological system or breast (7628) and endometriosis (7629) were added. • Section 4.116 was amended and included the revised diagnostic code for surgery of the breast (7626) at 67 FR 6872, Feb. 14, 2002.
Hemic and Lymphatic	• The entire body system was revised at 60 FR 49225, Sept. 22, 1995. • A new diagnostic code for aplastic anemia (7716) was added. • The diagnostic codes for secondary anemia (7701) and secondary adenitis (7713) were removed because they are symptoms of other, more specific diseases. • The diagnostic codes for axillary (7711) and inguinal (7712) tuberculous adenitis were removed and included under the diagnostic code for active or inactive tuberculous adenitis (7710).
Skin	• The entire body system was revised at 67 FR 49590, July 31, 2002. • New diagnostic codes 7820–7833 were added. • The diagnostic codes for pinta (7810) and verruga peruana (7812) were removed because they are so unusual as to no longer warrant a separate category; if these do occur, they may be rated under the diagnostic code for infections of the skin not listed elsewhere (7820). • The preamble was corrected at 67 FR 62889, Oct. 9, 2002. • NPRM 67 FR 65915, Oct. 29, 2002, proposed to revise section 4.118 and the diagnostic codes for disfigurement and scars (7800–7804), except for the code for other scars (7805). The final rule for this proposal was anticipated in Dec. 2006; however, the NPRM was withdrawn on Dec. 29 (71 FR 78391).
Endocrine	• The entire body system was revised at 61 FR 20400, May 7, 1996. • New diagnostic codes 7916–7919 were added. • The diagnostic code for hyperadrenia (7910) was removed at 61 FR 20400, May 7, 1996, because it is so rare among service persons.

continued

APPENDIX TABLE 4-1 Continued

Body System	Revisions
Neurological Conditions and Convulsive Disorders	• Some revisions have been made since the 1970s. • Section 4.124a was amended at 43 FR 45348, Oct. 2, 1978, to reflect the addition of the diagnostic code for the brain, malignant new growths (8002), and at that time a note was added to the code. • A note was added to the diagnostic code for malignant new growths of the spinal cord (8021) at 43 FR 45348, Oct. 2, 1978. • Final rule corrections were made at 54 FR 49754, Dec. 1, 1989, diseases of the peripheral nerves, to correct previously published information for diagnostic codes 8520–8530, 8620–8630, and 8720–8730, because the table was inadvertently misrepresented. • An incorrect word was corrected for the diagnostic code paralysis of posterior tibial nerve (8525) at 55 FR 154, Jan. 3, 1990. • The diagnostic code for soft-tissue sarcoma (8540) was addressed at 56 FR 51651, Oct. 15, 1991, which described service connection based on exposure to herbicides containing dioxin. • Correcting amendments were made at 57 FR 24363, June 9, 1992, to reinstate diagnostic codes 8510–8730, which had been inadvertently omitted at 54 FR 49754, Dec. 1, 1989.

APPENDIX TABLE 4-1 Continued

Body System	Revisions
Mental Disorders	• The entire body system was revised at 71 FR 52695, Oct. 8, 1996. There were extensive revisions in the preamble section and in the diagnostic codes throughout this body system, including new categories, new codes, removed codes, and the incorporation of conditions from removed codes into existing or new codes. DSM-IV was the basis for many of the revisions made. • In the schizophrenia and other psychotic disorders category, diagnostic codes 9200, 9206, 9207, and 9209 were removed. • In the delirium, dementia, and amnestic and other cognitive disorders category, new diagnostic codes for dementia (9326) and organic mental disorder (9327) were added. Diagnostic codes 9302, 9303, 9306, 9307, 9308, 9309, 9311, 9315, 9322, 9324, and 9325 were removed. • A category for anxiety disorders was added, under which new diagnostic codes for panic disorder and/or agoraphobia (9412) and anxiety disorder not otherwise specified (9413) were added. Diagnostic codes 9401, 9402, 9405, 9408, and 9409 were removed. • A category of dissociative disorders was added, under which a diagnostic code for dissociative amnesia, fugue, and identity disorder (9416) and depersonalization disorder (9417) were added. • A category for somatoform disorders was added. Former codes 9402 and 9409 were moved into the new diagnostic codes for pain disorder (9422), conversion disorder (9424), and hypochondriasis (9425). A new code for undifferentiated somatoform disorder (9423) was also added. • A category for mood disorders was added, and the diagnostic codes for bipolar disorder (9432, previously 9206), dysthymic disorder (9433, previously 9405), and major depressive disorder (9434, pulled from codes 9207, 9209, and 9405) were placed in this category. New diagnostic codes for cyclothymic disorder (9431) and mood disorder not otherwise specified (9435) were added. • A category for chronic adjustment disorder, and a new code for the disorder (9440) were added. • The category of psychophysiologic skin reaction was removed, including diagnostic codes 9500–9511 based on DSM-IV guidelines that preclude the need for a separate code and evaluation criteria for this disorder. • A category for eating disorders was added, with new diagnostic codes for anorexia nervosa (9520) and bulimia nervosa (9521). • NPRM 67 FR 63352, Oct. 11, 2002, "A Definition of Psychosis for Certain VA Purposes," was anticipated to become final in August 2006, but has not yet been issued.

continued

APPENDIX TABLE 4-1 Continued

Body System	Revisions
Dental and Oral Conditions	• The entire body system was revised at 59 FR 2529, Jan. 18, 1994. • New diagnostic codes for loss of more than half of the maxilla (9914), loss of half or less of the maxilla (9915), and malunion or nonunion of the maxilla (9916) were added. The previous diagnostic code for loss of whole or part of substance, nonunion, or malunion of the maxilla (9910) was removed because of the addition of the new codes. • The conditions of carious teeth, treatable; missing teeth, replaceable; dento-alveolar abscess; pyorrhea alveolaris; and Vincent's stomatitis were determined to be nondisabling conditions; the new section 4.149 served as a replacement to address these conditions. • Section 4.149, "Rating Diseases of the Teeth and Gums," was revised at 62 FR 8201, Feb. 24, 1997.

5

The Medical Examination and Disability Rating Process

Processing claims for veterans disability compensation, including determining the ratings, is the responsibility of the Veterans Benefits Administration (VBA), one of the three major organizations within the Department of Veterans Affairs (VA).[1] VA established VBA in 1953 (then called the Department of Veterans Benefits) to administer the GI Bill and the compensation and pension program.

VBA's mission is "to provide benefits and services to the veterans and their families in a responsive, timely, and compassionate manner in recognition of their service to the nation" (VA, 2007e). According to VA's strategic plan, disability compensation is part of strategic goal 1: "Restore the capability of veterans with disabilities to the greatest extent possible, and improve the quality of their lives and that of their families." To achieve this goal, VA has set out specific program objectives in its strategic plan. The objective most relevant to the disability compensation program is objective 1.2: "Provide timely and accurate decisions on disability compensation claims to improve the economic status and quality of life of service-disabled veterans" (VA, 2006c).

Chapter 4 addressed the effectiveness of VA's Schedule for Rating Disabilities (Rating Schedule) in assessing degree of disability for impairment purposes, with a particular focus on whether it is medically up to date and whether it is constructed appropriately to measure severity of impairment, limitation of function, quality of life, or extent of disability. This chapter

[1]The other organizations are the Veterans Health Administration (VHA) and the National Cemetery Administration.

addresses the process by which the Rating Schedule is applied, focusing on the timeliness, accuracy, and consistency of decisions on veterans claims.

The key medical aspects of the disability claims process are

- development of medical evidence, such as information about degree of impairment, functional limitation, and disability, which usually includes a disability examination conducted by a VHA clinician or medical contractor;
- the rating process, in which the medical evidence is compared with the criteria in the Rating Schedule and a percentage rating is determined; and
- the appeal process, in which the adequacy and meaning of the medical evidence is often the central question.

ORGANIZATION OF THE VETERANS BENEFITS ADMINISTRATION

VBA is an organization of about 13,000 employees. Staffing in fiscal year (FY) 2006 was 12,810 full-time equivalents (FTEs) and is estimated to be 13,104 FTEs in FY 2007. Approximately half the staff (an estimated 6,425 in FY 2007) is directly devoted to administration of the disability compensation program (VA, 2007b). VBA has 57 regional offices, including at least one in every state in the nation (except Wyoming, which is served by the Denver, Colorado, regional office), as well as offices in Puerto Rico and the Philippines, and additional locations in Korea and Germany.

Within VBA, the Compensation and Pension (C&P) Service administers the disability compensation program. C&P Service also administers the dependency and indemnity compensation, death compensation, disability pension, death pension, burial benefits, automobile allowance/adaptive equipment, clothing allowance, and specially adapted housing programs.[2]

Each regional office includes a veterans service center (VSC), which is the component that processes disability compensation claims. These centers function under a standardized structure called the claims process improvement (CPI) model, which was recommended in 2001 by the Claims Processing Task Force appointed by the VA secretary to address the growing backlog of claims.[3] The model was designed to increase efficiency in

[2]The other program components of VBA are the Vocational Rehabilitation, Education, Loan Guaranty, and Insurance Services.

[3]These descriptions of the organization and structure of a VSC are based on information provided to the Institute of Medicine (IOM) staff by the Baltimore, Maryland, Regional Office, as well as VA's *Compensation and Pension Adjudication Procedure Manual*, M21-1MR, Part III, Subpart I, Chapter 1. http://www.warms.vba.va.gov/admin21/m21_1/mr/part3/subpti/ch01.doc (accessed February 28, 2007).

processing compensation and pension claims and to reduce the number of errors. The model was fully implemented in 2002, and it established a consistent organizational structure and standard work processes across all regional offices.[4] The model

- requires triage of incoming mail and analysis of incoming claims;
- emphasizes the importance of complete and accurate development of claims by veterans service representatives (VSRs) specially trained to do the work; and
- promotes specialization that improves quality and the expeditious handling of claims, while at the same time allowing management the flexibility to adjust resources to meet the demands of changing workload requirements.

Specialized Team Structure

Each VSC uses six separate teams specialized to handle specific steps in the compensation claim process.

Public Contact Team

The public contact team handles personal interviews and telephone inquiries. Team members assist walk-ins, answer telephones, answer routine correspondence (including e-mails), respond to veterans assistance inquiries, and address outreach and fiduciary issues.

VSRs on the public contact team interview veterans and collect as much information as possible to complete a veteran's claim. If the veteran provides a birth certificate and the master record indicates an award can be prepared immediately, a VSR on the public contact team can prepare the veteran's award. If additional records are needed, such as from a VA medical center, or if the veteran was recently released from the military and his or her service medical records and separation examination are on record, the public contact team will forward the claim to the triage team.

The public contact team's regular outreach activities include contacts with veterans service organizations (VSOs), nursing homes, state fairs, stand-downs, and benefit clinics.

Personnel on the public contact team include a

- coach (GS-13);
- assistant coach (GS-12);
- VSR (rotational) (GS-11);

[4]Prior to this, regional offices had more latitude to vary their organization and procedures.

- public contact and outreach specialist (GS-10);
- public contact specialist (GS-9);
- field examiner (GS-10);
- legal instrument examiner (GS-9); and
- intake specialist (GS-7).

One of the primary objectives of the public contact team is to promote a bilateral exchange of information with the triage team.

Triage Team

The triage team helps coordinate the work of the other specialized teams. Team members review, control, and process all incoming mail. They also process actions that can be completed with little or no review of the claim folder.

Personnel in the triage team include a

- coach (GS-13);
- assistant coach (GS-12);
- rating VSR (GS-12);
- senior VSR (GS-12);
- VSR (GS-11);
- claims assistant (GS-6);
- file bank coach (GS-6); and
- file clerk/program clerk (GS-4).

Predetermination Team

The predetermination team's primary role is to develop evidence necessary for a rating to be made. This team is responsible for most of the medical development activity in the following cases:

- original and reopened compensation;
- compensation claimed due to injury or death caused by VA medical care or evaluation;
- original and reopened disability pension;
- original and reopened dependency and indemnity compensation (DIC); and
- basic eligibility issues requiring a rating decision.

Staff on the team also prepare administrative decisions, including decisions on

- character of discharge;
- line of duty;
- willful misconduct;
- deemed valid marriage (death claims); and
- common law marriage (live claims).

Personnel in the predetermination team are the same as in the triage team.

Rating Team[5]

The rating team makes decisions on claims that require consideration of medical evidence. Rating VSRs (RVSRs) on the rating team rate claims that have been certified by the predetermination team as "ready to rate." They may prepare a rating for partial grant if there is insufficient evidence to rate all of a veteran's medical conditions (referred to as *issues*), but there is sufficient evidence to make an award on one or more issues. In such a case, the rating specialist rates the issue(s) ready to be rated, prepares a separate deferred rating for the unresolved issues, and returns the claims file to the predetermination team for further development.

Personnel on the rating team include a

- coach (GS-13);
- assistant coach (GS-12);
- RVSR (GS-12); and
- claims assistant (GS-6).

Postdetermination Team

The postdetermination team develops evidence for non-rating issues, processes awards, and notifies claimants of decisions. This team also completes entitlement determinations for issues that do not require a rating, such as

- accrued benefits;
- apportionment decisions;
- competency issues;
- income changes;
- original pension;
- dependency issues;
- burials;

[5]The rating process, which involves the interpretation and application of VA's *Schedule for Rating Disabilities*, is described in more detail later in this chapter.

- death pension;
- hospital adjustments;
- specially adapted housing; and
- the Civilian Health and Medical Program.

Personnel on the postdetermination team include a

- coach (GS-13);
- assistant coach (GS-12);
- senior VSR (GS-12);
- VSR (GS-11); and
- claims assistant (GS-6).

Appeals Team

The appeals team handles decisions with which claimants have formally disagreed (i.e., appealed). The appeals team processes both appeals submitted by veterans and cases returned by the Board of Veterans' Appeals (BVA) for further development, called *remands*. The appeals team is also responsible for development of remands, which may involve returning the case to VHA for a medical examination or opinion and for making a decision on the basis of the additional information. If the adjudicator reaffirms the original denial of the case, the case is sent back to BVA for review and decision. The team is intended to increase the level of accountability and maintain control over the appeal workload.

Personnel on the appeals team include a

- coach (GS-13);
- decision review officer (GS-13);
- senior VSR (GS-12);
- RVSR (GS-12);
- VSR (GS-11);
- claims assistant (GS-6); and
- file clerk/program clerk (GS-4).

Role of the VSR and RVSR

VSRs on the public contact, triage, predetermination, postdetermination, and appeals teams perform a vital role in the compensation claim adjudication process. They conduct interviews, identify issues, gather relevant evidence, adjudicate certain claims, authorize payments, and input data for award generation and notification of the veteran. However, the key staff person in the actual disability rating is the RVSR, who is on the rating team. The rating team and the disability rating produced by that team is the central component of the veterans disability compensation claims process.[6]

The RVSR serves as the decision maker for most claims involving rating decisions. He or she analyzes claims, applies the Rating Schedule, and prepares rating decisions that inform the VSR or claimant of the decision and the basis for the decision. There is routine collaboration between the RVSR and the other members of a given team, which includes VSRs and the decision review officer (DRO). The RVSR is also available to discuss claims with VSO representatives. In addition, the RVSR may directly interact with the veteran and his or her representative or advocate.

An RVSR is required to analyze claims to determine

- if diseases and injuries were incurred or aggravated by military service in the line of duty for purposes of compensation, hospital and outpatient treatment, provision of prosthetics, vocational training, and related employment and compensation benefits;
- a need for examination, reexamination, and hospitalization for observation of veterans and their dependents and the character of these examinations; and
- the competency of veterans, their dependents, and beneficiaries, and the permanent incapacity of a veteran's children or widow or widower for self-support, as well as testamentary capacity for insurance purposes.

As needed, the RVSR may ask the VSR to initiate action to obtain evidence needed to support a veteran's claim. In some cases, the RVSR monitors the claim to eliminate unnecessary delays.

The RVSR determines

- service connection;
- percentage of disability;
- permanent and total disability;
- entitlement to compensation, pension, and vocational training;
- medical and dental treatment;
- automobiles or other conveyances;
- insurance;
- specially adapted housing;
- dependent education allowances; and
- other ancillary benefits.

[6]There are also RVSRs on the triage and predetermination teams because those teams perform a limited number of the ratings in certain circumstances and also assess whether the medical evidence is sufficient to support a rating decision.

He or she is fully accountable for proper analysis, appropriate development, proper application of the Rating Schedule, and final rating determinations.[7]

MEDICAL EVALUATION PROCESS

Claims for disability compensation are initiated when a veteran files an application, either online or at a regional office. VA rules require that "[a] specific claim in the form prescribed by the Secretary must be filed in order for benefits to be paid to any individual under the laws administered by VA."[8] However, any communication or action indicating an intent to apply for benefits from a claimant or his or her representative may be considered an informal claim.[9]

In 1998, VA and the Department of Defense (DoD) established a program called Benefits Delivery at Discharge (BDD) to help servicemembers initiate a disability compensation claim at their military bases prior to being discharged. The program is in effect in 140 locations in the United States, Korea, and Germany. It currently operates under a 2004 memorandum of agreement between VA and DoD to create a cooperative separation medical examination process to ease the transition from service to veteran status. The BDD program "enables separating service members to file disability compensation claims with VA staff at military bases, complete physical exams, and have their claims evaluated before, or closely following, their military separation" (U.S. Congress, House of Representatives, Committee on Veterans' Affairs, 2007a). In FY 2006, 40,600 claims were filed through the BDD program (about 5 percent of the compensation claims for that year) (VDBC, 2007). BDD sites took in 30,000 claims in FY 2004 and 35,000 in FY 2005 (U.S. Congress, House of Representatives, Committee on Veterans' Affairs, 2005c). VA reports that the BDD process reduces the average time for an adjudication decision to approximately 60 days (compared with 160–180 days for processing regular claims) (U.S. Congress, Senate, Committee on Veterans' Affairs, 2007). VA's goal is to have 65 percent of the original claims made by veterans within the first year after release from active duty filed at a BDD site (the actual percentage in FY 2006 was 50 percent) (VA, 2006). In 2005, VBA consolidated the rating of BDD claims in two regional offices to "bring greater consistency of decisions on claims filed by newly separated veterans" (U.S. Congress, House of Representatives, Committee on Veterans' Affairs, 2005a).

---

[7]Based, in part, on Position Description, Veteran Service Representative (Rating), RFSR, GS-996-12.

[8]38 USC 5101(a) and 38 CFR 3.151.

[9]38 CFR 3.155.

In addition to BDD, which is not available to wounded or injured servicemembers being considered for separation for inability to perform their duties, DoD provides VA a monthly list of servicemembers referred to a physical evaluation board by a medical evaluation board.[10] The list enables VA to contact servicemembers likely to be separated while they are still in the service to facilitate their transfer to VA health care and benefits when they separate. In spinal cord injury cases, DoD and VA have a memorandum of understanding under which active duty servicemembers can be treated in VHA's specialized spinal cord injury centers. More recently, a similar arrangement was made for treatment of traumatic brain injury (TBI) and polytrauma cases in VHA's TBI and polytrauma centers. As of the end of FY 2006, DoD had sent VA contact information for 13,622 individuals (U.S. Congress, Senate, Committee on Veterans' Affairs, 2007).

On receipt of a "substantially complete application" (which includes the claimant's name, his or her relationship to the veteran, sufficient service information for VA to verify the veteran's service and claimed medical condition or conditions), VA will begin to process the claim. In accordance with the Veterans Claims Assistance Act (VCAA) of 2000, VA has a "duty to assist" the claimant. VA must give the claimant written notification of the evidence necessary to substantiate the claim. It must also tell the claimant whether VA or the claimant is responsible for obtaining that evidence. VA must make reasonable efforts to obtain relevant records not in the custody of the federal government, and it must make as many requests as necessary to obtain relevant records within the custody of federal departments or agencies, including the veteran's service medical records and VA records of examination or treatment. However, VA encourages applicants to submit copies of their own medical records to expedite the claim (Box 5-1).

The evidence development phase of disability claims processing is often the most time-consuming part of the entire process. Multiple requests may be necessary to obtain needed information. This phase of the claims process is managed by the predetermination team in the VSC. The team sets diaries (deadline dates) for receipt of requested information, then determines the need for a VA medical examination to assess the current level of disability or to provide a medical opinion about whether the current disability is related to the veteran's military service (referred to as "medical nexus").

---

[10]As part of DoD's disability evaluation system, medical evaluation boards refer individuals deemed unable to carry out their duties to a physical evaluation board, which usually results in separation from service.

BOX 5-1
Excerpt from VA Publication:
Understanding the Disability Claim Process

What VA Does After It Receives Your Claim

After VA receives your Application for Compensation, it sends you a letter. The letter explains what VA needs in order to help grant your claim. It states how VA assists in getting records to support your claim. The letter may include forms for you to complete, such as medical releases. They help VA obtain pertinent medical records from your doctor or hospital. You should try to complete and return all forms VA sends within a month. Your claim can often be processed more quickly if you send a copy of your own medical records.

What Records VA Obtains to Support Your Claim

VA then attempts to get all the records relevant to your claimed medical conditions from the military, private hospitals or doctors, or any other place you tell us. The person who decides your claim (called a Rating Veterans Service Representative) may order a medical examination. This examination is free of charge. It is extremely important that you report for your examination at the scheduled time to avoid delaying your claim.

SOURCE: VA (2007f).

Compensation and Pension Examinations

According to VA, "The purpose of C&P examinations is to provide the medical information needed to reach a legal decision about a veteran's entitlement to VA monetary benefits based on disability" (Brown, 2003). Obtaining a C&P medical examination is part of VA's duty to assist the applicant. An examination is required

- when a veteran files a claim for service connection and submits evidence of disability;
- when a service-connected veteran asserts a worsened condition;
- to provide medical nexus;
- to reconcile diagnoses;
- as directed by BVA; and
- as required by regulation (Pamperin, 2006).

VA may accept a medical report from a private physician if it is "adequate for rating purposes."[11] However, C&P examinations are ordered in most disability compensation claims for several reasons:

- to obtain current medical information;
- to obtain information relevant to disability (such as functional impacts of an impairment) rather than the diagnostic and treatment information sought in a standard medical examination; and
- to have information from someone more independent than the applicant's treating physician might be.

In FY 2005 VA obtained more than a half million C&P examinations. VHA performed 84 percent of these examinations in its own medical facilities, and the remaining 16 percent were obtained from a contract examination provider (QTC, 2006). Examinations from VHA generally take about 35 days to complete, and those from the contract provider take about 38 days (Pamperin, 2006).

Generally, the predetermination team in the regional office's VSC determines the kind of examination needed based on the available medical records and uses one or more of 58 examination worksheets (referred to as AMIE worksheets, after the Automated Medical Information Exchange system for which they were originally developed in 1997) to describe for the examiner the specific requirements of the examination. There are separate worksheets for specific diagnoses (e.g., diabetes mellitus, hypertension, cold injury, posttraumatic stress disorder [PTSD]) and for certain body systems (e.g., eye, genitourinary, dental and oral, mental, hemic disorders). There is one sheet for a general medical examination. Although there are 58 different examination worksheets, the 10 most frequently requested examinations account for 67 percent of C&P exams (Brown, 2006b) (Table 5-1).

The first 57 examination worksheets were last thoroughly revised (by a workgroup with representation from VHA, VBA, and BVA) when they were incorporated in the AMIE system in 1997. Using the AMIE system, they can now be downloaded by examiners in the VA medical centers. The 58th worksheet, for social and industrial assessments surveys, was added in 2004, and the diabetes mellitus worksheet was updated the same year. In 2005, the worksheets for eating disorders; initial evaluation of PTSD; review examination for PTSD; joints; mental disorders except PTSD and eating disorders; nose, sinus, larynx, and pharynx; prisoner of war (POW) protocol examinations; and spine were updated (VA, 2007d).

In 2002, another VHA/VBA/BVA workgroup developed the *C&P Service Clinician's Guide* (VA, 2002a). The guide includes the worksheets and

[11] 38 CFR 3.326, "Examinations."

TABLE 5-1 The 10 Most Requested Medical Examinations

	Examination Worksheet	Percent of Exams
1	General medical examination	18.9
2	Joints (shoulder, elbow, wrist, hip, knee, and ankle)	11.7
3	Audio	8.7
4	Spine (cervical, thoracic, and lumbar)	8.4
5	Mental disorders (except initial PTSD and eating disorders)	5.7
6	Eye	3.5
7	Initial evaluation for PTSD	2.8
8	Feet	2.7
9	Review examination for PTSD	2.7
10	Skin diseases (other than scars)	2.7
	Cumulative total	67.2

SOURCE: Brown (2006b).

additional information on conducting each kind of examination. VA has also developed two more detailed guides for particular examinations: *Best Practice Manual for Posttraumatic Stress Disorder (PTSD) Compensation and Pension Examinations* (VA, 2001b) and *Handbook of Standard Procedures and Best Practices for Audiology Compensation and Pension Examinations* (VA, 2004b).

In 2004, VA began fielding online examination templates for each of the AMIE worksheets in graphical user interface format. These "intelligent," point-and-click templates are designed to structure the information gathering and reporting process, thus increasing completeness, consistency, and timeliness of examination reports. As of April 2005, a version of each of the automated templates was installed in all examination sites (U.S. Congress, House of Representatives, Veterans' Affairs Committee, 2005b). The templates had been used 290,000 times as of the end of February 2007 and accounted for about 28 percent (21,125 of 75,000) of the C&P examinations performed by VHA that month. Of 102 sites using the templates, 59 completed more than 1,000 in January 2007. According to the director of the Compensation and Pension Examination Program (CPEP), VA is committed to mandating template use, and key stakeholder feedback and refinement activities are underway prior to taking that step (Brown, 2007).

The regional office requesting an examination is responsible for specifying the type of examination required and any special reports or studies needed. The VHA health-care facility decides who will perform the examination and where and how the examination will be conducted. The regional office may request specific specialist examinations, but the physician examiner may also decide if a specialist examination is necessary on a case-by-case basis (VA, 2006b). If the examination is being conducted on a remanded case, BVA usually requires the examiner to review the entire claims file, including service records, medical records, and previous C&P examination reports.

In addition to medical information, such as the results of tests or examinations, the examiner may be asked to provide an expert opinion on such questions as whether a condition is related to a specific event during service in the military, or a preexisting condition was aggravated in service, or a condition may be a secondary manifestation or consequence of a condition that previously was service connected. In these cases, the examiner is asked to use the following terminology:

- *is due to* (100% sure);
- *more likely than not* (greater than 50%);
- *at least as likely as not* (equal to or greater than 50%); and
- *not at least as likely as not* (less than 50%) (VA, 2002a).

The VSC uses the Compensation and Pension Record Exchange (CAPRI) system (the successor to AMIE) to order C&P examinations from VHA. This system still relies on the AMIE worksheets for examination specifications. CAPRI allows more efficient communication between VBA and VHA by directly linking their information systems and thereby providing VBA with direct, online access to VHA medical data (VA, 2005a).

VHA C&P examiners are supposed to conduct the examination in accordance with the format of the AMIE worksheets and the *C&P Service Clinician's Guide* (VA, 2002a), but they are not required to use the worksheets to report the examination, as long as they provide

- an up-to-date, brief medical and industrial history from the date of discharge or the last examination;
- a record of subjective complaints;
- a complete description of objective findings stated in concrete terms;
- a diagnosis of all described conditions;
- answers to any questions specifically requested in the examination request;
- opinions specifically requested in the examination request;
- a diagnosis or notation that a chronic disease or disability was ruled out for each disability, complaint, or symptom listed on the examination request; and
- the clinical findings required by the rating schedule for the evaluation of the specific disability being claimed (VA, 2006b).

The VSC orders examinations from the contract examination provider, QTC, using the Veterans Examination Request Information System (VERIS). The VSR or other authorized employee enters examination requests on a daily basis. An encrypted file is transferred to QTC. After the examination is complete, the VSR or other authorized employee logs directly into QTC's secure website to download the completed examinations in batches (Pamperin, 2006). QTC examiners are provided with a template for online reporting but are not required to use it as long as they provide the required information.

If an examination report does not include sufficiently detailed information to support the diagnoses or about the effects of diagnosed conditions on functioning, the RVSR is instructed to return the report as inadequate for rating purposes.

VHA Examiner Qualifications, Training, and Quality Assurance

Training and qualifications of examiners who perform C&P examinations in VHA are monitored by CPEP, a joint initiative between VHA and VBA established in 2001 to improve the C&P examination process. CPEP focuses on the 10 most frequently requested examinations.[12] It first establishes baseline performance for examiners, then develops performance improvement initiatives, monitors performance, and provides feedback. It relies on a quality indicator approach, focusing on selected important and representative elements (rather than a comprehensive audit of all possible elements). Core quality indicators apply to all examination types, but there are additional examination-specific quality indicators as well. CPEP has produced regular reports of the top 10 examination types since 2003, based on data collected starting in 2001 (Brown, 2006a,b).

In May 2006, VA's under secretary for health and under secretary for benefits initiated a mandatory certification procedure for clinicians who perform C&P examinations, directing CPEP to

> provide every clinician who performs C&P exams for VHA, whether employee or contractor, the necessary training to have a full understanding of the requirements of the process. . . . Individuals who meet the training requirements for certification will be tracked, and this data will be made available to the credentialing and privileging authority for their respective healthcare facility.

[12]In FY 2007, the audio examination, which had demonstrated consistently high performance, was replaced by the diabetes examination, as one of the 10 examinations being monitored for quality performance (Brown, 2007).

Although this certification program is still under development, the program will consist of educational content, videotape and web-based training, and testing (Brown, 2006a,b, 2007).

For most examinations, VHA decides on a case-by-case basis the appropriate level of training the examiner must have. However, for initial mental disorder examinations (including PTSD examinations) the examination must be conducted by a board-certified or board-eligible psychiatrist or licensed doctorate-level psychologist or, under their close supervision, by a psychiatry resident, doctorate-level mental health provider, or clinical/counseling psychologist with a completed one-year internship or residency (VA, 2006e). Auditory examinations must be performed by licensed audiologists.

QTC Examiner Qualifications, Training, and Quality Assurance

QTC Medical Group, Inc. currently provides C&P examinations for 10 VA regional offices and 26 BDD sites, using a network of approximately 1,600 contracted private practitioners. QTC also has clinics in California, Texas, and Virginia, in which examiners are QTC employees. Examiners who perform C&P examinations for QTC must be

- graduates of an accredited medical school (M.D. or D.O.);
- licensed to practice medicine in the location(s) where they conduct examinations;
- board certified or board eligible;
- clear of Medicare, Medicaid, and any other federal exclusions; and
- covered by malpractice insurance.

QTC trains its examiners and monitors performance in an internal quality assurance program, which includes a probationary period with review and quality feedback. QTC has full-time quality assurance personnel who review all reports for quality before they are released, ensuring that they adhere to AMIE worksheet requirements. Quality assurance personnel also identify any negative trends, and retrain or dismiss problematic providers (QTC, 2006). The 150 contract psychiatrists who perform PTSD examinations are given additional training (Shahani, 2005).

QTC developed a training manual for its examiners, which was approved by the VBA medical director. It trains examiners either in person or during several conference calls. QTC's policy is to monitor examiners' work closely for the first three months. If the work is not satisfactory (that is, examination reports do not meet AMIE worksheet requirements), he or she is released. QTC has a quality control person on each administrative team who works with examiners to scrutinize each report before it goes to VA.[13] As noted above, reports of new examiners are analyzed in detail for the first three months and feedback is provided. To ensure QTC examination quality, the C&P Services' medical director reviews a random sample of 384 reports each quarter. At least 92 percent of the reports must be complete, and there are financial penalties for failing to meet, and incentives for exceeding, that figure.[14]

According to the VA inspector general, "There is little difference between the quality of contractor-produced C&P examinations and VA [VHA] examinations and their impact on the degrees of disability that are eventually awarded to the veterans." This finding was based on a comparison of a set of examination reports from each organization and the results of a survey of raters (VA, 2005b).

THE DISABILITY RATING PROCESS

After all development actions are complete, the VSC predetermination team refers the claim to the rating team for a rating. The rating team reviews all the evidence associated with the claim, makes decisions on issues raised by the claimant, and identifies any inferred issues that should be addressed. The team documents the rating decision in a standard format, using an automated rating preparation system called Rating Board Automation (RBA) 2000. After completing the rating decision, the team routes the claim to the postdetermination team.

The postdetermination team implements the rating decision by preparing either a monetary award or a denial. It also prepares notification letters for the claimant and representative.

When performing a rating evaluation, RVSRs consider all evidence associated with the claim. This includes service medical records, VA medical examination records, clinical summaries from VA medical centers where treatment has been provided to the veteran, and evidence provided from private sources, such as the veteran's treating physician.

Primary guidance for performing rating evaluations are contained in the Rating Schedule itself, the *Compensation and Pension Adjudication Procedures Manual,* M21-1MR, and internal program guides. Underlying principles that provide the philosophical base for rating evaluations include (but are not limited to) the following:

---

[13]QTC has administrative teams, each of which works with a set of contract examiners. Each team consists of a case coordinator, quality assurance coordinator, and case technician.

[14]Information provided by Bonnie Miranda, assistant director for training, Compensation and Pension Services, VBA, in response to committee staff questions, dated August 18, 2006.

- Each disabling condition shown by a veteran's service records, or for which he seeks a service connection must be considered on the basis of the places, types and circumstances of his service. . . . Determinations as to service connection will be based on review of the entire evidence of record, with due consideration to the policy of VA to administer the law under a broad and liberal interpretation consistent with the facts in each individual case (38 CFR 3.303).
- The veteran will be considered to have been in sound condition when examined, accepted and enrolled for service, except as to defects, infirmities, or disorders noted at entrance in service, or where clear and unmistakable (obvious or manifest) evidence demonstrates that an injury or disease existed prior thereto and was not aggravated by such service. Only such conditions as are recorded in examination reports are to be considered as noted (38 CFR 3.304b).
- Rating agencies will handle cases affected by change of medical findings or diagnosis, so as to produce the greatest degree of stability of disability evaluations consistent with the laws and VA regulations governing disability compensation and pension. It is essential that the entire record of examinations and the medical-industrial history be reviewed to ascertain whether the recent examination is full and complete, including all special examinations indicated as a result of general examination and the entire case history (38 CFR 3.344).
- It is the responsibility of the rating specialist to interpret reports of examination in the light of the whole recorded history, reconciling the various reports into a consistent picture so that the current rating may accurately reflect the elements of disability present. Each disability must be considered from the point of view of the veteran working or seeking work (38 CFR 4.2).
- Every element in any way affecting the probative value to be assigned to the evidence in each individual claim must be thoroughly and conscientiously studied (38 CFR 4.6).
- Where there is a question as to which of two evaluations shall be applied, the higher evaluation will be assigned if the disability picture more nearly approximates the criteria required for that rating (38 CFR 4.7).

As illustrated by this (partial) list, the RVSR must assess several areas in order to develop a rating decision. All the guiding principles in the Rating Schedule must be considered, as they apply, for each decision component of the rating. These basic decision components include

- a determination that the veteran has a disabling condition or conditions;
- a determination as to whether each disability is service-connected;

- a determination on the evaluation level (10 percent, 20 percent, etc.) to be assigned for each service-connected disability (done through referral to sections 4.71a to 4.150 of the Rating Schedule, where specific disabilities are listed, along with diagnostic criteria and associated evaluation levels); and
- an effective date for entitlement to payment for each service-connected condition.

RVSRs assign evaluation levels based on the tables, diagnostic codes, and the percentages provided in the Rating Schedule, correlating the medical evidence in the individual case to the criteria and percentages provided in the Rating Schedule.

When multiple conditions have been evaluated, a combined rating evaluation is performed according to a "combined rating table" found in 38 CFR 4.25.

To the extent that the Rating Schedule reflects current medical diagnostic knowledge, assessment of disability, and treatment, the resultant rating evaluation should accurately reflect disability. To the extent that the Rating Schedule is outdated, the resultant rating evaluation will be subject to distortions and imprecision.

The standard rating evaluation decision format contains the following sections: Introduction, Decision, Statement of Evidence, and Reasons and Bases for the Decision. It also includes a section called Coded Conclusion, containing statistical information about the veteran, the specific evaluations, and the combined evaluation. The RVSR signs the completed rating decision.

The discussion above shows that the rating process is complicated and multifaceted. The technicians who execute the ratings are expected to have substantial expertise in VA law and the medical aspects of the Rating Schedule. Rating team personnel are generally grouped together in a section or sections of the VSC. The RVSRs do their evaluations individually, however. They do not have routine access to medical practitioners or legal experts as they conduct their assessments. They have only their training guides and regulations to interpret.

Quality Review Process

VBA's primary means of assessing the quality of the rating process is a program called Statistical Technical Accuracy Review (STAR). The STAR program was developed in the late 1990s in response to concerns about the accuracy of C&P claims adjudications. In FY 2006, the program was staffed with 18 senior, experienced VSRs and RVSRs from within VBA (VA, 2006). These employees are recruited and managed by the C&P Service.

Most employees are located in Nashville, Tennessee, although some STAR staff work from the VA central office (VACO).

STAR reviews are done based on a standard protocol that asks questions in the following areas:

- Were all issues in the claim addressed, including inferred issues?
- Was evidentiary development done properly and thoroughly in accordance with the Veterans Claims Assistance Act?
- Were decisions on grant or denial, and percentage evaluation assigned, correct?
- Were payment dates and rates correct?
- Were decisions properly documented?
- Were notifications of decisions sent and appropriate?

STAR reviews are conducted by the national staff in Nashville, usually several weeks after the rating decision has been completed.

VA also began a new program, Statistical Individual Performance Assessment, in 2002 to offer immediate feedback on claims processing, including ratings, and to promote accuracy and consistency of claims adjudication. It also was intended to provide performance management results at the individual employee level. The original plan was to have supervisors review 10 cases from each technician every month, correcting errors before decisions were made. The program was absorbed into the employee performance management system.

APPEAL PROCESS[15]

A veteran (or other applicant, such as a surviving spouse, child, or parent of a veteran) who disagrees with a VA regional office's decision can file an appeal either to the local regional office (for reconsideration of the original decision) or to BVA. If the veteran chooses to appeal to the regional office, but is still dissatisfied with the decision, he or she may then appeal to BVA. If still dissatisfied, the veteran may file additional appeals (in sequential order) to

- the U.S. Court of Appeals for Veterans Claims (CAVC);
- the U.S. Court of Appeals for the Federal Circuit; and
- the U.S. Supreme Court.

Although a veteran can appeal for any reason, issues frequently appealed include disability compensation, pension, education benefits,

[15]For a detailed description of the appeal process, see BVA (2000a).

recovery of overpayments, and reimbursement for unauthorized medical services. The two most common appeals are made by veterans who feel that (1) the VA regional office denied them benefits for an impairment (i.e., it was declared not to be service connected) that they believe began while they were in service, and (2) the severity rating assigned to the impairment was too low and an increase in the rating level is warranted (BVA, 2002a).

Appeal Steps

To begin the appeal process, a veteran files a written notice of disagreement (NOD) with the field office from which the disputed decision was issued. For most compensation cases, the appeal must be filed within one year from the date of the decision.

If more than one claim is at issue (e.g., a claim for compensation based on an orthopedic condition and claim for compensation on a respiratory condition), the NOD must be specific about which issue or issues are being appealed. If a veteran is appealing to the local regional office (rather than BVA), he or she may choose to have the case handled in the traditional appellate review process (in which an RVSR handles the appeal) or to have the file be reviewed by a DRO. DROs provide a second review of an appellant's entire file, and they can hold a personal hearing about an appellant's claim. DROs are authorized to grant the contested benefits based on the same case record that the local office used to make the initial decision.

After completing any additional development or proceedings, the RVSR or DRO (as appropriate) sends the veteran either a favorable decision on all issues, or a statement of case explaining the reasons for the decision not to allow the appeal, along with VA Form 9, the substantive appeal form, which the veteran may use to ask for a BVA review of the decision. VA Form 9 must be filed within 60 days of the mailing of the statement of case, or within one year from the date VA mailed its decision, whichever is later. (The 60-day period for filing a substantive appeal can be extended for "good cause.")

On VA Form 9, the veteran states the desired benefit, notes perceived mistakes in the statement of case, and comments on anything with which he or she disagrees. If the veteran submits new evidence or information with the substantive appeal, such as records from recent medical treatments or evaluations, the VA local office prepares a supplemental statement of case, which is similar to the statement of case, but addresses the new information or evidence submitted.

The local VA office sends a letter to the veteran who is appealing when the claims folder is transferred to BVA in Washington, D.C. Generally, the appellant has 90 days (from the date of the letter) or until BVA decides his or her case, whichever comes first, during which to submit more evidence, request a hearing, or select or change a representative.

At personal hearings, veterans meet with either a DRO at the regional office or a BVA member (at BVA hearings). Personal hearings are informal. Appellants in most areas of the country can choose to hold a BVA hearing, commonly called a *travel board hearing*, either at the regional office or at the BVA office in Washington, D.C. Some regional offices are also equipped to hold BVA hearings by videoconference with the appellant at his or her regional office and the board member in Washington, D.C., which is considered the most expedient choice. BVA held 2,700 hearings by videoconference in FY 2006, up from 1,300 in FY 2000, and expects this number to continue to rise (BVA, 2006).

After the hearing, a BVA board member will review a transcript of the hearing (if applicable) and the appellant's file and make a decision either allowing or denying the case. Appeals may be dismissed in certain limited circumstances. However, if BVA cannot make a final decision, it may remand the case (i.e., send the claim back to the regional office) for additional development and a new determination. If after completing the additional development, the local office is again unable to allow the claim, the case is returned to BVA for a final decision.

Board of Veterans' Appeals

BVA is a quasi-judicial, organizationally independent component of VA that reports directly to the VA secretary and makes final agency decisions with respect to claims for veterans benefits. BVA reviews all appeals for entitlement to veterans benefits on behalf of the VA secretary, including appeals involving claims for service connection, increased disability ratings, individual unemployability, pension, insurance benefits, educational benefits, home loan guaranties, vocational rehabilitation, and dependency and indemnity compensation, and also determinations of duty status, marital status, dependency status, and effective dates of benefits. In FY 2005, 94 percent of the cases were appeals of compensation decisions by regional offices (Terry, 2006a).

The law requires BVA to decide cases on a "first come, first served" basis. To do that, BVA assigns cases a docket number in the order in which cases are received. A veteran may file a motion to advance the case if he or she believes that his or her appeal should be decided sooner than the appeals of others.

BVA decides cases *de novo* (that is, it makes an entirely new decision, rather than reviewing the prior decision), so it gives no deference to the regional office decision being appealed. Decisions are based only on the law, VA's regulations, precedent decisions of the courts, and precedent opinions of VA's general counsel. BVA performs an analysis of credibility and probative value of evidence and considers all potentially applicable provisions of law and regulations. Final decisions must include

- findings of fact;
- conclusions of law;
- analysis of the reasons and bases for the decision on each material issue of fact and law; and
- an order granting or denying the appeal (Terry, 2006a).

BVA Organization and Staffing

BVA consists of a chairman, vice chairman, senior deputy vice chairman, 56 veterans law judges (VLJs), 4 of whom are deputy vice chairmen and 8 of whom are chief judges, 248 staff counsel, and other administrative and clerical staff (Terry, 2006a). Staff is organized into four decision teams with jurisdictions covering four geographical regions—the Northeast, Southeast, Midwest, and West (including the Philippines). Each decision team includes

- 1 deputy vice chairman;
- 2 chief judges;
- 11 VLJs;
- 2 senior counsel; and
- 60 counsel and associate counsel.

Each VLJ works with five to six attorneys (counsel and associate counsel) as a small team. The attorneys

> review the claims file, research the applicable law, and prepare a comprehensive draft decision or remand document that details the relevant law and evidence. The document and the claims folders are then forwarded to the assigned VLJ for review, approval, revision, and signature (Terry, 2006b).

When an appellant's docket number is reached, the file is prepared by staff and the decision approved by a VLJ. Each VLJ is expected to complete a minimum of 752 decisions per year as his or her "fair share" of BVA's total workload and conduct three one-week travel boards to regional offices. Counsel, who draft decisions, are asked to draft at least 156 decisions per year (Terry, 2006b).

BVA Workload

In FY 2006, BVA received 41,802 appeals and issued 39,076 decisions (BVA, 2006). These included 37,295 decisions on compensation cases, of which

- 20 percent involved a grant on at least one issue;
- 46 percent involved a denial of all issues;
- 32 percent involved a remand to the agency of original jurisdiction, meaning the regional office; and
- 2 percent were classified as "other" (BVA, 2006).

Sources of Medical Expertise in BVA

Prior to passage of the Veterans Judicial Review Act of 1988, BVA had always used expert panels to adjudicate claims. Each three-person section of BVA had a physician member "whose medical judgment often controlled the outcome of an appeal" (BVA, 1996b:32).[16] BVA physician members acted as adjudicators and as providers of expert advice and medical opinions, and they also helped train BVA's attorneys (BVA, 1996b).

The 1988 act changed BVA from functioning as a panel of experts to one in which independent judges weigh and consider only the evidence of record. A subsequent series of opinions by the CAVC barred BVA physicians from acting as adjudicators:

> In the cases of *Gilbert v. Derwinski*, *Colvin v. Derwinski*, and *Hatlestad v. Derwinski*, the Court held, in essence, that the Board could no longer base its decisions on its own medical expertise, including that of physicians then serving as Board members (BVA, 1996a:18).

Since then, all board members have been lawyers, although there is no requirement that they be lawyers.

In response to the court decisions, BVA converted some of its physicians (two full-time and three part-time) from board members to advisors who provided expert medical opinions on the record when needed to adjudicate a case. They also provided informal advice to attorneys and VLJs, gave educational lectures on medical topics, and reviewed requests for VHA and outside medical advisory opinions "to ensure accuracy in the way in which the evidence is reported and the questions are framed" (BVA, 1997:14). However, using BVA physicians to provide expert opinions was soon barred by court decisions that questioned the fairness and impartiality of BVA's

[16]The three-person panels with a physician member reflected the composition of the rating boards at regional offices at that time (BVA, 1994).

own medical advisers (BVA, 2001).[17] Because BVA cannot use its own expertise to "fill in the blanks," it is very reliant on adequate development of medical evidence in the case by the regional office to render a decision, according to BVA's chairman. It also increases the time BVA attorneys need to analyze the medical evidence in the record, conduct research, and explain the medical principles on which their decisions rely, including citations of independent authority, such as medical treatises, texts, journals, and epidemiological studies (Terry, 2006a).

Currently BVA has a single medical advisor position, filled by a physician:

> The medical advisor's duties are to review draft outside medical opinions for the purpose of advising the originating VLJ as to the proper medical specialist to address the opinion request and whether the questions posed are adequate to elicit a meaningful response from that specialist.
>
> The Medical Advisor also provides training on medical issues to the Board's VLJs and staff counsel. Additionally, he is available to consult with staff counsel and VLJs to read medical records and provide background information and training on medical issues encountered in review of particular claims. He is not involved in the adjudication of the appeal (Keller, 2007).

BVA also began to obtain expert medical advice from VHA clinicians and, occasionally, the Armed Forces Institute of Pathology (AFIP). It also used its authority to obtain advisory medical opinions from independent experts more frequently:

> In an effort to alleviate the need for BVA to remand cases for additional medical information, we established a VHA medical opinion program. The board maintains a list of participating hospitals and their specialty, if any. When a case requires a medical opinion, a hospital is selected according to the particular need, and a specialist prepares an opinion answering the board's questions. This program cuts the cost and time—sometimes six to nine months—to obtain an independent outside medical opinion (VA, 2000:29).

In FY 2006, for example, BVA requested 643 outside medical opinions (464 from VHA, 4 from AFIP, and 175 from independent medical examiners). This was more than was requested from those sources in 2004 and 2005 (560 and 513, respectively).[18]

---

[17]See *Austin* v. *Brown*, 6 Vet. App. 547 (1994); *Williams* v. *Brown*, 8 Vet. App. 133 (1995); and *Perry* v. *Brown*, 9 Vet. App. 2 (1996).

[18]From Veterans Appeals Control and Locator System data provided by BVA for FY 2004–FY 2006. Previously, it requested between 200 and 500 outside medical opinions a year, according to annual reports of the chairman of BVA.

Medical opinions are generally sought for establishing medical nexus, differential diagnosis, unusual or complex issues, and legal issues, such as injury of the veteran being examined by VHA. Medical opinion may be needed to establish service connection when a veteran's record

- contains competent evidence of current disability, or persistent or recurrent symptoms of disability;
- contains supporting evidence of an in-service event, injury, or disease, or presumptive disease or symptoms;
- indicates claimed disability symptoms may not be associated with service; or
- does not contain sufficient competent medical evidence to decide the claim (Terry, 2006a).

No specific formula exists to use in weighing medical opinions. BVA may favor the opinion of one competent medical expert over that of another when adequate reasons or bases are provided. Factors weighed include

- competency of the medical professional or medical evidence provided;
- use of the correct factual history;
- adequacy of supporting analysis or basis provided for opinion;
- consideration of a review of the claims file or a full history of the disability;
- whether the clinician is the veteran's treating physician and familiar with his or her medical records and history;
- level of thoroughness and detail of opinion;
- equivocality of the opinion;
- personal interest in the case on the part of the opinion provider;
- special qualifications or expertise of the opinion provider;
- contradictory or internally inconsistent statements;
- differentiation among multiple opinions based on rationale or analyses; and
- consideration of the benefit of doubt rule if there are multiple conflicting medical opinions (Terry, 2006a).

U.S. Court of Appeals for Veterans Claims

In the event that a claimant is dissatisfied with a final BVA appeals decision, he or she has several options:

- Accept the decision and take no further action, in which case the decision becomes final;

- Go back to the regional office and try to reopen the claim;
- File a motion for reconsideration or to vacate (i.e., an attempt to have the same court withdraw or modify its decision) with BVA;
- Ask for a rereview of the case because there was a clear and unmistakable error in the BVA decision; or
- File an appeal with the U.S. Court of Appeals for Veterans Claims.

If BVA denies requested benefits, or it grants less than the maximum benefit available under the law, and the veteran decides to appeal to the CAVC, he or she must file the appeal within 120 days after BVA mailed its decision. Unlike BVA, the court may not receive new evidence. It considers only

- the BVA decision;
- briefs submitted by the veteran and VA;
- oral arguments, if any; and
- the case record that VA considered and BVA had available.

In cases decided on merit (cases not dismissed on procedural grounds), the court may (1) reverse the BVA decision (i.e., grant contested benefits); (2) affirm the BVA decision (i.e., deny contested benefits); or (3) remand the case back to BVA for rework.

U.S. Court of Appeals for the Federal Circuit and the U.S. Supreme Court

Under certain circumstances, a veteran who disagrees with a decision of the CAVC may appeal to the Federal Circuit Court of Appeals and then to the U.S. Supreme Court.

The court reviews the same record that was considered by BVA; that is, the court does not receive new evidence nor does it hold a trial. Appellants themselves or their lawyers or approved agents may serve as representatives before the court; however, the court directs whether oral argument is held. Either party may appeal a decision made by the CAVC to the Federal Circuit Court of Appeals, and may seek further review in the U.S. Supreme Court.

BVA Quality Assurance and Training

BVA's Office of Quality Review, headed by the senior deputy vice chairman, oversees a formal quality review (QR) program. The quantitative program began in 1998 with the collection of baseline data, and an ongoing QR process started at the beginning of 1999. Staffing of the QR unit was increased and the positions made permanent in 2002, including a permanent full-time training coordinator position.

The program reviews every 20th original VLJ decision and every 10th VLJ decision on cases remanded by the CAVC to BVA. This sample size, chosen to achieve a confidence level of 95 percent with a margin of error ±5 percent, is reviewed on an ongoing basis. The review evaluates decisions in five areas:

- identification of issues;
- findings of fact;
- conclusions of law;
- reasons and bases for decisions; and
- due process.

A deficiency or error in any of the five areas constitutes a failure. The standard is whether a deficiency or error exists that would be expected to result in a reversal by or remand from the CAVC or a change in the outcome (Terry, 2006a).[19]

The results of the QR program are the basis for training activities:

- quarterly "Grand Rounds" training sessions for all VLJs and staff counsel to stay current with changes in the law;
- training on specific legal issues, conducted by the full-time training coordinator, usually twice a month;
- periodic "Quality Review Tips," provided to legal staff;
- detailed monthly QR statistics for managers;
- referral of QR errors back to the originating VLJ; and
- a variety of team-level mentoring and training programs and online indexes and legal research tools for staff (Terry, 2006a).

Medical training occurs on an ongoing basis, and the BVA medical advisor is available for consultation and informal training. BVA training sessions held during the past two years on medical and legal topics involving medical matters included

- introduction to medical terminology;
- secondary service connection/Allen cases;
- presumption of service connection and applying rating criteria when there has been a change in the law;

[19]This standard was adopted in 2002 after the Government Accountability Office (GAO) suggested it; previously, non-substantive errors, such as using the wrong format, were counted against the accuracy rate (GAO, 2002a, 2005c).

- radiation claims;
- presumption of soundness;
- POW claims adjudication and medical matters;
- Agent Orange/herbicide exposure;
- rating spine disabilities;
- education and vocational rehabilitation;
- rating musculoskeletal disabilities—functional limitation and pain (*DeLuca* criteria);
- rating disabilities involving injuries to multiple muscle groups (gunshot and shrapnel wounds);
- multiple opinions—assigning credibility and weight of the evidence when reviewing;
- special monthly compensation and adaptive equipment;
- respiratory disorders;
- rating knee disabilities;
- total disability ratings based on individual unemployability; and
- hearing loss and tinnitus.

DISABILITY CLAIMS PROCESS ISSUES: TIMELINESS, ACCURACY, AND CONSISTENCY

Veterans deserve a claims process that is efficient and fair. They should not have to wait long for decisions on disability compensation and other benefits. The decisions should accurately determine eligibility to minimize the number of false negatives (veterans incorrectly denied benefits) and false positives (veterans granted benefits for which they are not eligible). Veterans with similar levels of disability should be treated the same even if they are dealing with different regional offices. And if they appeal, they should receive an accurate decision within a reasonable amount of time.

The VA claims process has long struggled with timeliness, accuracy, and consistency. The importance of adequate medical examinations in achieving timeliness, accuracy, and consistency has been recognized since the early 1990s. But, the most important factor affecting VA's ability to produce timely, accurate, and consistent decisions is the disability claim workload.

Medical Examination Quality

In 1996, BVA reported that about 70 percent of the cases remanded by BVA to the regional offices included a request for a C&P examination to obtain incomplete or missing medical information (BVA, 1996b). This followed a 1994 VA inspector general's report critical of C&P medical examinations services, and VBA and VHA were already working to improve the adequacy of medical examinations (VA, 1994). The VA Office of Inspector

General (OIG) reported that 24 percent (95,000 of 405,000) of the C&P examinations had been incomplete in FY 1993, a percentage that had not improved much in FY 1996, when 22 percent were incomplete (VA, 1997b). A C&P examination task force, on which BVA was represented, led to a 2001 memorandum of agreement between VBA and VHA on C&P examination standards and procedures to improve quality, expedite decisions, and reduce remands. The memorandum also established the CPEP program.

CPEP has monitored the quality of C&P examinations performed by VHA clinicians on a monthly basis since October 2003. Earlier, CPEP had identified the 10 most commonly requested C&P examinations and developed quality indicators, some applying to all examinations, some specific to each examination. The indicators were used to assess 110 randomly selected examinations of each type that had been performed in the last quarter of FY 2001. The resulting quality indicator score was 85 percent, but it varied across examination types from 72 percent for joint examinations to 94 percent for mental disorder examinations (VA, 2002c). Overall, 59 percent of the examinations scored 90 percent or better (met or exceeded 90 percent of the quality indicators) and 37 percent scored 100 percent. Most of the errors were omissions of specific data elements, whereas some were omissions of entire worksheets (Brown, 2003). CPEP then analyzed examinations by using the Veterans Integrated Service Network (VISN), finding differences in the percentage of A-level examinations, defined as those that meet 90 percent or more of the quality indicators, which are discussed in the next section, on "consistency." As a group, the percentage of A-level examination in this first, baseline study was 53.5 percent (Brown, 2006b).

Since 2001, CPEP has led a number of initiatives to improve the percentage of A-level examinations. The initiatives include onsite training sessions, video and computer-based training on the examinations, establishment of the percentage of A-level examinations as a performance goal for the directors of each VISN, and the development of online examination templates with structured data input. In 2006, CPEP was directed to establish a training and certification program for C&P examiners, which is currently under development. Web-based training modules have been developed for some body systems (musculoskeletal, mental, PTSD). Certification tests are in final testing, and audio and eye training modules are next to be developed (Brown, 2007). Deployment of the training and certification program is scheduled for FY 2008.[20]

In FY 2004 and FY 2005, the VISN performance target for A-level examinations was 64 percent. The average score across VISNs was 82 per-

[20]An executive directive describing roles and responsibilities for the certification process was prepared and was undergoing review by VA unions at the time this report was prepared (Brown, 2007).

cent in February 2006, compared with 77 percent in February 2005 and 58 percent in February 2004. All 21 VISNs met the performance target for A-level exams in September 2005, up from 18 in September 2004 (up from 1 in October 2003) (Brown, 2006b). When the target for A-level exams was increased from 64 percent to 83 percent for FY 2006, the number of VISNs meeting the target initially dropped to 9 but improved to 21 in December 2006. The average score across VISNs was 86 percent in January 2007, although the consistently high scoring audio examination had been replaced by the lower scoring diabetes examination among the 10 examinations being scored in October 2006 (Table 5-2) (Brown, 2007). Accuracy of examination reports is a performance measure for VISN directors (VA, 2006d).

CPEP randomly samples 1,470 examination reports each month—7 reports from each of the 10 examination types from each of the 21 VISNs. The sample size is set to produce statistically valid error rates for each VISN on a quarterly basis (VA, 2006d).

CPEP is also addressing the adequacy of regional office requests for C&P examinations. It has been conducting monthly reviews of these requests since early 2004, finding that many were incomplete or inaccurate, as noted in a 2005 GAO report:

> For example, of the spine exams requested during the second quarter of fiscal year 2005, 32 percent of the exam requests had at least one error such as:
>
> - not identifying the pertinent condition;
> - not requesting the appropriate exam;

TABLE 5-2 Rates of A-Level Compensation and Pensions Examinations, by Type of Examination, January 2007

	Examination Type	Percent of A-Level Exams
1	Initial PTSD	97
2	Eye	95
3	Mental disorders	94
4	Diabetes	89
5	General medical	88
6	Skin	85
7	Review PTSD	82
8	Feet	79
9	Joints	78
10	Spine	71
	All 10 examinations	86

SOURCE: Brown (2007).

- not providing clear or useful information in the remarks section of the request;
- not identifying the specific joint or part to be examined; or
- not explaining instances in which the exam request contained no telephone number for the veteran who was to be examined (GAO, 2005b).

In August 2005, CPEP revised the set of indicators of examination request quality to focus on content accuracy and exclude non-substantive process errors. It planned to track them for six months to establish a baseline, then provide the regional offices with the results (Mansfield, 2005).

Disability Claims Workload and Timeliness

In FY 2006, VA received 806,000 disability-related claims. Most of these (654,000) were from veterans for compensation for service-connected injuries and diseases.[21] Compared with the FY 2000 workload, this was a 38 percent increase in disability-related claims and a 56 percent increase in compensation claims (VA, 2006). In addition, the number of claims involving eight or more issues (i.e., medical conditions), each of which must be evaluated separately, has more than doubled, from about 21,000 (20 percent of the original claims) in 2000 to about 51,000 (22 percent of original claims) in 2006 (Figure 5-1). This means that the number of rating decisions that must be made was a multiple of the 654,000 disability compensation claims filed in FY 2006.

VBA has been unable to track total number of issues adjudicated until recently, with the advent of the current tracking system, RBA 2000. According to data provided to the committee by VBA, adjudicators made more than 1.8 million rating decisions on compensation for disabilities during calendar year 2006, while adjudicating 628,000 disability compensation claims, indicating that the average number of issues (disabilities) per claim was just under three.

As the annual number of rating-related claims filed has increased, so have the number of decisions on rating-related claims (Figure 5-2).

However, new claim receipts continue to exceed case dispositions, resulting in an increasing backlog of pending claims. Nearly 380,000 rating-related claims were pending at the end of FY 2006, compared with 228,000 at the end of FY 2000 (Figure 5-3).

From the point of view of the veteran, the average length of time a claim is pending action by a regional office has been about four months in recent years (down from six months in FY 2001–FY 2002). Subsequent

---

[21]The other disability-related claims were for disability pension, dependency and indemnity compensation for survivors, hospitalization reviews, and future examination reviews.

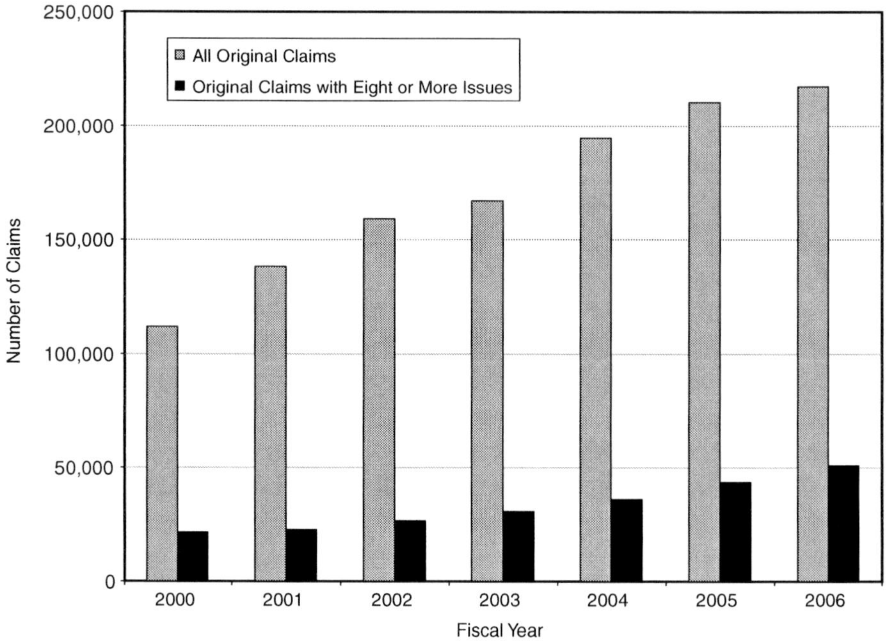

FIGURE 5-1 Number of original compensation claims from veterans and number of original compensation claims from veterans containing eight or more issues, end of fiscal years 2000–2006.
SOURCE: VA (2007b:6B-7, 6B-18).

processing by the regional office has averaged just under six months since FY 2000, except in FY 2002, when it was eight months (GAO, 2007). Accordingly, a veteran can expect to wait an average of about 10 months to receive a decision on his or her claim. This is two and one-half months more than the time period VA is trying to achieve. VA's current performance target for average days pending of rating-related actions on compensation claims is 100 days. Its target to process rating-related claims is 125 days on average (VA, 2007b:6B-24).

In 1993, the deputy under secretary for benefits appointed a blue ribbon panel on claims processing to find ways to decide disability decisions more quickly. GAO issued a series of reports on problems with claims processing at VA between 1992 and 1996. VA's Office of Inspector General also issued a series of reports on claims timeliness and accuracy during the

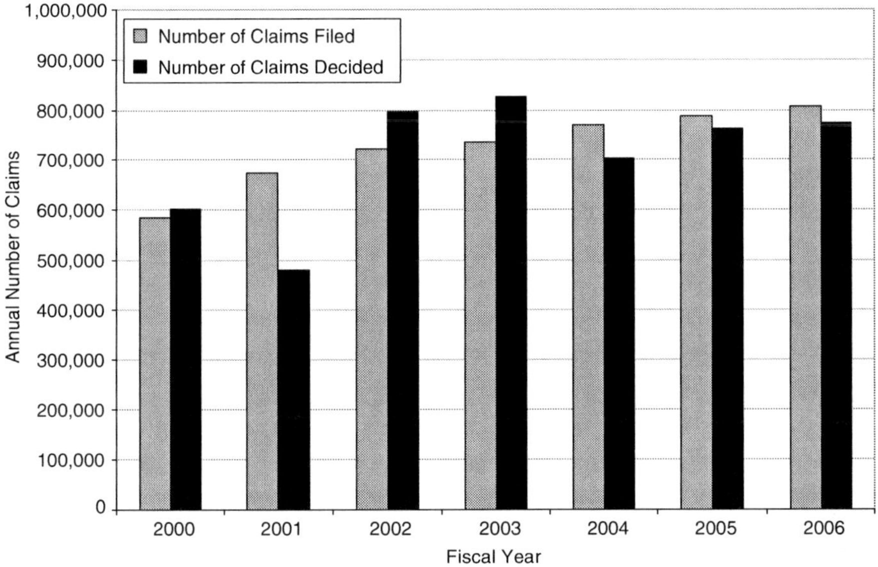

FIGURE 5-2 Number of rating-related claims filed and decided, FY 2000–FY 2006.
SOURCES: VA (2000, 2001a, 2002b, 2003, 2004c, 2005c, 2006a, 2007b).

1990s.[22] Congress established the Veterans' Claims Adjudication Commission, which reported in 1996, and the Senate Appropriations Committee mandated a study of VBA by the National Academy of Public Administration (NAPA), which reported in 1997.[23]

VBA regional offices were reorganized along case management lines, to ensure that someone was accountable for each case as it went through the decision-making process, and a major effort to improve the timeliness and quality of C&P examinations was launched (discussed earlier). Implementation of the case management model reduced production in the short run, however, while the number of claims increased substantially because of legislation (e.g., VCAA of 2000), court decisions, and regulatory changes (e.g., VA decision to make diabetes mellitus presumptive for Vietnam vet-

[22]VA's Office of Inspector General summary report reviews the recommendations of the blue ribbon panel, GAO, OIG, Veterans' Claims Adjudication Commission, and National Academy of Public Administration (VA, 1997a).

[23]During the same time period, there were similar studies of claims decision-making timeliness at BVA.

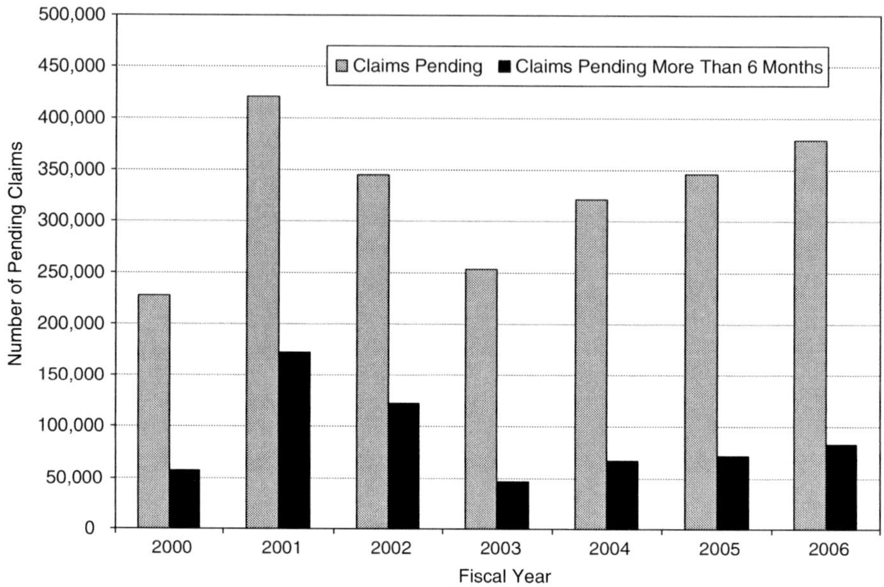

FIGURE 5-3 Number of rating-related claims pending and number pending more than six months, end of FY 2000–FY 2006.
SOURCES: VA (2000, 2001a, 2002b, 2003, 2004c, 2005c, 2006a, 2007b).

erans and to expand the list of radiation-related diseases with presumptive service connection).[24]

In 2001, the VA secretary appointed the Claims Processing Task Force. The task force not only recommended the major changes in the organization of the field offices described earlier (i.e., establishment of veterans service centers with staff units specializing in different parts of the claims process), but also a number of other steps to reduce the backlog of pending claims. These included

- creation of "tiger teams" in the Cleveland regional office and establishment of nine resource centers to focus on processing cases of claimants over age 70, and then claims older than a year;
- establishment of appeals claims processing teams in all regional offices;
- faster record recovery from the VA Records Management Center;
- better training;

[24]Additional factors slowing production were the time needed for staff to learn RBA 2000 and for training a substantial number of new VSC staff (GAO, 2002b).

- updated performance standards for VSRs, RVSRs, DROs, and regional office directors;
- consolidation of pension maintenance processing in three centers;
- temporary shifting of staff from the Education Service to work on compensation claims; and
- shifting of cases among regional offices to even out the workload.

VBA succeeded in substantially reducing the backlog by the end of FY 2003; after that, however, it began to climb again. The number of pending cases increased from 254,000 to 378,000 at the end of FY 2006, the number of cases pending more than 6 months increased from 47,000 to 83,000 (Figures 5-3), and the average number of days a case was pending increased from 111 to 127 (VA, 2006a).

VA points to several trends that affect the disability claims workload in terms of the number of claims and effort required to evaluate them. These include a larger share of claims with eight or more issues, more reopened claims submitted by veterans with chronic progressive conditions, additional claims submitted by the aging veteran population, and the claims submitted by veterans of Operation Iraqi Freedom (OIF) in Iraq and Operation Enduring Freedom (OEF) in and around Afghanistan.

In addition to the increasing number of disabilities claimed, VA reports that the nature of the disabilities has become more complex. VA cites PTSD, complex combat injuries, diabetes and related conditions, and environmental diseases as examples (VA, 2007b).

Another factor in timeliness is the adequacy of VA's capacity to process the claims. In its FY 2008 budget submission, VA is asking for 475 more FTEs for direct compensation work in FY 2008 than in FY 2006, because "current staffing levels do not enable VA to reduce the pending claims inventory and provide timely service to veterans" (VA, 2007b:6B-4).[25]

Cases remanded by BVA also add to the workload and increase claim processing time. The inventory of remanded cases was 21,200 at the end of FY 2006 (VA, 2007b). Remands are discussed more fully below.

Appeal Workload and Timeliness

As discussed earlier, veterans dissatisfied with the decision made by the regional office may file an appeal by submitting an NOD contesting the denial of service connection, rating level given, or effective date of the grant. According to BVA, the appeal rate on disability determinations has historically been about 7 percent. More recently that rate has climbed from about

---

[25]VA had 6,407 staff for direct work on compensation in FY 2006; it has 6,425 in FY 2007, and is asking for 6,882 in FY 2008.

11 to 14 percent. In FY 2006, the appeal rate was about 13 percent—down from a high of 16 percent in FY 2004, but still well above historical averages. During the same period, the rate of formal appeals (based on number of VA Form 9s filed after the veteran receives the statement of the case from VBA) was 6 percent in FY 2006, down from 7 percent in FY 2004, but more than double the rate in FY 2002 (Figure 5-4).

As a result of this increasing workload, BVA has struggled to process appeals within a reasonable time period. The annual number of NODs, the first step in the appeal process, nearly doubled from FY 2000 to FY 2003, from 60,000 to 115,000. This increase was caused in part by the increased number of cases decided that *could* be appealed, but it is also caused by the greater propensity of veterans to appeal.[26] The number of NODs has decreased since FY 2003, but was still 101,000 in FY 2006 (Figure 5-5). If current trends hold, VA is expecting between 90,000 and 110,000 appeals (NODs) a year in FY 2007 and FY 2008 (VA, 2007b:6B-14).

Many NODs are resolved by the regional office or when the veteran does not pursue the appeal, but the number of formal appeals was still higher in FY 2006 than in FY 2000. Veterans filed 46,100 formal appeals in FY 2006 by submitting VA Form 9, compared with 32,600 formal appeals in FY 2000. The annual number of BVA decisions, however, has not increased. As a result, the number of cases pending at BVA at the end of FY 2006—40,265—was almost double the number at the end of FY 2000. This does not include the substantial number of appeals being worked on by the appeals teams in regional offices and the Appeals Management Center, which was established by VBA in 2003 to consolidate expertise in processing remands from BVA (Figure 5-6).

The average number of days it took to resolve appeals, either by VBA or BVA, was 657 in FY 2006. This continued a steady increase since FY 2003, but was an improvement from the 731 days it took in FY 2002 (Figure 5-7).

Most appeals (72 percent in FY 2006) are resolved without a hearing before BVA. In FY 2006, 22,000 cases were resolved at the field office level after the NOD was received but before a formal appeal was filed on VA Form 9. In 42,200 cases, the veteran decided not to appeal further after reading the field office's statement of the case. Another 11,000 were resolved at the field office level after VA Form 9 was submitted. That left 29,000 appeals, of which BVA resolved 25,000 and remanded 4,000 to the field offices for further development (VA, 2007b:6B-15).

BVA decided 39,100 cases involving disability compensation specifically in FY 2006. It upheld the field office denials 46 percent of the time,

[26]The rate of NODs as a percentage of claims decided by VBA was 10 percent in FY 2000, 15.5 percent in FY 2004, and 13.1 percent in FY 2006.

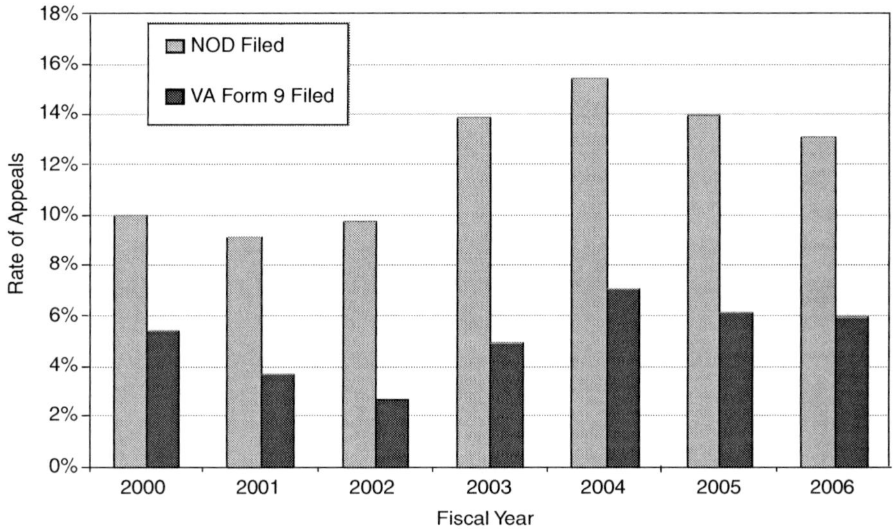

FIGURE 5-4 Rate of appeals (NODs), FY 2000–FY 2006.
SOURCES: BVA (2000b, 2001, 2002b, 2003, 2004, 2005, 2006), number of NODs; and VA (2000, 2001a, 2002b, 2003, 2004c, 2005c, 2006a), number of C&P claims decided.

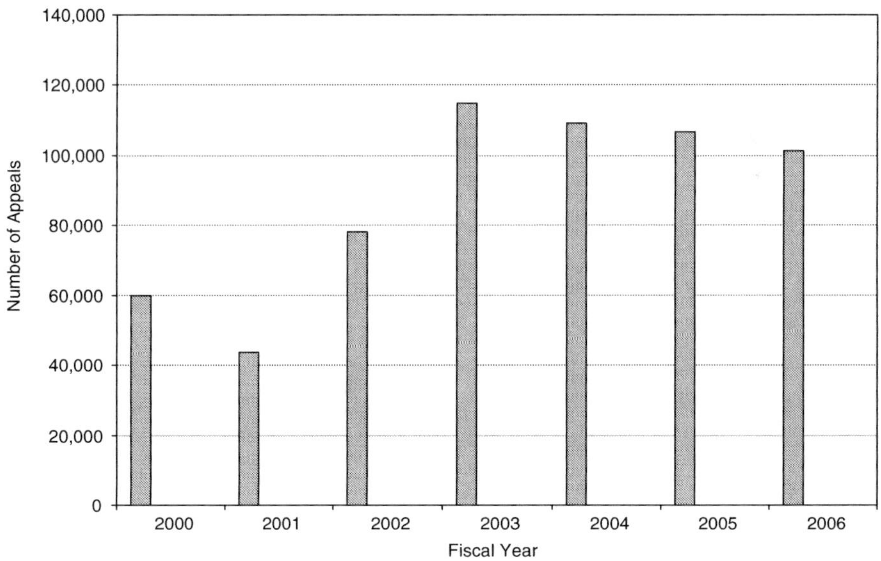

FIGURE 5-5 Number of appeals (NODs), FY 2000–FY 2006.
SOURCES: BVA (2003, 2006).

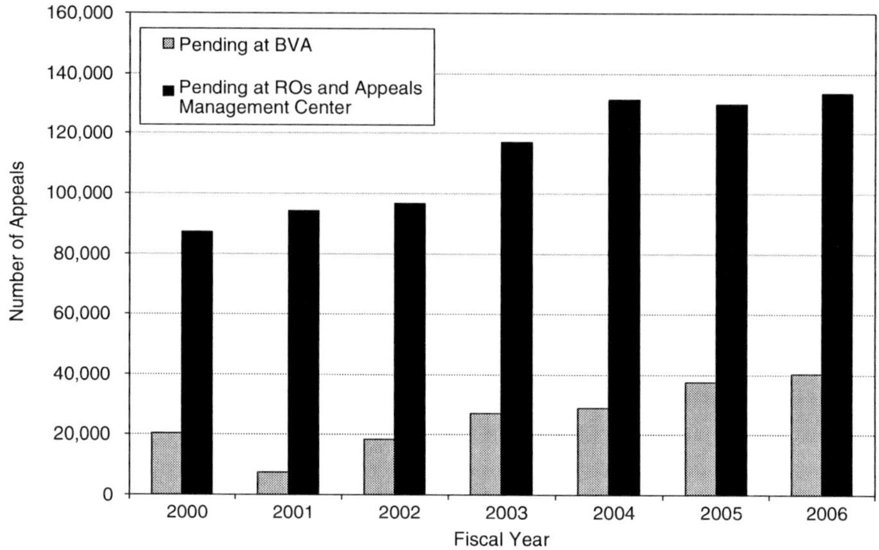

FIGURE 5-6 Number of appeals pending at BVA and at regional offices and the Appeals Management Center, FY 2000–FY 2006.
SOURCES: BVA (2001, 2003, 2004, 2006), cases ending at BVA; and VA (2007c), total appeals requiring adjudication.

reversed the field office decision on one or more of the issues 20 percent of the time, and remanded the case to the originating field office 32 percent of the time for further development of one or more issues (VA, 2006a:19).

The number of appeals to the CAVC averaged between 2,000 and 2,500 a year before FY 2005, when it jumped to 3,500 (Figure 5-8). The court received 3,700 appeals in FY 2006. It affirmed the BVA decision in full or in part in 11 percent of the cases in FY 2004, 16 percent in FY 2005, and 25 percent in FY 2006. During the same three years, the same court reversed the BVA decision or remanded the case for further development 50–60 percent of the time (U.S. Court of Appeals for Veterans Claims, 2006).[27]

There were 382 appeals to the federal circuit court in FY 2006, the highest since FY 2002, when 410 appeals were filed (Figure 5-8).

[27]Another 25–35 percent were dismissed on procedural grounds.

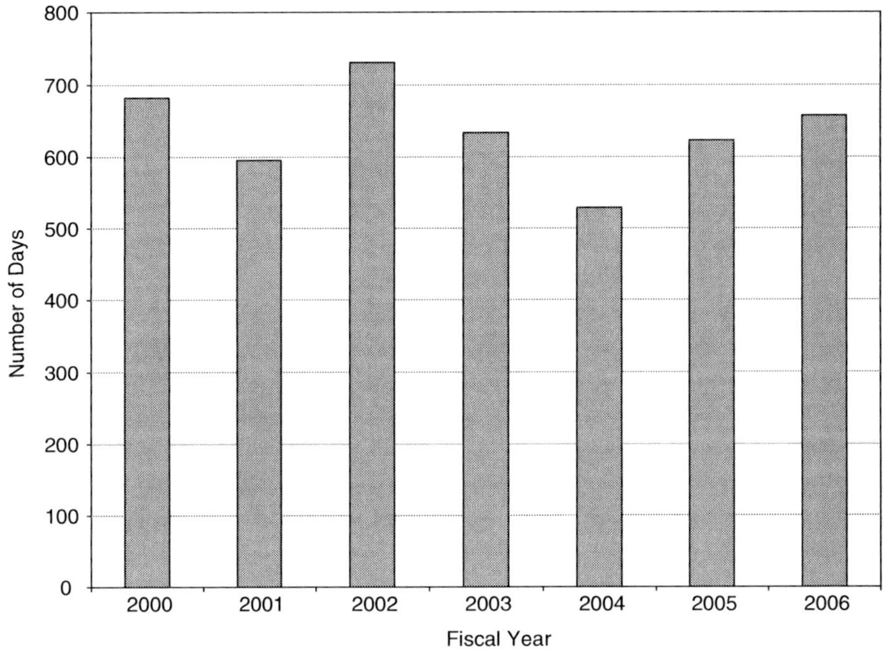

FIGURE 5-7 Average number of days to resolve appeals (i.e., appeals resolution time), FY 2000–FY 2006.
NOTE: Appeals resolution time is a joint BVA-VBA measure of time from receipt of an NOD by VBA to a final decision by VBA or BVA. Remands are not considered to be final decisions in this measure. Also not included are cases returned as a result of a remand by the CAVC.
SOURCES: VA (2000, 2001a, 2002b, 2003, 2004c, 2005c, 2006a).

Remands and Timeliness

Remands are of concern because not only do they increase the time it takes for a decision on the individual veteran's claim by at least a year, but they also increase the overall workload and slow the resolution of appeals of other veterans (VA, 2000:29). By law, BVA must decide on appeals in the order in which they were entered on the docket. If BVA remands a case to the regional office, and that case is subsequently returned to BVA for a decision, which happens about 75 percent of the time (Terry, 2006b), the returned case takes precedence over appeals currently before BVA. During FY 2006, BVA remanded 32 percent (12,500) of the cases it decided. At the end of FY 2006, 16 percent (21,200 of 133,600) of the rating-related claims pending at regional offices and the VBA Appeals Management Cen-

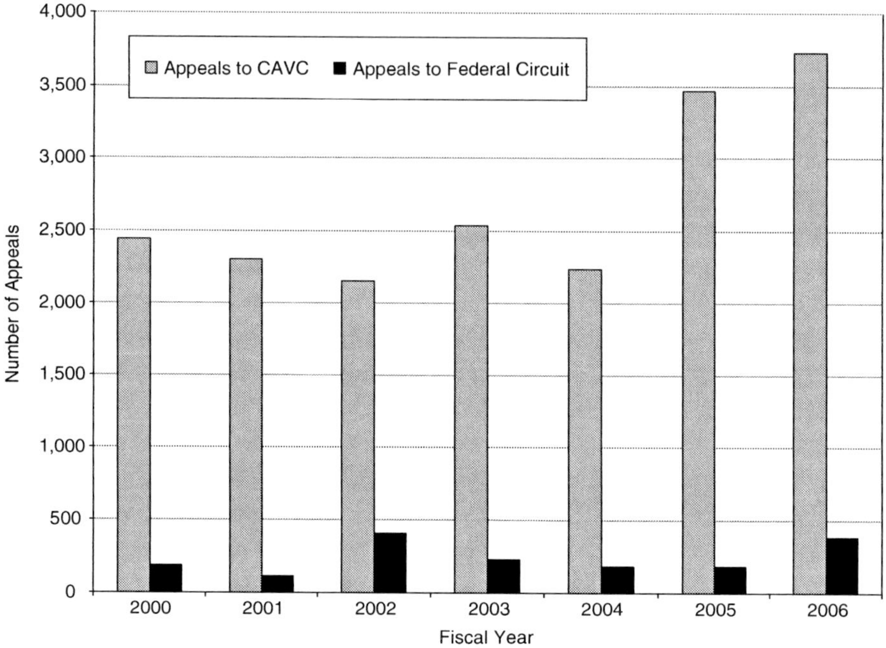

FIGURE 5-8 Annual number of appeals of BVA disability decisions to the courts, FY 2000–FY 2006.
SOURCE: U.S. Court of Appeals for Veterans Claims (2006).

ter were remands. If, as expected, 75 percent of the remands are returned to BVA after further development, they will constitute 30–40 percent of the 35,000–40,000 cases decided by BVA each year (in FY 2006, for example, BVA received 14,400 remands returned by the Appeals Management Center and regional offices for decision, equal to 37 percent of BVA decisions that year) (VA, 2007a:7C-4).

The percentage of BVA dispositions remanded jumped from 30 percent in FY 2000 to 49 percent in FY 2001. In 2002, in response to a recommendation of the 2001 Claims Processing Task Force, BVA established an evidence development unit to develop evidence needed to make a final decision or correct a procedural error in cases that otherwise would have to be remanded. The remand rate fell to about 15 percent "within a matter of months" (BVA, 2004:2).

When evidence development by BVA was barred by the CAVC, VBA created the Appeals Management Center in July 2003 to specialize in developing the cases that have been remanded by BVA and to review regional office decisions (U.S. Congress, House of Representatives, Committee on Veterans' Affairs, 2005d).

The remand rate began to increase again, from 19 percent in FY 2002 to 43 percent the next year to 57 percent in FY 2004. In 2004, the VA deputy secretary charged the under secretary for benefits and the chairman of BVA with developing a comprehensive plan to reduce the number of avoidable remands. As part of that effort, a joint working group analyzed a representative sample of explanations for past remands and began to track them prospectively. The reasons given were separated into "before certification" and "after certification," on the grounds that the causes of avoidable remands that happened before they were certified and transferred by regional offices to BVA should be in the control of, and therefore could be prevented by, regional offices. The initial analysis of 200 remand cases identified 379 precertification reasons for the remands. About a quarter of these (99) were for deficiencies involving C&P medical examinations and opinions; 9 percent (34) were for lack of an initial request for service medical records, VA medical records, or private medical records; and 6 percent (24) were for lack of an additional request for VA medical records or private medical records. Deficiencies in C&P examinations included lack of an examination, lack of a required medical opinion or an inadequate opinion, incomplete examination findings, and lack of current findings (VA, 2004a).

The remand rate dropped from 57 percent in FY 2004 to 32 percent in FY 2006 (BVA, 2006:20).[28] The number of remands involving precertification problems with C&P examinations and other medical evidence also fell (Figure 5-9). Missing and inadequate C&P examinations and opinions constituted a third of the remand reasons in all three years, and failures to obtain other medical records remained at about 19 percent of the remand reasons.

In addition to efforts by BVA and VBA to reduce avoidable remands, primarily by training, and to improve the adequacy of C&P examinations, BVA is trying to address the backlog of appeals by increasing productivity. These steps include

- having VLJs and counsel write shorter, more concise decisions;
- having VLJs draft some decisions;
- increasing the use of travel boards to decide cases and provide regional office training;
- expanding employee incentive, mentoring, and training programs;

[28]The absolute numbers of remands in FY 2004, FY 2005, and FY 2006 were 21,797, 13,179, and 12,487, respectively.

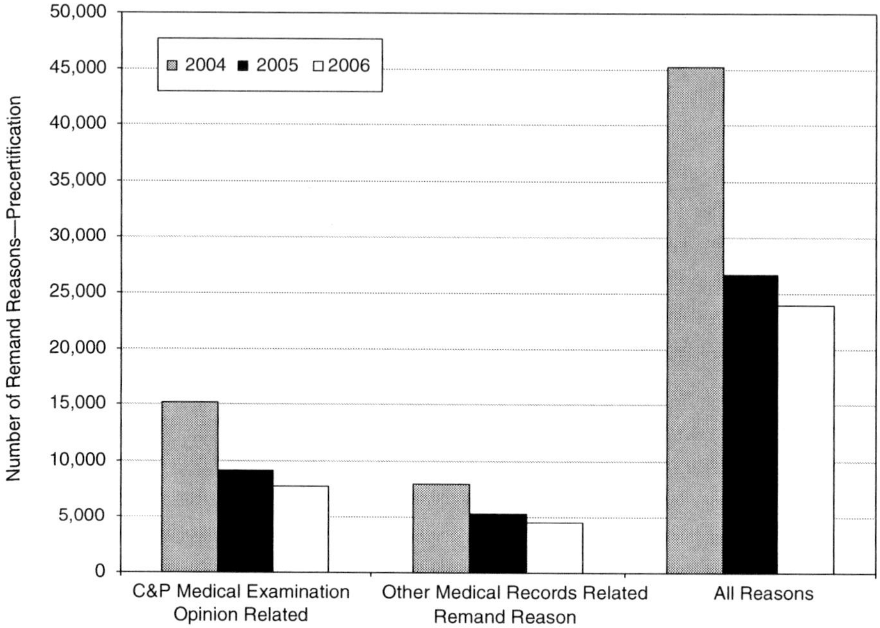

FIGURE 5-9 Number of remands by reason, FY 2004–FY 2006.
NOTE: Other medical records include military service, VA, and private medical records that should have been requested but were not, or if requested but not forthcoming, were not followed up. Nonmedical reasons for remands have to do with duty to notify (lack of, incorrect, or inadequate notices to appellants), duty to assist (not obtaining nonmedical service and other records), and due process (not following procedural rules).
SOURCE: Keller (2007).

- increasing paralegal assistance;
- increasing use of overtime;
- providing improved online legal and medical research tools; and
- focusing training on problems revealed through the quality assurance process (Terry, 2007).

Accuracy

VA has made accuracy of disability benefit decisions one of the key measures in its annual performance and accountability plans. As noted previously, VA has used the STAR process to measure technical accuracy since 1998. STAR review of a rating-related case determines if the benefit entitlement decision process addresses all issues claimed (including inferred issues), provides assistance in obtaining evidence as required by the Veterans Claims Assistance Act, and results in correct decisions, including correctness of the decision to grant or deny benefits, percentage rating, payment rate, and effective dates. If the adjudication of the case fails any of these standards, it is classified as incorrect in the accuracy rate calculation. STAR review also determines if there is adequate and correct decision documentation and proper notification of the decision, although these scores are not in the performance and accountability plan.

During the year ending May 31, 2006, VBA reviewed 6,458 rating cases and found the national benefit entitlement accuracy rate to be 88 percent and the decision documentation and notification rate to be 90 percent (VA, 2006a:172). The entitlement accuracy rate was less than 60 percent in FY 2000. It improved steadily to 87 percent in FY 2004, leveling off at approximately the same rate in FY 2005 (84 percent) and FY 2006 (88 percent) (Figure 5-10).

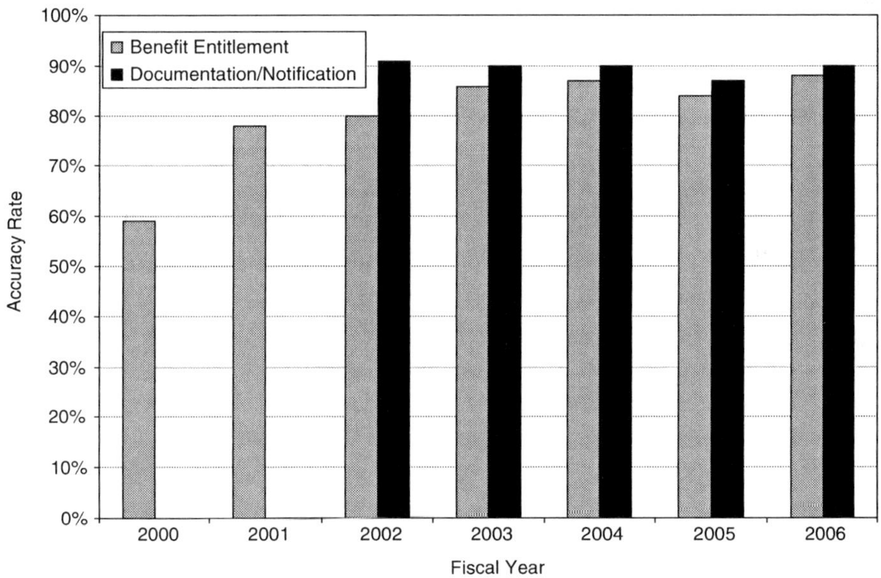

FIGURE 5-10 Accuracy of compensation and pension entitlement decisions, FY 2000–FY 2006.

NOTE: Documentation and notification were included in the entitlement accuracy rate until FY 2002. The 2001 Claims Processing Task Force recommended that VBA measure them separately so that the benefit entitlement accuracy rate would only include items that, if inadequate, could result in remand from BVA.

SOURCES: VA (2000, 2001a, 2002b, 2003, 2004c, 2005c, 2006a).

The STAR program began to determine annual accuracy rates for each regional office in FY 2002, which required a larger sample size and more staff (GAO, 2001). The original plan was to review approximately 10,000 cases annually in order to achieve a confidence level of 95 percent with a margin of error range of ±6 percent for best performing regional offices and ±9 percent for regional offices with the lowest performance rates. The actual number of cases reviewed has been less—6,458 in FY 2006. VBA randomly samples 120 rating cases per regional office each year, except it conducts 240 annual rating reviews for the four largest regional offices and the six regional offices with the lowest overall accuracy (VA, 2006d).

VBA requires regional offices to certify that appropriate action was taken on errors found in the STAR process. Offices with low accuracy rates are required to implement corrective action plans. Trends in error types are used to design national training programs and to identify needed regional office-specific training, which is offered during site visits (VA, 2007a).

Another indicator of accuracy problems is the percentage of initial decisions that are either reversed or remanded by BVA. In FY 2006, BVA reversed the initial regional office denial decision on at least one issue claimed by the appellant in 19 percent of cases and remanded another 32 percent of the cases, suggesting problems with just over half the cases reviewed. Although this is lower than the historical rate of about 60 percent, it still represents a substantial portion of the decisions (BVA, 2006).

BVA also has a quality assurance program that analyzes a sample of its own decisions to determine the percentage that have substantive or procedural deficiencies that would be expected to result in a reversal or a remand by the court. Deficiencies are identified in five areas: issues, findings of fact, conclusions of law, reasons and bases, and due process. BVA also uses the results to determine areas of training emphasis.

BVA's deficiency-free decision rate improved from 86 percent in FY 2000 to 93 percent in FY 2004. It fell to 89 percent in FY 2005, but increased again to 93 percent in FY 2006 (Figure 5-11).

Consistency

VA has only recently undertaken an effort to assess consistency of decision making across regional offices and adjudicators. It is not a new issue. In a 1997 report on VA claims processing (mentioned earlier), NAPA concluded that consistency would be difficult, at best, to achieve across 58 field offices.[29] NAPA recommended increasing consistency by reducing the number of regional offices. It also found that the quality assurance process did not address consistency:

[29]Currently, there are 57 regional offices.

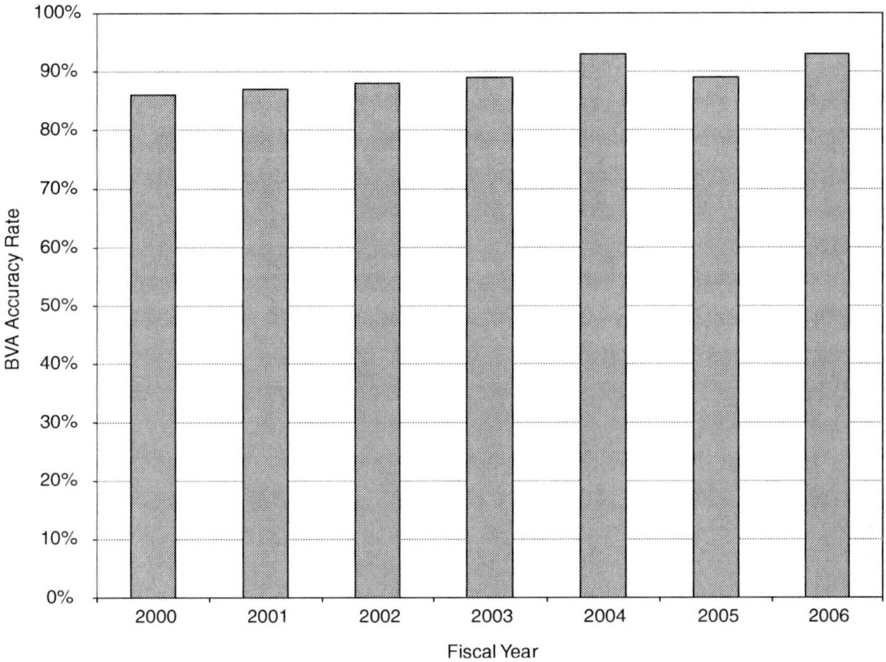

FIGURE 5-11 BVA accuracy rate, FY 2000–FY 2006.
NOTE: As recommended by the 2001 Claims Processing Task Force, BVA excluded deficiencies that would not be considered by the court, such as incorrect formatting, beginning in FY 2002.
SOURCES: VA (2003, 2006).

> There is no current measure of decision consistency within the system, and on data collected to inform management regarding to what extent consistency may be a problem. Given the differing types of medical issues and cases within the system which in many cases require subjectivity (such as psychiatric cases as compared with orthopedic cases), there is need to bound types of medical issues and the degree of subjectivity, set consistency standards, measure this as part of a QR process (or through blind testing of a control case by several regions), and accumulate data (NAPA, 1997:128).

The 2001 VA Claims Processing Task Force recommended that VBA evaluate and address inconsistencies among regional offices. The task force noted the large disparities in average compensation payments across states, differences in appeal rates and results of appeals in terms of reversal and remand rates from state to state, and lack of uniform guidance on interpretation of court decisions, any or all of which might indicate inconsistent decision making. GAO identified lack of consistency as a problem in a series of reports:

> Even though available evidence provides indications that variations in decision making may occur across all levels of VA adjudication, VA does not conduct systematic assessments to determine the degree of variation that occurs for specific impairments and to provide a basis for determining ways, if considered necessary, to reduce such variation (GAO, 2002a:2).
>
> VA's disability decision quality review program—known as Systematic Technical Accuracy Review (STAR)—assesses the overall accuracy of all disability decisions, but not the consistency of decisions overall or for specific impairments (GAO, 2005a:6).
>
> . . . variation is an inherent factor in the decision-making process. This makes it crucial that VA have a system for routinely identifying variations among its 57 regional offices so that such variations can be studied to determine if they are within the bounds of reasonableness and, if not, how to correct the problem. Also . . . VA must deal with issues involving not only its regional offices but also its 157 medical centers that conduct most of the disability examinations that regional offices rely on to provide the medical information they need to make disability decisions (GAO, 2006:2).

In 2005, VA's Office of Inspector General investigated the differences in average compensation payments from state to state, which ranged from $7,000 in Illinois to $12,000 in New Mexico in FY 2004 (VA, 2005b). The report also looked at the differences in the percentages of veterans receiving compensation across states, which ranged from 6.9 to 19.2 percent. The inspector general examined a number of explanations for the variation in payments besides inconsistencies in disability ratings among regional offices, including demographic differences (such as the percentage of veterans in a state's population, their period of service, and their average age) and process factors (such as percentage of claimants with representation, percentage of raters with more than two years of experience, and appeal rates). The inspector general could not analyze variations in grant rates, however, because VBA did not track them at that time. The report looked at correlations of explanatory factors with average payments one by one; a multivariate analysis was not done with average payment as the dependent variable or with other dependent variables of interest, such as percentage of veteran population receiving compensation or average combined rating degree. The report concluded that

> VBA should develop a comprehensive and systematic method for collecting data on factors impacting variance in payments that will enable VA to model the compensation claims process and predict outcomes. Such

information would help program managers evaluate issues such as variances in disability ratings or payment patterns (VA, 2005b:34).

In the course of the study, the inspector general collected information on state differences in the average number of service-connected disabilities per veteran, average combined degree of disability, average ratings for each of the 14 body systems, percentage of veterans service connected for PTSD, percentage of veterans with ratings of 100 percent and with individual unemployability, and STAR error rates, each of which shows substantial state-to-state variability. The average number of service-connected disabilities, for example, ranges from 2.1 to 3.4 across states. The average combined rating degree ranged from 33 to 45 percent across the states. The rate of service connection for PTSD also varies by state, ranging from 4.1 per thousand resident veterans to 25.5 per thousand resident veterans. The results for individual unemployability (IU) were similar to those for PTSD. The number of veterans service connected for IU ranged from 2.5 to 28.2 per thousand resident veterans in FY 2004. Overall STAR accuracy rates varied from 76 to 96 percent, while the median rate was 88 percent (see Figure 5-12).

BVA data for FY 2006 also shows wide geographical variation in appeal reversal and remand rates. Depending on the regional office from which cases originate, BVA remanded appeals between 22 and 65 percent of the time. Appeal allowance rates by region varied from 7 to 34 percent. BVA upheld the original denial in 63 percent of appeals from one office but in only 15 percent of appeals from another office (BVA, 2007).

Concerns with consistency are not limited to geographic variations. BVA's disposition of appeals also varies depending on the specific medical condition involved. Regional office decisions on some conditions are much more likely to be reversed or remanded on appeal than are others. Data for the first eight months of FY 2006 show that BVA was much more likely to either reverse (i.e., allow) or remand cases for individuals with certain medical conditions, and much more likely to deny cases for others. Table 5-3 lists the diagnostic codes present in cases that VLJs were most likely to reverse or remand, and those diagnostic codes present in cases that they were least likely to reverse or remand.[30]

Differences in judgment are inevitable in evaluating impairment and functional capacity, more for some conditions than others, depending on how subjective are the criteria; therefore, some degree of variation is inevitable. However, wide variation may be an indicator of inconsistent decision making. In addition, high reversal or remand rates may also indicate that the evaluation criteria are not as clear or appropriate as they should be.

[30]Medical conditions that occur infrequently are not included.

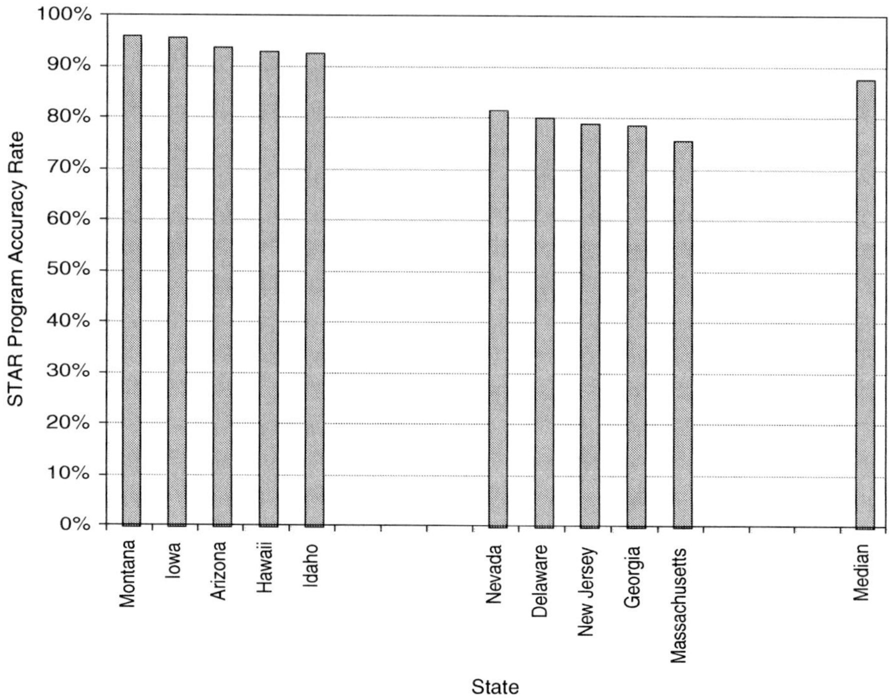

FIGURE 5-12 STAR program accuracy rates, 5 highest and 5 lowest states, FY 2004.
SOURCE: VA (2005b).

Another area of variability is C&P examination quality, which is critical to the accuracy of the rating process. Overall C&P examination quality was discussed earlier, but it also varies from region to region. For example, according to GAO, CPEP reported that only 78 percent of joint and spine examinations in FY 2004 included examiner discussions of pain now required due to the 1995 court case, *DeLuca* v. *Brown*. However, the extent to which examinations complied with these requirements varied considerably across VHA's 21 VISNs, ranging from 57 to 92 percent compliance (Figure 5-13) (GAO, 2005b).

In 1997, NAPA pointed out that the large number of regional offices was a source of inconsistency and inefficiency. In 1999, the Congressional Commission on Servicemembers and Veterans Transition Assistance suggested that consolidation of claims adjudication in fewer offices should be part of an effort to modernize VBA's benefits delivery processes (Congressional Commission, 1999). The 1991 Claims Processing Task Force

TABLE 5-3 Medical Conditions Most and Least Likely to Be Allowed or Remanded on Appeal by BVA (Minimum of 100 Appeals), October 1, 2005–May 31, 2006

Diagnostic Code	Issue	Number of Appeals	Number Allowed or Remanded	Percent Allowed or Remanded
5025	Fibromyalgia	122	75	61.5
9411	PTSD	3,796	2,245	59.1
5242	Degenerative arthritis of the spine	191	112	58.6
9203	Schizophrenia, paranoid type	234	134	57.3
5237	Lumbosacral or cervical strain	597	341	57.1
9434	Major depressive disorder	605	345	57.0
↓	↓	↓	↓	↓
6079	Partial blindness in one eye . . .	177	70	39.5
6099	Other eye disability	246	97	39.4
7305	Ulcer, duodenal	211	82	38.9
5024	Tenosynovitis	163	63	38.7
7338	Hernia, inguinal	159	51	32.1

NOTE: The percentages are of BVA dispositions and do not include disposition of appeals by VBA regional and other offices.
SOURCE: BVA Diagnostic Code Distribution Report, October 1, 2005–May 31, 2006.

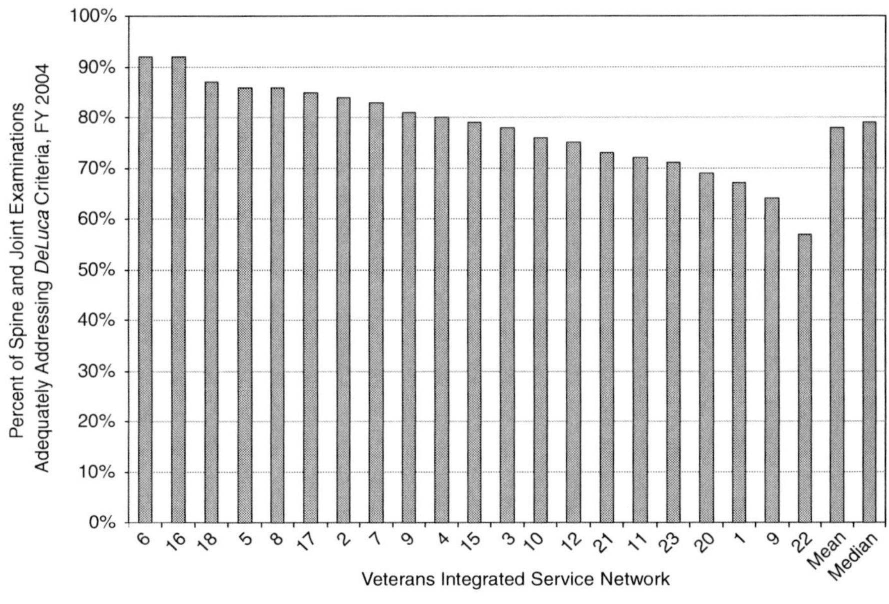

FIGURE 5-13 Percentage of spine and joint examinations adequately addressing *DeLuca* criteria, by VISN, FY 2004.
SOURCE: GAO (2005b).

reported that apparent inconsistencies in claims decisions from state to state should be addressed.

In 1995, a VBA task force on field office restructuring recommended some consolidations of compensation and pension functions, citing the following advantages:

- allowing VBA to assign the most experienced and productive adjudication officers and directors to the consolidated offices;
- facilitating increased specialization and as-needed expert consultation in deciding complex cases;
- improving the completeness of claims development, the accuracy and consistency of rating decisions, and the clarity of decision explanations;
- improving overall adjudication quality by increasing the pool of experience and expertise in critical technical areas; and
- facilitating consistency in decision making through fewer consolidated claims processing centers (NAPA, 1997).

During the 1990s, VBA consolidated loan guaranty work in four regional centers, education benefits in four regional processing centers, and insurance in one national service center. More recently, VBA consolidated the income and eligibility verification work of the pension program in three regional offices, and is planning to consolidate all pension work in these offices. To deal with the 2001 jump in pending claims, VBA established the tiger team unit at one regional office and established resource centers at nine regional offices to specialize in claims of older veterans. In 2003, as discussed previously, VBA established the Appeals Management Center to help process remands. VBA centralized dependency and indemnity compensation claims by survivors of servicemembers who die on active duty in a casualty assistance unit in the Philadelphia regional office. BDD claims are also handled in a few regional offices. VBA established two "development centers" in Phoenix and Roanoke to assist regional offices in developing all radiation claims and centralized the processing of radiation claims in the Jackson regional office. Just recently, the VA secretary designated the two development centers and three of the nine resource centers as a special tiger team for processing OIF/OEF claims. The two development centers are developing the evidence, and the three resource centers are rating OIF/OEF claims for regional offices with the heaviest workloads (U.S. Congress, House of Representatives, Committee on Veterans' Affairs, 2007b). Medical examinations for OIF/OEF veterans claims are also being expedited.

Nevertheless, the VSOs do not favor consolidating regional offices because they do not want to lose access to adjudicators or make it more difficult for veterans to appear in person before DROs who are reconsidering initial denials of their claims.

FINDINGS AND RECOMMENDATIONS

The Medical Evaluation Process

The quality and completeness of the medical information needed to apply the criteria in the Rating Schedule are critical to the disability compensation claims process for veterans. Obtaining needed medical information affects the timeliness, accuracy, and consistency of adjudication decisions. It requires the predetermination team to request the correct information needed from the medical examiners, examiners to conduct thorough examinations and report the results completely and accurately, and raters to interpret the medical information in light of the criteria in the Rating Schedule. It also requires VHA to ensure that the expertise of the examiner or examiners is appropriate for the condition or conditions being evaluated, especially for complex conditions such as PTSD, TBI, and polytrauma encountered in veterans of the current wars in Iraq and Afghanistan.

Need for Regular Updating of Examination Worksheets

VA has made a great deal of progress during the past 10 years in upgrading the medical evaluation process. Examination worksheets—two- to three-page outlines of the elements that must be addressed—for the most common conditions encountered in disability claims were developed. They were made available to examiners online to view and download. Currently, VA is developing intelligent interactive examination templates that structure the input needed in each case, which increases completeness and timeliness. VA does not, however, have a regular process for updating the worksheets, most of which date from 1997. Committee members evaluated some of the worksheets in light of the criteria in the Rating Schedule and current medical knowledge and found problems with outdated tests and examinations. Some of the problems stem from outdated criteria in the Rating Schedule. For example, rating of intervertebral disc syndrome relies on the duration of incapacitating episodes to assign 10 percent (1–2 weeks), 20 percent (2–4 weeks), 40 percent (4–6 weeks), or 60 percent (6 weeks or more). Incapacitating episodes are defined as bed rest prescribed by a physician, although bed rest is not the standard treatment for back problems.

Recommendation 5-1. VA should develop a process for periodic updating of the disability examination worksheets. This process should be part of, or closely linked to, the process recommended above for updating and revising the Schedule for Rating Disabilities. There should be input from the disability advisory committee recommended above (see Recommendation 4-1).

Use of the Examination Templates

VA does not require examiners to use printed-out examination worksheets and, consequently, many examiners do not use them. Although use of the online examination templates has increased rapidly (presumably because of their ease of use), VA also does not require their use—although it is considering such a mandate.

In an October 2005 report on C&P examinations, VA's inspector general noted progress being made in developing the templates, but expressed concern about their limited use:

> While VA, through the development and implementation of CPEP report templates, is making an effort to standardize C&P medical examinations, use of the templates is not yet required of VHA facilities. VBA rating personnel have seen only a limited number of examination reports submitted in the template format. We spoke with personnel at seven VAROs [VA regional offices] and were informed that use of the templates at VHA facilities is not yet common. VSC personnel at five of the seven VAROs indicated that they either have not seen any examination reports completed in the template format or they have only seen a limited number completed by one medical center in their area. Use of the templates was more frequent at medical centers serving the other two VAROs. Rating personnel at two VAROs who have seen the results of C&P examinations presented in the template format stated that they believed the examination reports need to be improved and that it was difficult to locate the information needed for rating purposes. According to VBA management, they are engaged in an effort to review and approve the report templates (VA, 2005b:69).

In the same report, the inspector general went on to recommend that the examination report templates be made mandatory, and that VA needed to ensure that medical and rating staff are familiar with the templates and that they are used consistently. The VA undersecretary for benefits concurred with this recommendation, and stated:

> We will continue to work with the Veterans Health Administration to improve the quality of medical examinations performed to support disability compensation evaluations. We will work with the CPEP Office to ensure that all automated examination report templates thoroughly and accurately solicit the medical evidence needed to consistently evaluate the disability. We will also work with VHA to establish a formal approval process for the templates and to obtain agreement on the mandatory use of approved templates (VA, 2005b:189).

By June 2006, more than 128,000 examinations had been completed using the report templates, but they were still not mandatory, despite the fact that early results had shown template examination reports to have higher quality than dictated reports, often significantly. In addition, template reports were released from 7 to 17 days sooner than dictated reports. "High-level" discussions were still underway within VA about whether to mandate use of the templates (Brown, 2006b,c).

> **Recommendation 5-2. VA should mandate the use of the online templates that have been developed for conducting and reporting disability examinations.**

Assessing and Improving Quality and Consistency of Examinations

As noted previously, VA established CPEP in 2001 to develop and administer a QR program, and it has integrated the QR results into the performance plans of the VISN directors. Improvement in meeting the quality indicators has been rapid since 2002 when the effort began. The percentage of examinations meeting 90 percent of the quality indicators was 86 percent in January 2007, much better than the 58 percent achieved three years earlier. However, this percentage is still too low.

Another concern is that the quality indicators used in the QR process are more procedural rather than substantive. They are measures of the presence or absence of a particular worksheet item in the report, not of whether the examination was good. Independent examinations of a sample of claimants to assess inter-rater reliability are not performed.

Recently, CPEP began to assess the quality of the examination requests, which is critical. Previously, if the examiner provided 100 percent of the information requested, but the request was not correct, the QR system counted it as a quality examination. The next step would be for VA to make the quality of examination requests part of the performance program for predetermination teams and regional office directors.

In addition, the QR program currently does not directly assess consistency among examiners. It relies on improving accuracy to narrow the differences among examiners and VISNs.

> **Recommendation 5-3. VA should establish a recurring assessment of the substantive quality and consistency, or inter-rater reliability, of examinations performed with the templates, and if the assessment finds problems, take steps to improve quality and consistency, for example, by revising the templates, changing the training, or adjusting the performance standards for examiners.**

This substantive assessment should be part of the QR audit and include a mechanism for random sampling. The training program should include examples of well-done and complete reports.

The Rating Process

Quality of Rating Decisions

VBA's QR program, STAR, was implemented in 1998 and substantially revised and expanded to monitor individual regional office accuracy in 2001. The accuracy rate has improved from 64 percent in 1998 to 80 percent in FY 2002, and to 88 percent in FY 2006. Although this represents substantial improvement, it still shows that one of every nine rating decisions is incorrect, and this leaves considerable room for further improvement.

In addition, the STAR accuracy rate is based on a relatively small sample—only large enough to determine the aggregate accuracy rate of regional offices. It does not assess accuracy at the body system or diagnostic code level, and it does not measure consistency across regional offices. In 2005, in response to findings of inconsistencies by GAO and VA's Office of Inspector General, VBA announced an effort to identify high rates of variability in claims adjudication by diagnostic code, to be followed by an assessment of decision consistency among and between regional offices for those conditions. The results would be used to identify needs for additional training, better guidance, procedural changes, or regulatory changes (U.S. Congress, House of Representatives, Committee on Veterans' Affairs, 2005a).[31]

In 2005, VBA chose three conditions to assess for inconsistency: hearing loss, PTSD, and knee conditions. Ten subject-matter specialists were assigned to review 1,750 regional office decisions, followed by studies of additional conditions. These analyses were not made public.

According to VA's latest strategic plan

> VA will analyze ratings and claims data to track any unusual patterns of variance for further consistency review. Integrated systems and better data sharing will improve the quality of decision making by providing more accurate information to claims adjudicators. We will also develop systems and programs to evaluate employees' information needs and deliver training to address those needs (VA, 2006c).

There are many sources of variability in decision making that, if not addressed and reduced to the extent possible, make it unlikely that veterans

[31] In 2007, VA's deputy under secretary for benefits made a similar statement: "We are also identifying unusual patterns of variance in claims adjudication by diagnostic code, and then reviewing selected disabilities to assess the level of decision consistency among and between regional offices. These studies are used to identify where additional guidance and training are needed to improve consistency and accuracy, as well as to drive procedural or regulatory changes. Site surveys of regional offices also address compliance with procedures" (U.S. Congress, House of Representatives, Committee on Veterans' Affairs, 2007b).

with similar disabilities are being treated the same. VA should identify conditions subject to a great deal of decision variability, understand the reasons for the variability, and act to reduce that variability. Variability cannot be totally eliminated in evaluating most disabling conditions. There will be cases in which raters with the same information and criteria reach different conclusions, especially conditions with large subjective elements such as mental disorders and back pain. Still, sources of variability that can be controlled, such as training, guidelines, and rater qualifications, should be addressed.

> **Recommendation 5-4. The rating process should have built-in checks or periodic evaluations to ensure inter-rater reliability as well as the accuracy and validity of rating across impairment categories, ratings, and regions.**

For example, VA could have a sample of claims rated by two or more RVSRs and analyze the degree of consistency in the ratings given. Or the same claims could be analyzed by RVSRs using standard procedures and information sources and by raters with access to medical advisers, and the results compared to assess whether having medical advisers for raters improves decision making. A comparison of raters with a medical background, such as nurses and physician assistants, and raters without medical backgrounds would inform decisions about the qualifications of raters. These comparisons could be done using hypothetical or actual cases. BVA might do the same with appeals.

VA could sample claims involving the rating of a particular diagnostic code across field offices and analyze inter-rater and inter-regional differences. Presumably these would be diagnostic codes of conditions that are relatively numerous or costly. A next step could be to determine the degree to which regulations, the adjudication manual, and other forms of guidance could be revised to reduce variability, or training or the QR system could increase consistency.

Another approach to reducing unwanted variability in the rating process is the use of best practices. The adoption of the CPI model by all regional offices in 2001–2002 is an example of this approach, but there is still evidence of considerable variation across regional offices in decision outcomes, such as grant rates, rating levels, and rates of appeals. VA should study these variations and identify best practices for all offices to adopt.

Better Access to Medical Expertise

In some cases, disability evaluators can use an authoritative medical finding, such as a particular test score of a certain degree, to make a rating decision. In most cases, however, the evidence is less direct, more complex, and perhaps conflicting. The evaluator must understand the medical evidence and use judgment, for example, in weighing conflicting medical opinions. The evaluators are not usually medical professionals themselves. Other major disability programs either involve physicians or other appropriate clinicians in the adjudication decision or have medical experts readily available to review cases, for example, to interpret medical information for disability evaluators or advise on missing information that should be requested (see Appendix D). These are in addition to arrangements for independent medical examinations where needed to provide missing or inconsistent medical information. For example, Social Security disability determinations are generally made by two-person teams, one member of which is a physician or other appropriate medical professional (e.g., audiologist). At DoD, physical evaluation boards—which also use and apply the VA Rating Schedule—have at least one physician among the three members. The Federal Employee Compensation Act program and civil service disability retirement programs have physician consultants on staff. Private disability insurance carriers have a variety of arrangements to provide disability evaluators with advice.

The separation between medical examiners and rating specialists at VA is artificial and based on a misunderstanding of the role of physicians in adjudication. The U.S. Court of Appeals for Veterans Claims barred the participation of physicians in rating decisions on the grounds that they should not substitute their own clinical judgment because they represent the agency. In fact, the role of a physician-adjudicator differs from that of a physician performing a disability examination. They do not examine the claimant. They evaluate the evidence in the claimant's file to confirm that a diagnosis was made and is adequately documented, weigh conflicting evidence in the medical records, and apply other aspects of the adjudication process. RVSRs can probably adjudicate many or most cases without physician involvement, but physician advice is helpful in complex cases. The Social Security Administration experimented successfully with having disability evaluators decide cases alone and only bring in medical consultants when, in their judgment, they needed the expert advice.

Currently, RVSRs do not have readily available medical consultants. If there is a question, they have to send the case back to VHA, which adds time to the process. VBA should have medical consultants accessible to RVSRs in the regional office VSCs. With modern communications technology, these consultants could be in a national or in regional centers, and have access to the claims file, the C&P examination report, and VA medical records, if any. This would not obviate the need for C&P examinations but would expedite the adjudication decision process.

Recommendation 5-5. VA raters should have ready access to qualified health-care experts who can provide advice on medical and psychological issues that arise during the rating process (e.g., interpreting evidence or assessing the need for additional examinations or diagnostic tests).

These health-care experts could come from VHA or outside contractors, or VBA could hire health-care providers to serve on its own staff. If they were VHA staff, arrangements would have to be made to ensure that the C&P examiner of a veteran was also not the consultant on his or her case, and training on the appropriate adjudication consultant role would have to be provided.

Training of Examiners and Adjudicators

VA is well along in developing a training and certification program for C&P medical examiners, and it is scheduled to be developed during FY 2007 and deployed during FY 2008. It is to be mandatory, although a date by which examiners must be certified has not yet been set.

VBA has also developed an extensive training program for case adjudicators. This is critical because VBA hired approximately 1,180 new VSRs and RVSRs in FY 2006, and plans to hire many more in FY 2007 and FY 2008 to make up for attrition and to meet the increase in caseload (VA, 2006a). A centralized two-week training course is given every quarter to new VSRs. This is followed by a national standardized training 23-week curriculum given at their home regional offices, which includes full lesson plans, handouts, student guides, instructor guides, and slides for classroom instruction. Newly-hired RVSRs are also provided a nationally consistent training program. VBA gives a week-long instructor development course to trainers in the regional offices. A computer-based training program, the Training and Performance Support System, has a set of modules on rating-related topics, including evaluation of disability conditions by body system. BVA also has an extensive training program, part of which is given by an on-staff medical adviser, a physician who also acts as an informal adviser to VLJs and counsel in a role somewhat like the medical consultant role recommended in Recommendation 5-4. The QR programs of both VBA and BVA are used to identify training needs, whether on particular topics or at particular regional offices.

In FY 2006, the VA under secretary for benefits directed regional offices to provide all claims adjudicators with a mandatory 70 hours of job-specific training, increasing to 80 hours in FY 2007 (U.S. Congress, House of Representatives, Committee on Veterans' Affairs, 2006). VBA is not evaluating the effectiveness of its training programs, however.

VBA has developed a certification program for VSRs and plans to extend it to RVSRs and DROs. The test was developed and validated for VBA by the Human Resources Research Organization (HumRRO), a national nonprofit organization that specializes in certification testing. As of September 2006, VBA had promoted 633 VSRs to the GS-11 level through the certification testing process. It is working with HumRRO on a test for the GS-12 RVSR position (U.S. Congress, House of Representatives, Committee on Veterans' Affairs, 2006).

> **Recommendation 5-6. Educational and training programs for VBA raters and VHA examiners should be developed, mandated, and uniformly implemented across all regional offices with standardized performance objectives and outcomes. These programs should make use of advances in adult education techniques. External consultants should serve as advisors to assist in the development and evaluation of the educational and training programs.**

REFERENCES

Brown, S. H. 2003. *Presentation on CAPRI C&P worksheet module*. VHA eHealth University class #145, May 14. http://www.vehu.med.va.gov/vehu/campcprs2003/ SessionCaptures/ Hands-On/145/145_files/frame.htm (accessed March 15, 2007).

Brown, S. H. 2006a. *Overview of CPEP and quality assurance improvement initiatives for C&P exams*. Presentation to the IOM Committee on Medical Evaluation of Veterans for Disability Compensation, Washington, DC, May 25.

Brown, S. H. 2006b. *Compensation and pension examination program overview*. Presentation to the Veterans' Disability Benefits Commission, Washington, DC. http:// www.1888932-2946.ws/vetscommission/e-documentmanager/gallery/ Documents/June_ 2006/CPEPBriefing_June2006.pdf (accessed March 2, 2007).

Brown, S. H. 2006c. *Examiner certification and exam templates update*. Presentation to the Veterans' Disability Benefits Commission, Washington, DC. http://www.1888932-2946. ws/vetscommission/e-documentmanager/gallery/Documents/September_2006/CPEP_ Presentation_09-15-2006.pdf (accessed March 16, 2007).

Brown, S. H. 2007. Written response to IOM request for most recent information on quality review of compensation and pension examinations, use of online examination templates, and training and certification of examiners, attached to April 9, 2007, e-mail from Steven H. Brown, director, VA Compensation and Pension Examination Program.

BVA (Board of Veterans' Appeals). 1994. *FY 1994 report of the chairman, Board of Veterans' Appeals*. Washington, DC: BVA. http://www.va.gov/Vetapp/ChairRpt/ BVA1994AR.pdf (accessed March 16, 2007).

BVA. 1996a. *FY 1995 report of the chairman, Board of Veterans' Appeals*. Washington, DC: BVA. http://www.va.gov/Vetapp/ChairRpt/BVA1995AR.pdf (accessed March 16, 2007).

BVA. 1996b. *FY 1996 report of the chairman, Board of Veterans' Appeals*. Washington, DC: BVA. http://www.va.gov/Vetapp/ChairRpt/BVA1996AR.pdf (accessed March 16, 2007).

BVA. 1997. *FY 1997 report of the chairman, Board of Veterans' Appeals*. Washington, DC: BVA. http://www.va.gov/Vetapp/ChairRpt/BVA1997AR.pdf (accessed March 16, 2007).

BVA. 2000a. *Understanding the appeal process*. VA Pamphlet 01-00-1. http://www.va.gov/ vbs/bva/y2000.pdf (accessed February 28, 2007).

BVA. 2000b. *FY 2000 report of the chairman, Board of Veterans' Appeals.* Washington, DC: BVA. http://www.va.gov/Vetapp/ChairRpt/BVA2000AR.pdf (accessed March 16, 2007).

BVA. 2001. *FY 2001 report of the chairman, Board of Veterans' Appeals.* Washington, DC: BVA. http://www.va.gov/Vetapp/ChairRpt/BVA2001AR.pdf (accessed March 16, 2007).

BVA. 2002a. *How do I appeal?* VA Pamphlet 01-02-02A. http://www.va.gov/vbs/bva/0102A.pdf (accessed February 28, 2007).

BVA. 2002b. *FY 2002 report of the chairman, Board of Veterans' Appeals.* Washington, DC: BVA. http://www.va.gov/Vetapp/ChairRpt/BVA2002AR.pdf (accessed March 16, 2007).

BVA. 2003. *FY 2003 report of the chairman, Board of Veterans' Appeals.* Washington, DC: BVA. http://www.va.gov/Vetapp/ChairRpt/BVA2003AR.pdf (accessed March 16, 2007).

BVA. 2004. *FY 2004 report of the chairman, Board of Veterans' Appeals.* Washington, DC: BVA. http://www.va.gov/Vetapp/ChairRpt/BVA2004AR.pdf (accessed March 16, 2007).

BVA. 2005. *FY 2005 report of the chairman, Board of Veterans' Appeals.* Washington, DC: BVA. http://www.va.gov/Vetapp/ChairRpt/BVA2005AR.pdf (accessed March 16, 2007).

BVA. 2006. *FY 2006 report of the chairman, Board of Veterans' Appeals.* Washington, DC: BVA. http://www.va.gov/Vetapp/ChairRpt/BVA2006AR.pdf (accessed March 16, 2007).

BVA. 2007. Data from the Veterans Appeals Control and Locator System on the disposition of claims by regional office during FY 2005, provided by BVA.

Congressional Commission (Congressional Commission on Servicemembers and Veterans Transition Assistance). 1999. *Final report of the Congressional Commission on Servicemembers and Veterans Transition Assistance.* http://www.vetbiz.gov/library/Transition%20Commission%20Report.pdf (accessed March 16, 2007).

GAO (General Accounting Office). 2001. *Veterans' benefits: Quality assurance for disability claims processing.* GAO-01-930R. http://www.gao.gov/new.items/d01930r.pdf (March 15, 2007).

GAO. 2002a. *Veterans' benefits: Quality assurance for disability claims and appeals processing can be further improved.* GAO-02-806. http://www.gao.gov/new.items/d02806.pdf (accessed February 28, 2007).

GAO. 2002b. *Veterans' benefits: Despite recent improvements, meeting claims processing goals will be challenging.* GAO-02-645T. http://www.gao.gov/new.items/d02645t.pdf (accessed March 15, 2007).

GAO. 2005a. *Veterans benefits: VA needs plan for assessing consistency of decisions.* GAO-05-99. http://www.gao.gov/new.items/d0599.pdf (accessed March 15, 2007).

GAO. 2005b. *Veterans' disability benefits: VA could enhance its progress in complying with court decision on disability criteria.* GAO-06-46. http://www.gao.gov/new.items/d0646.pdf (accessed March 15, 2007).

GAO. 2005c. *VA disability benefits: Board of Veterans' Appeals has made improvements in quality assurance, but challenges remain for VA in assuring consistency.* GAO-05-655T. http://www.gao.gov/new.items/d05655t.pdf (accessed February 28, 2007).

GAO. 2006. *VA disability benefits: Routine monitoring of disability decisions could improve consistency.* GAO-06-120T. http://www.gao.gov/new.items/d06120t.pdf (accessed March 15, 2007).

GAO. 2007. *Veterans' disability benefits: Long-standing claims processing challenges persist.* GAO-07-512T. http://www.gao.gov/new.items/d07512t.pdf (accessed May 28, 2007).

Keller, S. 2007. Written response to IOM request for information on BVA sources of medical expertise and statistics on reasons for remands, attached to March 21, 2007, e-mail from Steve Keller, senior deputy vice chairman, Board of Veterans' Appeals.

Mansfield, G. H. 2005. Letter to Cynthia A. Bascetta, director, Education, Workforce and Income Security Issues, GAO. GAO-06-46. http://www.gao.gov/new.items/d0646.pdf (accessed March 15, 2007).

NAPA (National Academy of Public Administration). 1997. *Management of compensation and pension benefits claim processes for veterans.* Washington, DC: NAPA.

Pamperin, T. 2006. *Overview of disability compensation and pension examinations.* Presentation to Veterans' Disability Benefits Commission. http://www.1888932-2946.ws/vetscommission/e-documentmanager/gallery/Documents/June_2006/ VBAPresentation_6-21-06.pdf (accessed March 2, 2007).

QTC. 2006. *QTC exam process and demo.* Presentation to the Veterans' Disability Benefits Commission. http://www.1888932-2946.ws/vetscommission/e-documentmanager/gallery/Documents/June_2006/QTCOverview_June2006.pdf (accessed March 2, 2007).

Shahani, M. 2005. *QTC medical services overview.* Presentation to VA's Advisory Committee on Women Veterans. http://www.va.gov/womenvet/docs/ACWV_Nov._05_meeting_web_version.doc (accessed September 5, 2006).

Terry, J. P. 2006a. *Briefing for the Institute of Medicine.* Presentation to the IOM Committee on Medical Evaluation of Veterans for Disability Compensation, Washington, DC, July 7.

Terry, J. P. 2006b. *Prepared statement of James P. Perry, Chairman, Board of Veterans' Appeals, before the Veterans' Disability Benefits Commission.* Washington, DC, January 20. http://www.1888932-2946.ws/vetscommission/e-documentmanager/gallery/Documents/January_2006/Statement_Terry_BVAChairman_Jan06.pdf (accessed February 28, 2007).

Terry, J. P. 2007. *Statement before the Committee on Veterans' Affairs, U.S. Senate, March 7, 2007.* http://veterans.senate.gov/index.cfm?FuseAction=Hearings.CurrentHearings&rID=943&hID=250 (accessed March 15, 2007).

U.S. Congress, House of Representatives, Committee on Veterans' Affairs. 2005a. *Prepared statement of Ronald R. Aument, Deputy Under Secretary for Benefits, VA.* 109th Cong., 1st Sess., December 7. http://veterans.house.gov/hearings/schedule109/dec05/12-7-05/raument.html (accessed March 5, 2007).

U.S. Congress, House of Representatives, Committee on Veterans' Affairs. 2005b. *Prepared statement of Steven H. Brown, Director, Compensation and Pension Examination Program, VA, on compensation and pension examination variability.* 109th Cong., 1st Sess., October 20. http://www.va.gov/OCA/testimony/hvac/sdama/051020SB.asp (accessed March 15, 2007).

U.S. Congress, House of Representatives, Committee on Veterans' Affairs. 2005c. *Statement of Gordon H. Mansfield, Deputy Secretary, VA.* 109th Cong., 1st Sess., September 28. http://veterans.house.gov/hearings/schedule109/sep05/9-28-05/gmansfield.pdf (accessed March 5, 2007).

U.S. Congress, House of Representatives, Committee on Veterans' Affairs. 2005d. *Testimony of Michael Walcoff, Associate Deputy Under Secretary for Field Operations, Veterans Benefits Administration.* 109th Cong., 1st Sess., May 5. http://www.va.gov/OCA/testimony/hvac/sdama/050505MW.asp (accessed May18, 2007).

U.S. Congress, House of Representatives, Committee on Veterans' Affairs. 2006. *Prepared testimony of Michael Walcoff, Associate Deputy Under Secretary for Field Operations, Veterans Benefits Administration, VA.* 109th Cong., 2nd Sess., September 13. http://veterans.house.gov/hearings/schedule109/sep06/9-13-06/MichaelWalcoff.html (accessed May 22, 2007).

U.S. Congress, House of Representatives, Committee on Veterans' Affairs. 2007a. *Testimony of R. James Nicholson, Secretary of Veterans Affairs.* 110th Cong., 1st Sess., February 8. http://veterans.house.gov/hearings/schedule110/feb07/02-08-07/JamesNicholson.html (accessed March 1, 2007).

U.S. Congress, House of Representatives, Committee on Veterans' Affairs. 2007b. *Prepared statement of Ronald R. Aument, Deputy Under Secretary for Benefits, VA.* 110th Cong., 1st Sess., March 13. http://veterans.house.gov/hearings/schedule110/mar07/03-13-07/3-13-07aument.shtml (accessed March 5, 2007).

U.S. Congress, Senate, Committee on Veterans' Affairs. 2007. *Prepared statement of David S. C. Chu, Under Secretary of Defense (Personnel and Readiness)*. 110th Cong., 1st Sess., January 23. http://veterans.senate.gov/index.cfm?FuseAction=Hearings.CurrentHearings&rID=891&hID=234 (accessed March 5, 2007).

U.S. Court of Appeals for Veterans Claims. 2006. *Annual reports of the U.S. Court of Appeals for Veterans Claims*. http://www.vetapp.uscourts.gov/documents/Annual_Reports.pdf (accessed May 15, 2007).

VA (Department of Veterans Affairs). 1994. *Timeliness of C&P medical examination services*. Report No. 4R1-A02-092. Washington, DC: Office of Inspector General, VA.

VA. 1997a. *Summary report on VA claims processing issues*. Report No. 8D2-B01-001. Washington, DC: Office of Inspector General, VA. http://www.va.gov/oig/52/reports/1998/8D2-B01-001.pdf (accessed March 12, 2007).

VA. 1997b. *Review of compensation and pension medical examination services*. Report No. 7R1-A02-114. Washington, DC: Office of Inspector General, VA. http://www.va.gov/oig/52/reports/1997/7R1-A02-114--C-PEXAM.PDF (accessed March 12, 2007).

VA. 2000. *Annual performance report, FY 2000*. Washington, DC: Office of Budget, Office of Management, VA. http://www.va.gov/budget/report/2000/PerfRpt2000.pdf (accessed March 16, 2007).

VA. 2001a. *Annual performance report, FY 2001*. Washington, DC: Office of Budget, Office of Management, VA. http://www.va.gov/budget/report/2001/PerfRpt2001.pdf (accessed March 15, 2007).

VA. 2001b. *Best practice manual for posttraumatic stress disorder (PTSD) compensation and pension examinations*. http://www.ptsdmanual.com/ptsd.pdf (accessed March 20, 2007).

VA. 2002a. *C&P Service clinician's guide*. Version 3.0, edited by L. R. Coulson, VHA. http://www.warms.vba.va.gov/Admin21/GUIDE/Cliniciansguide.doc (accessed March 4, 2007).

VA. 2002b. *Fiscal year 2002 performance and accountability report*. Washington, DC: Office of Budget, Office of Management, VA. http://www.va.gov/budget/report/2002/Perform_AccountRpt2002.pdf (accessed March 15, 2007).

VA. 2002c. *Quality measurement of compensation and pension examinations: National baseline performance, ten most common exam types*. Washington, DC: Compensation and Pension Examination Project Office, VA.

VA. 2003. *Fiscal year 2003 performance and accountability report*. Washington, DC: Office of Budget, Office of Management, VA. http://www.va.gov/budget/report/2003/Perform_AccountRpt2003.pdf (accessed May 20, 2007).

VA. 2004a. Avoidable remands agreement and implementation. VBA Letter 20-04-58. http://www.warms.vba.va.gov/admin20/letters/vba04_58.doc (accessed March 15, 2007).

VA. 2004b. *Handbook of standard procedures and best practices for audiology compensation and pension examinations*, edited by K. C. Dennis, L. B. Beck, D. W. Chandler, and J. Schafer. Washington, DC: Employee Education System, VA. http://www-nehc.med.navy.mil/downloads/Occmed/HCToolbox/Toolbox_files/VA%20Audiology%20Best%20Practices%20%26%20Procedures.pdf(accessed March 20, 2007).

VA. 2004c. *Fiscal year 2004 performance and accountability report*. Washington, DC: Office of Budget, Office of Management, VA. http://www.va.gov/budget/report/2004/9208DepVetAff_2004.pdf (accessed March 15, 2007).

VA. 2005a. *Department of Veterans Affairs compensation and pension record interchange user guide*. http://www.va.gov/vdl/documents/Financial_Admin/CAPRI/ capri_ug_dvba_2.7_91.pdf (accessed March 4, 2007).

VA. 2005b. *Department of Veterans Affairs Office of Inspector General review of state variances in VA disability compensation payments.* Report No. 05-00765-137. http://www.va.gov/oig/52/reports/2005/VAOIG-05-00765-137.pdf (accessed March 4, 2007).

VA. 2005c. *Fiscal year 2005 performance and accountability report.* Washington, DC: Office of Budget, Office of Management, VA. http://www.va.gov/budget/report/2005/VA-2005_FULL-WEB.pdf (accessed March 15, 2007).

VA. 2006a. *FY 2006 performance and accountability report.* Washington, DC: Office of Budget, Office of Management, VA. http://www.va.gov/budget/report/2006FullWeb.pdf (accessed March 16, 2007).

VA. 2006b. *VHA handbook 1601E.01, Compensation and pension (C&P) examinations.* http://www.va.gov/vhapublications/ViewPublication.asp?pub_ID=1400 (accessed March 15, 2007).

VA. 2006c. *VA strategic plan FY 2006-2011.* http://www.va.gov/op3/docs/VA_2006_2011_Strategic_Plan.pdf (accessed March 16, 2007).

VA. 2006d. Accuracy and accountability. Unpublished PowerPoint presentation. Washington, DC: C&P Service, VA.

VA. 2006e. *Qualifications for examiners performing compensation and pension (C&P) mental disorder examinations.* VBA Fast Letter 06-03, March 15. http://www.va.gov/vhapublications/ViewPublication.asp?pub_ID=1391 (accessed April 4, 2007).

VA. 2007a. *Veterans Administration fiscal year 2008 budget submission. Vol. 4, Summary.* http://www.va.gov/budget/summary/VolumeIVSummaryVolume.pdf (accessed February 28, 2007).

VA. 2007b. *Veterans Administration fiscal year 2008 budget submission. Vol. 2, National Cemetery Administration, benefit programs, and departmental administration.* http://www.va.gov/budget/summary/VolumeIINationalCemeteryAdministrationBenefits-ProgramsandDepartmentalAdmin.pdf (accessed February 28, 2007).

VA. 2007c. *Monday morning workload reports, end of the fiscal year: 2000–2006.* http://www.vba.va.gov/bln/201/reports/mmrindex.htm (accessed May 22, 2007).

VA. 2007d. *Index to disability examination worksheets.* http://www.vba.va.gov/bln/21/Benefits/exams/index.htm (accessed May 20, 2007).

VA. 2007e. *Mission statement of the Veterans Benefits Administration.* http://www.vba.va.gov/mission_vision.htm (accessed February 28, 2007).

VA. 2007f. *Understanding the disability claims process.* http://www.vba.va.gov/bln/21/Topics/claims.htm (accessed May 18, 2007).

VDBC (Veterans' Disability Benefit Commission). 2007. *Transition report.* http://www.1888932-2946.ws/vetscommission/e-documentmanager/gallery/Documents/2007_February/TransitionReport_Slides_2-21-2007.pdf (accessed March 3, 2007).

6

Medical Criteria for Ancillary Benefits

INTRODUCTION

Military veterans are generally eligible for a number of benefits through the Department of Veterans Affairs (VA) aimed at easing their reentry into and improving the quality of their civilian lives. These include health-care services, compensation for service-connected disabilities, means-tested pensions for nonservice-connected disabilities, education benefits under the GI Bill, home loan guaranties, life insurance, burial benefits, and survivor benefits.

Part 9 of VA's *Compensation and Pension Adjudication Procedure Manual* (M21-1MR) breaks down veterans benefits into two categories—ancillary and special. The Veterans' Disability Benefits Commission asked the committee to focus on the appropriateness of medical criteria for five specific ancillary benefits available to veterans with disabilities: vocational rehabilitation and employment (VR&E) services, automobile assistance and adaptive equipment, housing adaptation, and clothing allowances. (See Box 6-1 for the current medical eligibility criteria to qualify for these selected benefits.)

VA's special benefits—called *special* and *ratings for special purpose* benefits—for veterans with disabilities are therefore not discussed in this report. They include the Special Allowance under 38 U.S.C. 1312(a), Medal of Honor Pension (special benefits), and the following ratings for special purposes:

- rating determinations for dependents educational assistance, veteran's civil service disability preference, and discharge of liability for educational loans under 38 U.S.C. 3698;

BOX 6-1
Medical Eligibility Criteria to Qualify for Selected Benefits

VR&E assistance

- Ten percent rated disabled with a serious employment handicap and discharged or released from military service under other than dishonorable conditions
- Twenty percent or more rated disabled with an employment handicap and discharged or released from military service under other than dishonorable conditions
- Twenty percent rated disabled if pending medical separation from active duty if their disabilities are reasonably expected to be rated at least at 20 percent following their discharge

Automobile assistance

- Service-connected loss or permanent loss of use of one or both hands or feet
- Permanent impairment of vision of both eyes to a certain degree (i.e., permanent impairment of vision in both eyes with a central visual acuity of 20/20 or less in the better eye with corrective glasses, or central visual acuity of more that 20/200 if there is a field defect in which the peripheral field has contracted to such an extent that the widest diameter of visual field has an angular distance no greater than 20 degrees in the better eye)
- Ankylosis (immobility) of one or both knees, or one or both hips

Adaptive equipment allowance

Anyone who qualifies for the automobile allowance also qualifies for adaptive equipment.

- To be eligible to receive only adaptive equipment (as opposed to the automobile allowance), the veteran or serviceperson must be entitled to disability compensation for ankylosis of one or both knees or hips based on:
  - the establishment of service connection, or
  - entitlement under 38 U.S.C. 1151 as the result of
    - VA treatment or examination,
    - compensated work therapy, or
    - vocational training under 38 U.S.C. Chapter 31.

- ratings for dental treatment, medical care, service connection for psychosis under 38 U.S.C. 1702, insanity determination, insurance purposes, and Polish and Czechoslovakian Armed Forces under 38 U.S.C. 109(c); and
- rating to extend the delimiting dates for educational assistance.

Table 6-1 describes the full complement of veterans benefits by service-connected disability rating percentages.

Specially adapted homes

- $50,000 grant for permanent and total service-connected disability due to one of the following:
  1. Loss or loss of use of both lower extremities, such as to preclude locomotion without the aid of braces, crutches, canes, or a wheelchair
  2. Loss or loss of use of both upper extremities at or above the elbow
  3. Blindness in both eyes, having only light perception, plus loss or loss of use of one lower extremity
  4. Loss or loss of use of one lower extremity together with (a) residuals of organic disease or injury, or (b) the loss or loss of use of one upper extremity which so affects the functions of balance or propulsion as to preclude locomotion without the use of braces, canes, crutches, or a wheelchair
- $10,000 grant for permanent and total service-connected disability due to:
  1. Blindness in both eyes with 5/2000 visual acuity or less, or
  2. Anatomical loss or loss of use of both hands
- Supplemental financing: Veterans with available loan guaranty entitlement may also obtain a VA-guaranteed loan or a direct loan to supplement the grant to acquire a specially adapted home. The VA maximum direct loan from a private lender varies; the VA maximum is $33,000.
- Special Home Adaptation Grant for veterans who do not qualify for special adaptive housing, for actual cost up to a maximum of $10,000. May be applied for if the veteran is permanently and totally disabled due to blindness in both eyes with visual acuity of 5/200 or less or the loss or permanent loss of use of both hands.

Clothing allowance

- Service-connected disability for which a veteran uses prosthetic or orthopedic appliances
- Service-connected skin condition that requires prescribed medication that irreparably damages the veteran's outer garments
- Paid annually

SOURCES: Adapted from VA (2006b), and VA's *Compensation and Pension Adjudication Procedure Manual,* M21-1MR, Part 9.

Perhaps the most important benefit provided to veterans with service-connected disabilities is priority access to free health care for all medical care needs from the Veterans Health Administration (VHA). They are not required to enroll for the health-care benefits, but are urged to enroll for better planning of health resources (VA, 2006a). Veterans with disabilities receive health care if they (1) have a service-connected disability rated 50 percent or higher; (2) need care for a disability the military determined was incurred or aggravated in the line of duty, but which VA has not yet

TABLE 6-1 Veterans Benefits by Service-Connected Disability Rating Percentages

If a veteran has a service-connected disability rating percentage of . . .	Additional Benefits[a]
10 percent with an effective date of October 1, 1993, or after	Veteran may be entitled to vocational rehabilitation services if the veteran either • originally applied for vocational rehabilitation before November 1, 1990, reapplied after that date, and has an employment handicap; or • did not originally apply for vocational rehabilitation before November 1, 1990, applied on or after October 1, 1993, and has a serious employment handicap.
0 to 20 percent	• Home loan guaranty fee exemption • Vocational rehabilitation and counseling under title 38 U.S.C. Chapter 31 (must be at least 10 percent) • Service-disabled veterans' insurance (maximum of $10,000.00 coverage), must file within 2 years of date of new service connection • 10-point civil service preference (10 points added to civil service test score) • Clothing allowance for veterans who use or wear a prosthetic or orthopedic appliance (artificial limb, braces, wheelchairs) or use prescribed medications for skin condition which tend to wear, tear, or soil clothing
30 percent (in addition to the above)	Additional disability compensation for dependent spouse, child(ren), stepchild(ren), helpless child(ren), full-time student between the ages of 18 and 23 and parent(s)
40 percent (in addition to the above)	Automobile grant and/or special adaptive equipment for an automobile provided there is loss or permanent loss of use of one or both feet, loss or permanent loss of use of one or both hands, or permanent impaired vision of both eyes with central visual acuity of 20/200 or less in the better eye. Special adaptive equipment may be applied for if there is ankylosis of one or both knees or one or both hips.
50 percent (in addition to the above)	• Preventative health-care services • Hospital care and medical services in non-VA facilities under an authorized fee-basis agreement

TABLE 6-1 Continued

If a veteran has a service-connected disability rating percentage of . . .	Additional Benefits[a]
60 to 90 percent (in addition to the above)	Increased compensation (100 percent) based on individual unemployability (applies to veterans who are unable to obtain or maintain substantial gainful employment due solely to the service-connected disability)

100 percent (in addition to the above)	• Special adaptive housing for veterans who have
	  • loss or permanent loss of use of both lower extremities,
	  • blindness in both eyes, having light perception only, plus
	    • loss or permanent loss of use of one lower extremity or permanent loss of use of one upper extremity or the loss or permanent loss of use of one extremity together with an organic disease that affects the function of balance and propulsion as to preclude locomotion without the aid of braces, crutches, canes, or wheelchair
	• Special home adaptation grant (for veterans who do not quality for special adaptive housing). May be applied for if the veteran is permanently and totally disabled due to blindness in both eyes with visual acuity of 5/200 or less or the loss or permanent loss of use of both hands

100 percent permanent and total (in addition to the above)	• Civilian health and medical program for dependents and survivors (CHAMPVA) • Survivors and dependents educational assistance under Title 38 U.S.C. Chapter 35

[a]Service-connected veterans with current disability ratings by VA may be eligible for additional benefits as outlined.

SOURCE: Adapted from VA's *Compensaton and Pension Adjudication Procedure Manual*, M21-1MR, Part 9.

rated, during the 12-month period following discharge; or (3) need care for a service-connected disability only. Veterans with service-connected conditions rated at any percentage, from zero percent and higher, receive care for the condition(s) that are service connected, without requiring a copayment. Depending on the nature and degree of the veteran's service-connected disabilities, free VHA health-care benefits may include eyeglasses, hearing aids, cochlear implants, pharmacy services, dental treatment, prosthetic devices (e.g., artificial limbs, orthopedic braces, shoes), durable medical equipment (e.g., wheelchairs, crutches, canes), and other medical supplies. (It should be noted that some of these health-care benefits are also indicated as ancillary benefits, as described below.)

In 1999, in accord with the Veterans' Health Care Eligibility Reform Act of 1996, VHA developed a priority group system to balance demand for health care with available resources. Service-connected disability is an important factor in assigning veterans to higher priority groups. For example, first priority (group 1) is given to veterans with service-connected disabilities rated 50 percent or more and to veterans deemed unemployable because of service-connected conditions (see Table 6-2 for eligibility criteria by group). Priority groups 2 and 3 include veterans with service-connected disabilities rated 30 or 40 percent, or 10 or 20 percent, respectively. Group 8, in contrast, includes all other nonservice-connected veterans and zero percent, noncompensable service-connected veterans who agree to make copayments. As of January 2003, VHA stopped enrolling new veterans in priority group 8.

ANCILLARY BENEFITS

Ancillary benefits are secondary benefits considered when evaluating claims for disability compensation, pension, or dependency and indemnity compensation (DIC) entitlement. Eligibility for ancillary benefits depends on the veteran's type of disability entitlement, his or her degree of disability, or in the case of DIC, the circumstances of his or her death.[1] This report addresses ancillary benefits in compensation cases, and not such benefits as pensions for low-income veterans, VA's Civilian Health and Medical Program (geared toward dependents and spouses of both living and deceased veterans), loan guaranties for surviving spouses, and the entitlement program for survivors. The benefits addressed in this report are VR&E services, automobile and adaptive equipment allowances, specially adapted homes, special housing adaptation grants, and clothing allowance. In fiscal year

---

[1] VA's *Compensation and Pension Adjudication Procedure Manual*, M21-1MR, Part 3, Ch. 6, Topic 3.

TABLE 6-2 Priority Groups for Health-Care Benefits

Priority Groups	Criteria
1	• Veterans with service-connected disabilities rated 50 percent or more • Veterans determined by VA to be unemployable due to service-connected conditions
2	Veterans with service-connected disabilities rated 30 or 40 percent
3	• Veterans with service-connected disabilities rated 10 or 20 percent • Veterans who are Former Prisoners of War (POW) or were awarded a Purple Heart • Veterans awarded special eligibility for disabilities incurred in treatment or participation in a VA vocational rehabilitation program • Veterans whose discharge was for a disability incurred or aggravated in the line of duty
4	• Veterans receiving aid and attendance or housebound benefits • Veterans determined by VA to be catastrophically disabled • Some veterans in this group may be responsible for copayments.
5	• Veterans receiving VA pension benefits or eligible for Medicaid programs • Nonservice-connected veterans and noncompensable, zero percent service-connected veterans whose annual income and net worth are below the established VA means-test thresholds
6	• Veterans of the Mexican border period or World War I • Veterans seeking care solely for certain conditions associated with exposure to radiation or exposure to herbicides while serving in Vietnam • For any illness associated with combat service in a war after the Gulf War or during a period of hostility after November 11, 1998 • For any illness associated with participation in tests conducted by the Department of Defense (DoD) as part of Project 112/Project SHAD • Veterans with zero percent service-connected disabilities who are receiving disability compensation benefits
7	Nonservice-connected veterans and noncompensable, zero percent service-connected veterans with income above VA's national means-test threshold and below VA's geographic means-test threshold or with income below both the VA national threshold and the VA geographically based threshold, but whose net worth exceeds VA's ceiling ($80,000 in 2006) who agree to make copayments
8	All other nonservice-connected veterans and zero percent, noncompensable service-connected veterans who agree to make copayments. (Note: Effective January 17, 2003, VA no longer enrolls new veterans in priority group 8.)

SOURCE: VA (2006a).

(FY) 2005, more than 160,000 veterans received approximately $700 million for these benefits (VA, 2006b).

Vocational Rehabilitation and Employment Services

VR&E services are provided under Title 38, Chapter 31, by VA's Vocational Rehabilitation and Employment Service. VR&E Service, like the Compensation and Pension (C&P) Service, is part of the Veterans Benefits Administration (VBA). VR&E Service helps veterans with service-connected disabilities prepare for and find jobs within their physical, mental, and emotional capabilities. According to VR&E, strategic goal 1 is to "restore the capability of veterans with disabilities to the greatest extent possible and improve the quality of their lives and that of their families," and objective 1.3 is to "provide all service-disabled veterans with the opportunity to become employable and obtain and maintain employment, while providing special support to veterans with serious employment handicaps" (Steier, 2006).

VR&E services may include

- an evaluation of the individual's abilities, skills, and interests;
- help with resumes and other work readiness assistance;
- help finding and keeping a job;
- vocational counseling and planning;
- on-the-job training and work-experience programs;
- training, such as certificate, two-year, or four-year college or technical programs (including assistance with applications and preparation for preadmission testing);
- supportive rehabilitation services and additional counseling; and
- for veterans whose disabilities are so severe they cannot currently consider employment, a program of services to assist in achieving independence in daily living.[2]

To be eligible for VR&E services, a veteran must have a service-connected disability of at least 20 percent with an employment handicap or at least 10 percent service-connected disability with a serious employment handicap, and be discharged or released from military service under other than dishonorable conditions.[3] Servicemembers pending medical separation

[2]VA's *Compensation and Pension Adjudication Procedure Manual*, M21-1MR, Part 9, Subpart i, Ch. 1, Topic 1; and VA (2006a).

[3]See also VA's *Compensation and Pension Adjudication Procedure Manual*, M21-1MR, Part 9, Subpart i, Ch. 1, Topic 1.

from active duty may also apply if their disabilities are reasonably expected to be rated at least 20 percent following their discharge (VA, 2006a).

According to VA, "The term *employment handicap* means an impairment of the veteran's ability to prepare for, obtain, or retain employment consistent with the veteran's abilities, aptitudes, and interests" (emphasis added). The veteran's service-connected disability "must materially contribute to the impairment," although it does not have to be the sole or even the primary cause of the handicap.[4]

"The term *serious employment handicap* means a significant impairment of a veteran's ability to prepare for, obtain, or retain employment consistent with such veteran's abilities, aptitudes, and interests" (emphasis added). Also, "A veteran who has been found to have an employment handicap shall also be held to have a serious employment handicap if he or she has (1) a neuropsychiatric service-connected disability rated at thirty percent or more disabling; or (2) any other service-connected disability rated at fifty percent or more disabling." The determination of a serious employment handicap is made by a VR&E counseling psychologist.[5]

Veterans rated individually unemployable (IU) because of a service-connected disability may request an evaluation by VR&E and, if entitled, receive rehabilitation services and assistance in securing employment. If the veteran secures employment, the IU rating is protected from reduction for the first 12 months of continuous work. Currently, there is no requirement for people with an IU rating to participate in the VR&E program, although these services are available to any such veteran.

VA pays the cost of VR&E services and pays a subsistence allowance to veterans who participate in a training program. If the training takes place in a college or university, technical school, on-the-job training, or a specialized rehabilitation program (for individuals with severe disabilities), VA pays for tuition, books, supplies, and equipment, and may pay for other special services (e.g., transportation, tutorial assistance, adaptive equipment).[6]

VR&E Service offers a work-study program for veterans training at the three-quarter or full-time rate; this program is available to all veterans, not only those who are service-connected disabled. A portion of the annual work-study reimbursement equal to 40 percent of the total must be paid to the veteran in advance. Veterans in a work-study program may be employed to provide VA outreach services, prepare and process VA paperwork, work at a VA medical facility, or perform other VA-approved activities (VA, 2006a).

[4]38 CFR §21.51.

[5]38 CFR §21.52.

[6]VA's *Compensation and Pension Adjudication Procedure Manual*, M21-1MR, Part 9, Subpart i, Ch. 1, Topic 1.

Generally, veterans must complete a VR&E program within 12 years from their separation from military service, or 12 years from the date VA notifies them that they have a compensable service-connected disability. Veterans may be provided up to 48 months of full-time services or their part-time equivalent, depending on the length of program needed (these limitations may be extended in certain circumstances).[7]

VR&E Task Force

In 2004, the VA VR&E Task Force issued a report about the current VR&E program, based on a two-year study. According to the report,

> In general, the current VR&E service delivery system is out of date, data poor, and understaffed to meet the needs of today's veterans with service-connected disabilities. The current situation raises many questions about how to best serve the needs of these veterans. The Task Force's answers to those questions [are] a new employment-driven service delivery system, integrated services across agencies, and recommendations with implementation timeframes (VA, 2004:60).

The report contained a number of recommendations concerning the VR&E program itself. It also recommended that VA take a broader, integrated approach to helping veterans transition from military to civilian life, by coordinating its health, VR&E, and compensation programs.

According to the report, veterans receive a DoD discharge physical examination or a VA medical exam to support initial C&P disability determinations. However, veterans, when separating from active duty, are not systematically evaluated and given information to make informed career and employment decisions based on their vocational abilities at the time of the initial service-connected disability decision or subsequent disability decisions. If they are rated 20 percent or higher, they are informed of possible eligibility for VR&E services, but it is left to the veteran to initiate an application for services and be evaluated by a counselor.

The task force criticized the current process as a sequence of steps that each veteran must follow in order to receive services, which are unconnected and do not address the unique needs and skills of the individual with respect to his or her environment. In the view of the task force, a more appropriate approach would be one that considers rehabilitation potential based on a combination of education, vocational, and compensation needs together. The task force urged that early functional capacity assessments

---

[7]VA's *Compensation and Pension Adjudication Procedure Manual*, M21-1MR, Part 9, Subpart i, Ch. 1, Topic 1.

be done routinely by vocational experts and used as a basis for making disability compensation as well as vocational rehabilitation decisions. In addition, these evaluations should be repeated at specified intervals to determine the response to intervention or to identify the need for more or different treatment.

To implement its recommendations, the task force recommended the addition of 112 full-time equivalent (FTE) employment counselors in field positions (meaning 2 per field office). As a near-term priority, the task force recommended the design and implementation of pilot formal vocational assessment projects, and suggested that VBA program and technical capabilities be leveraged by colocating the pilot project office with VBA's C&P Examination Program (CPEP) in Nashville.[8] The goal of the recommended pilot projects would be to tailor off-the-shelf technology (systems, knowledge, and protocols for functional capacity evaluation) for VA to implement nationwide. CPEP could use existing electronic processes and infrastructure (e.g., the Compensation and Pension Record Interchange [CAPRI], the Automated Medical Information Exchange [AMIE], and the electronic record system called VistA) combined with electronic templates for functional capacity exams.

Five Tracks to Employment Model

VR&E Service currently uses what it calls the Five Tracks to Employment Model, which focuses on employment goals and on providing veterans with better information to help them make informed choices on employment options (U.S. Congress, House of Representatives, Committee on Veterans' Affairs, 2006). The Five Track Process

> . . . standardizes program orientation practices; integrates veterans, counselors and employment professionals through a comprehensive triage (evaluation) phase; and places the emphasis on employment up front and early on in the rehabilitation process (U.S. Congress, House of Representatives, Veterans' Affairs Subcommittee on Economic Opportunity, 2007:2).

This model encompasses five different rehabilitation plans intended to enable the veteran to find employment in a sustainable, high-level job.

[8]CPEP was established by VHA and VBA in 2001 to improve the quality and timeliness of the disability examination process, as well as veteran satisfaction with disability examinations, through examiner training videos, examination template training CDs, and satellite broadcasts. The program's headquarters are in Nashville.

The tracks include

- reemployment services to help a veteran return to a former civilian job and assistance in understanding rights under the Uniformed Services Employment and Reemployment Act;
- rapid access to employment, which entails assistance in finding a job with government agencies and private corporations that have positions reserved for veterans (e.g., Department of Labor ReaLifeLines, Army Materiel Command, Army Wounded Warrior Program, Marine For Life Injured Support Program, Military Severely Injured/Disabled Operations Center, Home Depot Initiative, YMCA & Armed Forces YMCA Initiative, Helmets to Hardhats Initiative, VA Coming Home to Work Initiative);
- employment through long-term services, such as specialized training and/or education, on-the-job training, apprenticeships, internships, job shadowing, higher education (about 80 percent of veterans in a current VR&E plan to attend college);
- independent living services, including comprehensive in-home assessment, assistive technology, independent living skills training, and connection to community-based support services; and
- self-employment for veterans with limited access to traditional employment and who need flexible work schedules or a more accommodating work environment because of the limitations caused by their disabilities and life circumstances (Steier, 2006). This program is intended primarily for veterans whose businesses collapsed because they were deployed for a period of time. The self-employment track assists the veteran in reestablishing a business through help with developing a business plan, fees and licenses, accounting and legal matters, and start-up supplies and building leases.

A pilot test of the model was successfully completed in FY 2005, and staff training on the new process and tools was completed in FY 2006. Job resource labs are being established in all regional offices, and the VetSuccess.gov website has been developed. In other recent developments, the position of vocational rehabilitation counselor (VRC) was established to combine the former roles of counseling psychologist and vocational rehabilitation specialist, which gave the VRC full responsibility for evaluating, planning, and managing a veteran's program from the beginning through rehabilitation. The position of employment coordinator (72 are currently assigned to 56 regional offices) was established to focus on employment for job-ready veterans in order to incorporate employment readiness, marketing, and placement (U.S. Congress, House of Representatives, Committee on Veterans' Affairs, 2006). Other referral services include medical, dental, optical, mental health treatment, veteran centers, specially adapted housing, vocational/educational counseling, and special hiring authority (Steier, 2006).

In response to written questions submitted at a 2005 congressional hearing on the IU program, the following data on the VR&E program were provided:

- The average number of days from the point of entering the evaluation/planning phase to the determination that the veteran has achieved rehabilitation is 933 days
- The top five occupational categories veterans are rehabilitated into are professional, technical, or managerial; clerical; services; structural (building trades); and machine trades
- The average salary of a suitably employed rehabilitated veteran in FY 2005 was $39,600
- As of September 30, 2005, the VR&E program had a total of 625 vocational rehabilitation counselors and counseling psychologists
- The average workload per counselor was 150 cases
- In FY 2005, 34,038 veterans received favorable VR&E entitlement determinations. Of that number, 25,400 entered a plan of rehabilitation. The rest either decided not to pursue the program at that time or were unable to pursue the program because the extent of their injuries or disabilities made it infeasible for them to obtain their vocational objective (U.S. Congress, Senate, Committee on Veterans' Affairs, 2005).

The Coming Home to Work (CHTW) program recently was established as an expanded outreach effort to provide civilian job skills, exposure to employment opportunities, and work experience for Operation Iraqi Freedom and Operation Enduring Freedom (OIF/OEF) servicemembers and veterans. These individuals work with a vocational rehabilitation counselor to gain work experience in a government facility that supports their career goals. According to testimony, in FY 2007 through the end of January 2007,

- 16 servicemembers are participating in active work experience programs with federal agencies while awaiting discharge or return to duty orders
- 121 servicemembers are receiving early intervention services in preparation for work experience programs, including vocational counseling, testing, and administrative support necessary for successful placement in a work experience program
- 24 servicemembers have returned to active duty following early intervention services
- 108 veterans participating in the CHTW program at a military treatment facility were referred to their local Regional Office for continuation of VR&E services

• 7 veterans have been hired directly by their work experience employers upon discharge from active duty (U.S. Congress, House of Representatives, Veterans' Affairs Subcommittee on Economic Opportunity, 2007:4-5)

As a further step to answer the needs of the OIF/OEF servicemembers and veterans, priority outreach and case management are provided for those who apply to the VR&E program. Vocational rehabilitation and employment case coordinators were recently established in regional offices to assist these individuals in addressing their needs (U.S. Congress, House of Representatives, Veterans' Affairs Subcommittee on Economic Opportunity, 2007).

Joint Efforts

Several joint efforts have been developed in recent years to enhance employment opportunities for veterans with disabilities:

> The VR&E Service has developed working partnerships and signed Memoranda of Understanding (MOU) with Federal, State, and private-sector employers who have agreed to train and hire veterans participating in the VR&E Program. The VR&E Service has also expanded its relationship with faith-based and community-based organizations for careers in a host of not-for-profit employment areas (U.S. Congress, House of Representatives, Veterans' Affairs Subcommittee on Economic Opportunity, 2007:2).

VA collaborates with the Department of Labor (DOL) in its efforts. Through an October 2005 memorandum of understanding, VA and DOL established a partnership in the Department of Labor Veterans' Employment and Training Services (DOL-VETS). A team approach to job development and placement activities is being made to improve vocational outcomes for program participants. Veterans who enter a program of vocational rehabilitation are provided information about this employment assistance through the DOL-VETS program and they are encouraged to register with their state workforce agency.

The services of DOL's Disabled Veterans Outreach Program (DVOP) specialists and the local veterans employment representatives (LVERs) have been combined, and a network of over 3,200 one-stop career centers have been established throughout the United States. VR&E staff in all regional offices and more than 100 outbased offices work with the DVOP specialists and LVERs. Currently, 71 DVOP specialists or LVERs are colocated with VBA staff in 38 VA regional offices and 26 outbased locations, and they share access to VA resources, and collaborate in the production of training resources (U.S. Congress, House of Representatives, Veterans' Affairs Subcommittee on Economic Opportunity, 2007).

Another joint effort with DOL is the Disabled Transition Assistance Program (DTAP), which involves intervening on behalf of servicemembers who may be released because of a disability or who believe they have a disability qualifying them for VR&E services. The DTAP customizes transition information to the needs of veterans with service-connected disabilities and provides assistance to servicemembers in filing applications for VR&E benefits and educational counseling services. In FY 2006, VA conducted 1,462 DTAP briefings with 28,941 participants. FY 2007 figures, through the end of January 2007, were 493 briefings with 9,407 participants (U.S. Congress, House of Representatives, Veterans' Affairs Subcommittee on Economic Opportunity, 2007).

In 2007, VA reported the following improvements in the DTAP program:

- Standardized PowerPoint presentations and a standardized video that provide information on the VR&E program and introduces the Five Track Process. The DTAP presentation is available online at http://www.vetsuccess.gov
- QuickSeries booklet on VR&E benefits and services distributed during DTAP briefings
- 80,000 DTAP CDs distributed to Military Transition Centers in FY 2006
- DTAP oversight visits for quality assurance and best practices
- One-on-one DTAP briefings provided to servicemembers receiving treatment at the Polytrauma SCI Centers
- An updated memorandum of agreement signed on September 19, 2006 between VA, DOL, DoD, and Department of Homeland Security (U.S. Congress, House of Representatives, Veterans' Affairs Subcommittee on Economic Opportunity, 2007:3-4)

A further improvement was the recommendation made by a White House Task Force (Task Force, 2007) and ordered by the President (The White House, 2007) that DoD increase attendance at the Transition Assistance Program (TAP) and DTAP sessions to 85 percent of those separating servicemembers and demobilizing National Guard and Reserve forces. VA and DoD are to ensure that an overview of the TAP program and the benefits and support available from DOL and VA are provided, and that the DTAP presentations include specific information and materials for injured or disabled servicemembers who are being demobilized, deactivated, or discharged. It was also recommended that the spouses of servicemembers of the Global War on Terror (GWOT) be invited to attend to expand the outreach effort. The primary recommendation was made to ensure that these individuals be given the tools to support their transition back into civilian lives (Task Force, 2007).[9]

In May 2005, VA and the National Guard Bureau signed an agreement to enhance access and services to veterans and to share information, and 54 National Guard state benefits advisors who act as statewide points of contact subsequently were trained. To assist VBA in its efforts to contact servicemembers eligible to apply for disability compensation, VA and DoD are collaborating to ensure that VA is notified of servicemembers referred to the physical evaluation board and who may be medically separated or retired. Partnerships with private and not-for-profit sectors are being promoted by VA to provide veterans with early access to competitive career opportunities and training (U.S. Congress, House of Representatives, Committee on Veterans' Affairs, 2006).

Statistics

About one in five veterans who reported receiving service-connected disability compensation also reported that at some point they received VA vocational rehabilitation services. At 14.4 percent, those veterans in military service between the World War II and Korean War eras represent the lowest proportion receiving these services, while those veterans serving in the post-Vietnam era and during the Gulf War received the highest proportions at 24.6 and 23.2 percent, respectively (VA, 2001).

According to the VA FY 2007 budget request, and based on actual 2005 numbers, 22,940 veterans received VR&E rehabilitation, evaluation, planning, and employment services with no monetary benefit payment. The number of veterans who received subsistence allowances was 55,725, for a total cost of about $228.6 million, while 14,038 veterans received benefits for books, tuition, supplies, fees, and other applicable expenses, for a total cost of $335.6 million (VA, 2006b). In summary, 92,703 veterans received services with or without monetary compensation, at a total cost of $564.3 million in compensation.

For the 12 months ending September 30, 2006, VA processed 63,286 VR&E applications, of which 60,084 were deemed eligible and 3,202 were disallowed. The number of IU cases processed for VR&E benefits was 495. Overall, in the 12 months ending August 31, 2006, 11,965 veterans successfully completed their rehabilitation plans and either became

[9]The target date for this outreach recommendation to be enacted is August 30, 2007. It applies to the (1) National Guard and Reserve TAP, (2) Injured/Disabled TAP, (3) Marketing TAP/DTAP, and (4) Turbo TAP. The lead agency is VA; however, the other agencies involved include DoD, DOL, the Department of Education, the Small Business Administration, and the Office of Personnel Management (Task Force, 2007).

employees or entered into independent living arrangements. For this same time period, veterans were provided VR&E services for graduate school (2,117); undergraduate school (43,195); vocational, technical, or nondegree study (3,683); work experience (498); and farm cooperative work-study (8) (Steier, 2006). It is difficult to determine from the data how many veterans successfully completed the program or how many of them subsequently became employed.

It was reported in March 2007 House testimony that there has been improvement in the rehabilitation rate, which is defined as the number of veterans with disabilities who achieve their VR&E goals and are declared rehabilitated compared with the number who discontinue or leave the program before achieving these goals. In FY 2006, 73 percent of program participants were reported to have achieved rehabilitation, while in FY 2007, the rate had risen to over 74 percent. Further, according to this testimony, improvement was seen in the number of days it takes a veteran to begin a program of services intended to lead to suitable employment, which is measured by the days a veteran spends in applicant status. It was reported that veterans spent an average of 54 days in applicant status in FY 2006, and an average of 53 days in FY 2007. Finally, the testimony indicated that in FY 2006, 9,335 veterans had achieved their rehabilitation employment goals, with the top five occupational categories being professional, technical, and managerial careers (6,632 veterans); clerical careers (660); services careers (439); machine trades (349); and building trades (226). VR&E is planning to hire additional staff in FY 2007, which would increase the number of employees to over 100, reduce the number of cases assigned to the counseling staff, and reduce case management workload by approximately 10 percent (U.S. Congress, House of Representatives, Veterans' Affairs Subcommittee on Economic Opportunity, 2007).

According to VA's budget request for FY 2008, the VR&E program constitutes less than 1 percent of the VA budget. In FY 2006, for example, VR&E expenditures were 0.8 percent ($573 million) of the total VA expenditures of $69,809 million, and VA expects this percentage to be about the same in FY 2007 and FY 2008 (VA, 2007).

Observations

The range and quality of the services made available to veterans impressed the committee, as did the potential for very positive outcomes for veterans who take advantage of VR&E services for improving employability, independence, income, and quality of life. On the other hand, the committee noted that relatively few eligible veterans with disabilities apply for VR&E services, and that the confluence of similar benefits could be confusing. Additional concerns raised during committee presentations and deliberations included the validation of the costs expended for the programs and their effectiveness, the insufficient number of trained personnel providing services, the coordination among the various benefits, and the limited benefit for those veterans who may be unmotivated to participate in the various VR&E programs.

Given the potential strong positive impact of VR&E services on a veteran's life, the committee feels VA should address concerns about the program's structure (e.g., interrelatedness of the benefits), socioeconomic reliability, and validity of the tests used to assess potential benefits from VR&E programs. VA should also address personnel issues, as well as seek out ways to encourage and provide incentives for the use of VR&E services by veterans with disabilities.

From a medical standpoint, medical intervention at as early a stage as possible is very important. However, VA's historical approach as far as VR&E services are concerned is that it occurs at a later step in the sequential process; that is, the veteran receives a rating determination and then is informed of his or her eligibility. The VR&E Task Force stated:

> In order for VA to fulfill its mission "to care for him who shall have borne the battle, and for his widow and his orphan," the delivery of vocational employment services for disabled veterans must be changed—and in fact, it must become a totally new program. Previous reforms of the VR&E Program have not been successful. This is due in large measure to the fact that the VR&E Service has been modifying a multi-step, serial process system that is wedded to an outdated, traditional view of vocational rehabilitation that emphasizes veteran training (VA, 2004:5).

Soldiers seriously wounded in Iraq and Afghanistan, who in the past would not have survived their wounds, have survived because of the wider use of improved body armor and protective equipment, better battlefield medical care, and improved evacuation techniques. These veterans, including those with amputations, hearing and vision losses, and other conditions, are returning home and are in need of both medical and vocational attention. Modern medicine and assistive technologies both can improve their health outlook and enable them to find gainful employment of various kinds. According to the task force:

> This sense of urgency has never been more acute than now. VR&E Service is facing a new challenge: the thousands of Guard and Reserve personnel who have been mobilized from their civilian jobs and who will return directly to employment or to college.
>
> Significant numbers of veterans—in war and during peacetime—will continue to experience illnesses or impairments that impact their lives forever. The advances in medical rehabilitation, biomedical technology, rehabilitation engineering, and assistive technology will enable many veterans with

disabilities who were not previously employable to now be employed and for veterans to be employed for longer periods of time after military service than in previous generations (VA, 2004:5).

The Government Accountability Office (GAO) reported:

> More than 10,000 U.S. military servicemembers, including National Guard and Reserve members, have been injured in the conflicts in Afghanistan and Iraq. Those with serious injuries are likely to be discharged from the military and return to civilian life with disabilities. The Department of Veterans Affairs (VA) offers vocational rehabilitation and employment (VR&E) services to help these injured servicemembers in their transition to civilian employment. GAO has noted that early intervention—the provision of rehabilitation services as soon as possible after the onset of a disability—is a practice that significantly facilitates the return to work (GAO, 2005:Summary).

An important part of a VA program shift is a change in focus from employability through education and training to employment services:

> There are also strong indicators pointing to the fact that the current VR&E program, organization, and traditional vocational rehabilitation process are stressed. These signs include high caseloads among the VR&E staff and increasing demand for both vocational rehabilitation training and independent living services. Essential functions of employment readiness, job placement, and marketing are not being performed either adequately or in a standardized way across the system, and veterans are dissatisfied with the current level of employment services (VA, 2004:6).

As an example of possible improvements in VR&E services, the longitudinal study of veterans mentioned by Judith Caden, director of VA's VR&E Service, looks promising, although the results had not been released during the time this report was being prepared:

> In FY 2003, VR&E Service entered into a contract for a longitudinal study of veterans who have been declared rehabilitated upon completing our program. This study will cover the years 1992 to 2002 and provide data in several key areas, such as how many veterans have sustained employment, their current salaries, work stability, educational history prior to disability, length of rehabilitation program, and other demographic information (branch of service, age, etc). The study results, which should be available by the end of FY 2005, are expected to provide VR&E empirical information that can be used to predict participants' potential for successfully completing a program of rehabilitation services (U.S. Congress, House of Representatives, Committee on Veterans' Affairs, 2005:5).

Further, Caden addressed future VR&E initiatives:

> The initiatives we have planned for the coming years will continue to have a positive impact on services to veterans. We are planning joint information technology initiatives with the Education Service that will allow VR&E to utilize existing web-based applications for enrollment verification and certification. We are also developing a formal mentoring program for newly selected VR&E and Assistant VR&E Officers. In addition to the one-on-one mentoring relationship with an established VR&E field manager, the newly selected managers will have an opportunity to learn from VR&E Central Office staff (U.S. Congress, House of Representatives, Committee on Veterans' Affairs, 2005:6).

Responding to the need to improve VR&E services will take a proactive approach that includes early intervention and monitoring of the medical improvements made by those who at first, understandably, were not ready to accept vocational rehabilitation when they returned home. While steps are being taken to facilitate the transition from military service to civilian employment, more remains to be done.

Automobile Assistance

Automobile assistance is a one-time payment of up to a statutory limit (currently $11,000) toward the purchase of a vehicle (e.g., automobile, van, jeep, truck, station wagon) or other conveyance by veterans with certain service-connected disabilities (VA, 2006a).[10] The payment must be made to the seller. To receive automobile assistance, a veteran must have acquired one of the following service-connected disabilities as a result of injury or disease incurred or aggravated during activity military service, or as a result of medical treatment or examination, vocational rehabilitation, or compensated work therapy provided by VA:

- loss, or permanent loss of use, of one or both feet; or
- loss, or permanent loss of use, of one or both hands; or
- permanent impairment of vision in both eyes with a central visual acuity of 20/20 or less in the better eye with corrective glasses, or central visual acuity of more that 20/200 if there is a field defect in which the peripheral field has contracted to such an extent that the widest diameter of visual field has an angular distance no greater than 20 degrees in the better eye; and
- ankylosis (immobility) of one or both knees or one or both hips.

[10]See also 38 CFR § 3.808 and VA's *Compensation and Pension Adjudication Procedure Manual*, M21-1MR, Part 9, Ch. 2. Under 38 U.S.C. 1151, veterans injured while receiving medical care or training and rehabilitation services from VA are eligible as if service connected. Active duty military personnel with these disabilities are also eligible for the automobile and adaptive equipment allowance.

Qualifying disabilities must be incurred or aggravated by service and not under 38 U.S.C. 1151.[11] An additional rating is not required to establish eligibility to either automobile or adaptive equipment (see section below) if a prior rating decision had already established service connection for qualifying disabilities. The rating decisions that initially established service connection for qualifying disabilities should address eligibility for automobile or adaptive equipment even though a specific claim for the benefit has not been filed.[12]

According to the VA FY 2007 budget request, 1,461 veterans received this benefit in FY 2005 at an average cost of $10,784, for a total cost of about $15.8 million (VA, 2006b).

Adaptive Equipment Assistance

Anyone who qualifies for automobile assistance also qualifies for adaptive equipment assistance. To be eligible to receive only adaptive equipment (as opposed to the automobile allowance), the veteran or serviceperson must be entitled to disability compensation for ankylosis of one or both knees or hips based on the establishment of a service connection, or entitlement under 38 U.S.C. 1151 as the result of VA treatment or examination, compensated work therapy,[13] or vocational training under 38 U.S.C. Chapter 31. It must be clear in rating decisions that grant eligibility for this benefit does not include the automobile.[14]

The adaptive equipment benefit may be paid more than once (no limit[15]), and it may be paid to either the seller or the veteran. Repair, replacement, or reinstallation of adaptive equipment may also be required because of the wear and tear caused through use over time and for the safe operation of a vehicle purchased with VA assistance. The adaptive equipment assistance pays for such items as an automatic transmission, power steering, power brakes, power window lifts, hand-operated gas and brake pedals, power seats, and special equipment necessary to assist the veteran in and out of his or her vehicle.[16]

---

[11] Title 38, Part II, Chapter 11, Subchapter VI, § 1151. Benefits for persons disabled by treatment or vocational rehabilitation.

[12] 38 CFR 3.808 and M21-1, Part IX, subpart 1, Ch. 2.

[13] The Veterans Industries/Compensated Work Therapy Program provides a structured environment where clients participate in vocational rehabilitation activities at least 30 hours per week. Clients for this program must have a primary psychiatric or medical diagnosis, be medically stable, and have a goal of competitive employment. http://www1.va.gov/VI-Dayton/page.cfm?pg=2 (accessed May 4, 2007).

[14] 38 CFR 3.808 and M21-1, Part IX, subpart 1, Ch. 2.

[15] 38 CFR 3.808 and M21-1, Part IX, subpart 1, Ch. 2.

[16] The application form (VA Form 21-4502) has a preapproved list of equipment matched with disabilities (e.g., loss of right foot– and left foot–operated gas pedal). Equipment not on the list must be approved by VA.

According to VA's FY 2007 budget request, 8,009 veterans received grants for specially adaptive equipment at an average cost of $4,714, for a total cost of about $37.8 million (VA, 2006b). These numbers were based on 2005 figures.

Specially Adapted Homes

According to the VA FY 2007 budget request, 668 veterans received grants for specially adapted homes at an average cost of $42,259, for a total cost of $28.2 billion (VA, 2006b). These numbers were based on 2005 figures. Before any improvement grant can be approved and before expenditure from the estate can be authorized, real estate must be titled in the veteran's name. Any purchase of real estate by a fiduciary requires court appointment (VBA, 2006).

The grants available to qualified veterans are described below.

$50,000 Grant

Veterans with certain service-connected disabilities are eligible for a grant to assist in building a new specially adapted home or in purchasing an existing home remodeled or modified to meet their disability-related needs (VA, 2006a).[17] VA may approve one-time grants for half the cost of building, buying, or adapting existing homes, or to pay down the mortgage on a previously owned house being adapted, up to $50,000. In some instances, the full grant amount may be applied toward the cost of remodeling. A veteran may qualify if he or she has a permanent and total service-connected condition or conditions that

- preclude locomotion without the aid of braces, crutches, canes, or a wheelchair due to the loss, or loss of use, of both lower extremities; or loss, or loss of use, of one lower extremity together with residuals of organic disease or injury, or one upper extremity, together with one lower extremity, which affects the functions of balance or propulsion;[18]
- result in the loss, or loss of use, of both upper extremities at or above the elbow; or
- cause blindness in both eyes, having only light perception, combined with the loss or loss of use of one lower extremity.

[17]See also 38 U.S.C. 2101(a), 38 CFR § 3.809, and VA's *Compensation and Pension Adjudication Procedure Manual*, M21-1MR, Part 9, Ch. 3.

[18]"Preclude locomotion" as defined by 38 CFR 3.809(d) permits occasional locomotion by other means as long as the use of aids is the *normal* means of locomotion. Thus, a veteran can *occasionally* walk unassisted and still qualify as long as the use of described aids is the *usual* method of locomotion. See 38 CFR 3.808, and M21-1, Part IX, subpart 1, Ch. 2.

$10,000 Grant

VA may approve grants for the actual cost, up to $10,000, for adaptations to a veteran's home or to help a veteran acquire a home already adapted with special features for his or her disability (VA, 2006a).[19] A veteran is eligible when he or she has a permanent and total service-connected condition that is due to blindness in both eyes with 5/200 visual acuity or less, or includes the anatomical loss or loss of use of both hands. This grant may be used in conjunction with the veteran's available loan guaranty entitlement (VBA, 2006).

Supplemental Financing

Veterans with available loan guaranty entitlement may also obtain a VA-guaranteed loan or direct loan to supplement the grant to acquire a specially adapted home. Amounts with a guaranteed loan from a private lender vary; however, the maximum VA direct loan is $33,000 (VA, 2006a).

Special Home Adaptation Grant

This one-time benefit is offered for veterans who do not qualify for special adaptive housing. If the veteran has received the special home adaptation grant and subsequently becomes eligible for the specially adapted homes grant (described above), payment more than once for the same type of adaptation, improvement, or structural alteration is not allowed by law. The grant for up to a maximum of $10,000 is offered for the actual cost of adaptations to a veteran's residence that VA determines as reasonably necessary and may be used in conjunction with the veteran's available loan guaranty entitlement. It may be used to help a veteran acquire a residence already adapted with special features to accommodate his or her disability (VBA, 2006). A veteran who is permanently and totally disabled due to blindness in both eyes with visual acuity of 5/200 or less or the loss or permanent loss of use of both hands may apply.[20]

Clothing Allowance

Veterans are eligible for an annual lump-sum clothing allowance if they have a service-connected disability that requires them to wear or use prosthetics or orthopedic appliances that tend to wear out or tear clothing or if their service-connected disability is due to anatomical loss or loss of use of

[19]See also 38 U.S.C. 2101(a), 38 CFR §3.809, and VA's *Compensation and Pension Adjudication Procedure Manual*, M21-1MR, Part 9, Ch. 3.

[20]38 CFR 3.808 and M21-1, Part IX, subpart 1, Ch. 2.

a hand or foot. VA will also pay a clothing allowance to a veteran if he or she uses medication prescribed by a physician for a service-connected skin condition that causes irreparable damage to the veteran's outer garments (VA, 2006a).[21] According to VA's FY 2007 budget request, 82,074 veterans received this benefit at an average cost of $615.42, for a total cost of $49.2 million (VA, 2006b). These numbers are based on 2005 figures.

TASK FORCE ON RETURNING GLOBAL WAR ON TERROR HEROES

In April 2007, President Bush approved the recommendations made by his Task Force on Returning Global War on Terror Heroes, which was appointed in March 2007 (72 FR 10589, based on Title 3—Executive Order 13426 of March 6, 2007; The White House, 2007; Task Force, 2007). Chaired by the secretary of Veterans Affairs, the membership consisted of the secretaries of Defense, Labor, Health and Human Services, Housing and Urban Development, and Education, and the director of the Office of Management and Budget, the administrator of the Small Business Administration, and the director of the Office of Personnel Management (Task Force, 2007). Regarding the Task Force report, President Bush announced a 45-day deadline for the pertinent agencies to report on the implementation of the recommendations issued by the Task Force:

> Today, Secretary of Veterans Affairs Jim Nicholson and members of the Interagency Task Force on Returning Global War on Terror Heroes released a government-wide action plan that sets out steps to improve our care for America's troops and veterans. The Task Force has proposed specific recommendations to immediately begin addressing the problems and gaps in services that were identified across the veterans and military healthcare systems. These recommendations include directing the Department of Defense and the Department of Veterans Affairs to develop a joint process for disability determination. . . . I commend the work of the Task Force, welcome its recommendations, and have directed Secretary Nicholson to work with all agencies involved in the recommendations and to report back to me within 45 days on how these measures are being implemented (The White House, 2007).

The Task Force made recommendations that could be implemented within agency authority and with existing resource levels, and the focus was

[21] 38 U.S.C. 1162, 38 CFR § 3.810, and VA's *Compensation and Pension Adjudication Procedure Manual*, M21-1MR, Part 9, Ch. 7. Under 38 U.S.C. 1151, veterans injured while receiving medical care or training and rehabilitation services from VA are eligible as if service connected.

on timeliness, ease of application, and efficient delivery of services. The services and benefits currently being provided to GWOT servicemembers were cataloged, and the Task Force found that no written or electronic single repository houses a comprehensive list. The Task Force made 15 process and 10 outreach recommendations (Task Force, 2007).[22]

Of particular interest for this report are Recommendations P-1 (develop a joint process for disability determinations),[23] P-11 (extend vocational rehabilitation evaluation determination time limit),[24] and P-12 (expedite adapted housing and special home adaptation grants claim).[25] The outreach recommendations were made to encourage the inclusion as widely as possible of GWOT servicemembers by making sure they are properly and efficiently notified of services and benefits for which they may qualify (Task Force, 2007).

Recommendation P-11 was formulated to allow a seriously injured GWOT servicemember sustained access to independent living services and to increase his or her ability to benefit from rehabilitation services and allow more time to determine whether he or she will be able to achieve an employment goal. Those severely disabled will have sustained access to independent living services for a period exceeding 12 months until a plan to achieve a suitable vocational rehabilitation goal can be formulated (Task Force, 2007).

Recommendation P-12 requires the specially adapted housing agent to contact the servicemember or veteran within 24 to 48 hours after the rating decision that awards eligibility for the grant is received, such that the grant process can be explained, the individual's immediate interest in using the grant can be determined, and, when appropriate, a face-to-face interview can be scheduled. The Task Force recommended that VA expedite service for GWOT servicemembers and veterans in all stages of the application process by both this more timely contact and frequent communication (Task Force, 2007).

---

[22]These include processes such as interagency disability determination, electronic health-care record sharing, health screenings, health benefits enrollment, care management, coordination of transfers, and assuring continuity of care (Task Force, 2007).

[23]This process was begun on April 3, 2007, and VA was to participate in an advisory council meeting on May 3, 2007; DoD is the lead agency, working with VA to develop an in-depth plan for a VA/DoD collaboration in the Medical Evaluation Board/Physical Evaluation Board (Task Force, 2007).

[24]The target date for this process was April 20, 2007, and allowed for the immediate extension of the 12-month limit on extended evaluation plans. VA is the lead agency.

[25]The target date for this process was April 30, 2007, with VA as the lead agency to develop and disseminate implementation procedures to VBA's field stations.

ISSUES

The VA benefits package for veterans is provided to compensate them for their service to their country and to enable them to better adjust to and function in the civilian world. The myriad benefits offered—including ancillary and special as described earlier in this chapter—and the eligibility requirements for each individually and as interconnected with other benefits in the network create a complex tapestry. The transition for a veteran leaving military service and reentering civilian life can be difficult for a number of reasons, but it is further complicated when a veteran has become disabled in the course of his or her military service. Disability compensation is one part of the benefits package aimed at increasing the ability of veterans to succeed in the civilian world and, if they have impairments, to compensate them for their loss of earning capacity (defined as the average loss of earnings of those with the same degree of impairment). An example of the interconnectedness of disability compensation with additional benefits is that of veterans with disabilities who are assisted by being able to obtain such items as hearing aids, prosthetics, and wheelchairs, and are eligible for automobile and adaptive equipment, a clothing allowance, and continuing medical care and health insurance.

The committee has been asked to consider, from a medical viewpoint, the difficult question of whether the ancillary benefits of vocational rehabilitation, and the automobile, adaptive equipment, housing, and clothing allowances, are appropriate for the conditions the veteran must have to receive them. Although the committee agrees that these benefits and others should be provided to veterans with service-connected disabilities, there are many issues to consider in determining the appropriate thresholds for the entitlements, including

- Should the focus of a benefit be the kind of impairments (e.g., current criteria for automobile benefits and housing) or the individual veteran's specific/actual needs in a given area (e.g., vocational rehabilitation)?
- Is it possible to determine with some degree of accuracy whether the current levels of benefits have improved veterans' medical or vocational outcomes? Without knowing the impact of the current benefits on those veterans receiving them, it is difficult to make judgments about the appropriateness of the current eligibility rules and benefit amounts. In addition, it is difficult to consider whether eligibility rules and benefits amounts should be changed without benchmark information on the efficacy of the current benefits.

To address such issues, it is imperative to have reliable and valid research data in such areas as the realized beneficial effect of the medical and vocational benefits in veterans' quality of life, reentrance into the workforce, and the ability to maintain gainful employment. These data should demonstrate sufficient improvement to support the existence and structure of the programs offered.

The same is true on the issue of the remuneration levels that have been set and how they were determined. Some of the benefits are indexed, while others are not, and some benefits have not been adjusted for many years. Although VA takes a national average approach, consideration should be given to adjusting the rate on a regional basis, taking into account differences in cost of living nationwide. The need for an automatic adjustment for inflation should also be considered, based on rising costs in recent years of owning a home, purchasing an automobile, and purchasing adaptive equipment in homes and automobiles. Reliable data are needed to inform these decisions.

The VR&E benefits are an integral part of the compensation package for many service-connected veterans. However, despite demonstrated improvements in the program in recent years, the current VR&E system was been found to be "out-of date, data poor, and understaffed" by the VA VR&E Task Force (VA, 2004). The task force recommended a new employment-driven service delivery system, integrated services across agencies, and implementation time frames for these specific suggestions. A broader, integrated approach to assist veterans in their transition from military to civilian life was recommended through the coordination of VA's health, VR&E, and compensation programs. An even more individualized approach was suggested by the task force, including

- continuing and systematic medical examinations of veterans for better informed career and employment decisions;
- early, routine functional capacity assessments by vocational experts for both disability compensation and rehabilitation decisions; and
- a change from a sequential series of required steps to a more individualized sequence taking into consideration the person's education, vocational rehabilitation, and compensation needs.

The committee agrees with these recommendations and has formulated other questions as well:

- What is the basis for the 12-year limit on eligibility for vocational rehabilitation services?
- What is the basis for the requirement that a veteran have a service-connected disability rated at 20 percent (if there is an "employment handicap") or a 10 percent rating (if there is a "serious employment handicap") in order to qualify for VR&E services? VR&E services are likely to enable

the veteran with disabilities to engage in substantial and fulfilling gainful employment and improve his or her quality of life. Over the long term, this appears to be a better solution than fostering dependence on the VBA system across the veteran's life span. The committee thus questions the current 20 percent or higher disability threshold for eligibility and encourages consideration of a lower threshold for entitlement to these services.

Again, one must have reliable data to make appropriate judgments. There are also difficult policy issues to be considered:

- Should every veteran be offered vocational rehabilitation, or should the current threshold be lowered, taking into consideration that veterans are reentering a workforce in which desired job qualifications may well have changed from their preservice period, sometimes significantly?
- Currently, VR&E counselors are not involved in determining whether a service-connected veteran is unemployable, but should this approach in the decision-making process change?
- Should age, an issue that has been raised in individual unemployability, be a factor in determining eligibility? Certainly, the cost-benefit ratio is lower (more favorable) for younger veterans who access VR&E services and improve job opportunities over the course of their working life than older veterans who are approaching typical retirement age. Also, with increasing age, individuals are likely to have more medical problems and normal decline in some faculties that may limit employability and ease of returning to a training program. VA should therefore consider age as one of several factors in providing VR&E services, particularly during time periods when resources limit the availability of these services to all veterans with disabilities.

FINDINGS AND RECOMMENDATIONS

The committee supports providing a comprehensive package of benefits for veterans reentering civilian life after serving their country in the military. However, data on the mitigating effects of each type of benefit on functional limitation or work disability or other forms of participation, or on improving quality of life, are lacking. A better approach to assessing the needs of individual veterans is needed, and severity of illness and quality of life should be taken into consideration throughout the processes of determining which benefits are appropriate and how the benefits should be administered.

An assessment of health-care and rehabilitation needs should be performed in conjunction with the assessment of compensation needs, so that veterans will benefit from all services VA provides to help veterans with disabilities succeed in civilian life. These include specialized research and rehabilitation centers for vision impairment, spinal cord injury, traumatic brain injury, polytrauma, and difficult-to-diagnose war-related illnesses. The assessment should also include the need for education, vocational rehabilitation, and other VA ancillary services and benefits, which, together, could enhance a veteran's ability to succeed in civilian life.

The most beneficial time for comprehensively evaluating a veteran's needs for VA services to maximize his or her success in civilian life is at the time of separation from the service, although separating servicemembers might be given a grace period of six months or a year to apply to VA for benefits. With several hundred thousand servicemembers who are leaving the service and applying for VA compensation each year, the workload of evaluating this group alone would be substantial. Accordingly, the recommendation of comprehensive multidisciplinary evaluations is not meant to be retroactive.

Recommendation 6-1. VA and the Department of Defense should conduct a comprehensive multidisciplinary medical, psychosocial, and vocational evaluation of each veteran applying for disability compensation at the time of service separation.

The Task Force indicated that the handling of adapted housing and special home adaptation grants claims needs to be expedited by notifying the returning GWOT applicant within 48 hours of his or her rating decision (Task Force, 2007). A larger issue than the important step of expedited notification is that VA does not systematically assess the needs of veterans or evaluate its ancillary service programs. Many ancillary benefits arose piecemeal, in response to circumstances of the time they were adopted, such as clothing allowances, automobile grants, and adaptive housing. The thresholds that have been set for ancillary benefits requirements were not based on research on who benefits or who benefits most from the services in terms of rating level. Therefore, it is not possible to judge their appropriateness. It is possible that these programs could be changed to serve veterans better or that there are other unaddressed needs.

Recommendation 6-2. VA should sponsor research on ancillary benefits and obtain input from veterans about their needs. Such research could include conducting intervention trials to determine the effectiveness of ancillary services in terms of increased functional capacity and enhanced health-related quality of life.

The President's Task Force recommended that the time limit in the VA VR&E program should be extended from 12 to 18 months to allow additional time for returning servicemembers to better understand their rehabilitation needs:

> VA Vocational Rehabilitation and Employment Service (VR&E) will authorize the immediate extension, to 18 months, for an Individualized Extended Evaluation Plan (IEEP) for those OIF/OEF participants whose severity of injuries warrant additional time to make the determination of current feasibility of achieving an employment goal while continuing to provide independent living services (Task Force, 2007:2).

While this time extension is applauded, the committee must point out another important aspect of rehabilitation policy that should be considered. The current 12-year limit on eligibility for vocational rehabilitation services is a policy decision with no medical basis, although there may be administrative convenience or fiscal control reasons. There are types of employment and training requirements that do not realistically adhere to a 12-year deadline. For example, emerging assistive and workplace technologies (e.g., computing) may provide training or retraining opportunities for veterans with disabilities through continuing education of various kinds. New types of work may also emerge for which veterans with disabilities could be trained. Advancements in medical knowledge and breakthroughs in medical technology also do not abide by a 12-year limit.

Recommendation 6-3. The concept underlying the extant 12-year limitation for vocational rehabilitation for service-connected veterans should be reviewed and, when appropriate, revised on the basis of current employment data, functional requirements, and individual vocational rehabilitation and medical needs.

The percentage of entitled veterans applying for VR&E services is relatively low. In FY 2005, about 40,000 veterans applied for VR&E services and were accepted. About 160,000 veterans began receiving benefits for service-connected disabilities that year, but the pool of those potentially eligible is much larger. Of those deemed eligible, between a quarter and a third have not completed the program in recent years. VA should explore ways to increase participation in this program.

Recommendation 6-4. VA should develop and test incentive models that would promote vocational rehabilitation and return to gainful employment among veterans for whom this is a realistic goal.

REFERENCES

GAO (Government Accountability Office). 2005. *Vocational rehabilitation: More VA and DOD collaboration needed to expedite services for seriously injured servicemembers.* GAO-05-167. http://www.gao.gov/new.items/d05167.pdf (accessed March 6, 2007).

Steier, F. 2006. *Vocational Rehabilitation & Employment Service.* Presentation to the IOM Committee on Medical Evaluation of Veterans for Disability Compensation, Washington, DC, September 21.

Task Force (Task Force on Returning Global War on Terror Heroes). 2007. *Task force report to the President: Returning global war on terror heroes.* Washington, DC: Task Force. http://www1.va.gov/task/force/docs/GWOT_TF_Report_042407.pdf (accessed April 25, 2007).

The White House. 2007. Statement by the President, April 24. Washington, DC: Office of the Press Secretary. http://www.whitehouse.gov/news/releases/2007/04/20070424-12.html# (accessed April 25, 2007).

U.S. Congress, House of Representatives, Veterans' Affairs Subcommittee on Economic Opportunity. 2007. *Statement of Bill Borom, Deputy Director, Vocational Rehabilitation and Employment Service, VA.* 110th Cong., 1st Sess., March 7. http://veterans.house.gov/hearings/schedule110/mar07/03-07-07/BillBorom.pdf (accessed May 2, 2007).

U.S. Congress, House of Representatives, Committee on Veterans' Affairs. 2006. *Statement of Gordon H. Mansfield, Deputy Secretary, VA.* 109th Cong., 2nd Sess., December 7. http://www.va.gov/OCA/testimony/hvac/seo/061207GM.asp (accessed May 4, 2007).

U.S. Congress, House of Representatives, Committee on Veterans' Affairs. 2005. *Statement of Judith Caden, Director, Vocational Rehabilitation and Employment Service, VA.* 109th Cong., 1st Sess., April 20. http://veterans.house.gov/ hearings/schedule109/apr05/4-20-05e/jcaden.pdf (accessed March 6, 2007).

U.S. Congress, Senate, Committee on Veterans' Affairs. 2005. *Statement of Daniel Cooper, Under Secretary for Benefits, VA.* 109th Cong., 1st Sess., October 27. http://www.va.gov/OCA/testimony/svac/05102720.asp (accessed May 4, 2007).

VA (Department of Veterans Affairs). 2001. *2001 National Survey of Veterans: Final report.* Washington, DC: Department of Veterans Affairs. http://www.va.gov/vetdata/docs/NSV%20Final%20Report.pdf (accessed June 22, 2007).

VA. 2004. *The Vocational Rehabilitation and Employment Program for the 21st century veteran: Report to the Secretary of Veterans Affairs.* Washington, DC: Vocational Rehabilitation and Employment Task Force. http://www.va.gov/op3/docs/VRE Report.pdf (accessed December 8, 2006).

VA. 2006a. *Federal benefits for veterans and dependents, 2006 edition.* Washington, DC: VA. http://www.va.gov/opa/vadocs/fedben.pdf (accessed December 8, 2006).

VA. 2006b. *FY 2006 congressional submission, summary, volume 4.* Washington, DC: VA. http://www.va.gov/budget/summary/HTML/ html_files/chapter_1.html (accessed December 8, 2006).

VA. 2007. *Department of Veterans Affairs, budget of the United States government: Fiscal year 2008.* http://www.gpoaccess/usbudget/fy08/pdf/budget/veterans.pdf (accessed March 6, 2007).

VBA (Veterans Benefits Administration). 2006. *Chapter 4: Reviewing entitlements.* LIE Program Guide. http://www.warms.vba.va.gov/admin21/guide/lie/ch04.doc (accessed May 4, 2007).

7

Individual Unemployability

"Individual unemployability," or IU, is a way for the Department of Veterans Affairs (VA) to compensate veterans at the 100 percent rate who are unable to work because of their service-connected disability, although their rating according to VA's Schedule for Rating Disabilities (Rating Schedule) does not reach 100 percent. IU is based on an evaluation of the individual veteran's capacity to engage in a substantially gainful occupation, which is defined as the inability to earn more than the federal poverty level, or about $10,000 a year, rather than on the schedular evaluation, which is based on the average impairment of earnings concept. IU takes occupational as well as medical factors into account. Age is expressly prohibited as a consideration, meaning that veterans beyond the normal age of retirement may secure benefits under the provisions of IU. The effects of nonservice-connected disabilities also are prohibited as a consideration.

BACKGROUND

IU is a fast-growing part of the disability compensation program. The number of recipients has increased from about 112,400 veterans in FY 2000 to about 228,500 in FY 2006, or 103 percent.[1] The overall number of veterans receiving any form of disability compensation increased by about 16 percent over the same period. At the end of FY 2006, 8.5 percent

[1]Figures from the VA FY 2008 budget request, pp. 2A1-2A12. http://www.va.gov/budget/summary/VolumeIINationalCemeteryAdministrationBenefitsProgramsandDepartmentalAdmin.pdf (accessed May 8, 2007).

of veterans receiving compensation were rated IU, compared with 4.9 percent at the end of FY 2000.

By service era, the largest group receiving IU is Vietnam veterans (113,956 in FY 2005, or 52 percent), followed by peacetime veterans (36,383, or 16.4 percent), and World War II veterans (36,153, or 16.3 percent). See Figure 7-1.

Currently, according to the Veterans Benefits Administration (VBA), 35 percent of IU beneficiaries have mental health conditions as their major diagnosis (of which more than two-thirds are posttraumatic stress disorder [PTSD] diagnoses), followed by musculoskeletal conditions (29 percent), and cardiovascular conditions (13 percent) (Flohr, 2006).

According to the Government Accountability Office (GAO), at the end of FY 2005, about 38 percent of all IU beneficiaries were age 65 or older, 13 percent were between the ages of 60 and 64, and 49 percent were age 59 or younger. Forty-six percent of those who were granted IU benefits from October 2004 to October 2005 were age 60 or older, and 19 percent were age 75 or older (for comparison, 46 percent of all living veterans are age 60 or older and 16 percent are age 75 or older) (GAO, 2006).

The VA Office of Inspector General reports that the rate of IU grants varies substantially by state. In FY 2004, veterans receiving compensation who were rated IU ranged from a low of 3.3 percent to a high of 20.1 percent (median of 7.6 percent) among the states. In terms of all resident veterans, not only veterans with disabilities, IU beneficiaries ranged across the states from 2.5 per thousand veterans to 28.2 per thousand (median of 7.8 per thousand) (VA, 2005).

Congress held hearings on IU in 2005, out of concern about the growth in the number of beneficiaries and the advanced age of many of them.

DEFINITION OF INDIVIDUAL UNEMPLOYABILITY

IU is regulatory, not statutory. The key section of the regulation reads:

> Total disability ratings for compensation may be assigned, where the schedular rating is less than total, when the disabled person is, in the judgment of the rating agency, unable to secure or follow a substantially gainful occupation as a result of service-connected disabilities. Provided that, if there is only one such disability, this disability shall be ratable at 60 percent or more, and that, if there are two or more disabilities, there shall be at least one disability ratable at 40 percent or more, and sufficient additional disability to bring the combined rating to 70 percent or more.[2]

---

[2] 38 CFR § 4.16a.

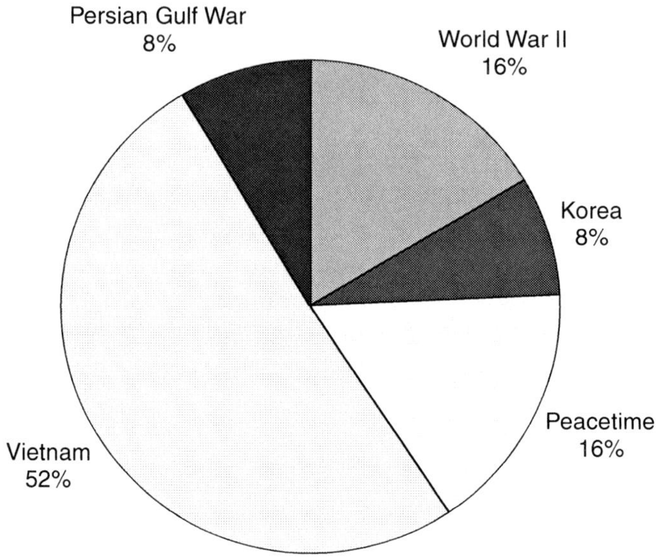

FIGURE 7-1 IU beneficiaries by period of service, FY 2006.
SOURCES: Computer Output Identification Number Control Point 501 for IU; and FY 2005 Performance and Accountability Report for all beneficiaries.

The regulation goes on to say: "Marginal employment shall not be considered substantially gainful employment" and defines marginal employment as earned income that does not exceed the poverty threshold for one person established by the Bureau of the Census. In certain circumstances, such as the protected environment provided by a family business or sheltered workshop, the veteran with higher earnings may be considered for IU by the director of the Compensation and Pension (C&P) Service.

If a veteran is rated 100 percent according to the medical criteria in the Rating Schedule, IU is not considered because, VA has reasoned, it is not needed. There is an advantage for the veteran in being rated 100 percent according to the Rating Schedule rather than extraschedularly for IU: a schedular 100 percent rating allows the veteran to engage in substantially gainful employment, while an extraschedular 100 percent rating based on IU does not.

If a rater finds that a veteran is unable to secure and follow a substantially gainful occupation because of his or her service-connected disability, but the veteran does not meet the minimum rating level of 60 percent for one disability or 70 percent for multiple disabilities, one of which is 40 percent, the case may be submitted to the director of the C&P Service to decide whether to grant an extraschedular 100 percent rating.[3]

ORIGIN AND HISTORY OF INDIVIDUAL UNEMPLOYABILITY

Authorization for IU was added to the 1933 Rating Schedule in 1934. Previously, the Rating Schedule said that total disability exists when any impairment makes it impossible for the average person to follow a substantially gainful occupation. The 1934 revision of the regulations authorized total disability ratings "without regard to the specific provisions of the rating schedule" if a veteran with disabilities is unable to secure or follow a substantially gainful occupation as a result of his disabilities (U.S. Congress, Senate, Committee on Veterans' Affairs, 2005).[4]

At that time, the ratings were determined by three-member rating boards consisting of a medical specialist, a legal specialist, and an occupational specialist (Griffith, 1945). Currently, the decision is made by a rating veterans service representative (RVSR), based on medical records, usually including a C&P disability examination by a physician or psychologist, and possibly including a "social and industrial" (occupational) evaluation by a VA clinical social worker. The RVSR, although a lay person, has medical and legal training, but not vocational training.

PROCEDURES FOR DETERMINING INDIVIDUAL UNEMPLOYABILITY

Before even considering IU, the veteran is evaluated for a schedular 100 percent evaluation. If he or she is evaluated at 100 percent according to the Rating Schedule, any pending IU claim is disregarded.

A veteran must be unable to secure or retain employment by reason of service-connected disability and either meet the requirements of 38 CFR 4.16 or have an extraschedular evaluation approved by the under secretary for benefits or the director of the C&P Service under 38 CFR 3.321.[5]

The requirements of 38 CFR 4.16 are such that, if there is only one service-connected disability, it must be rated at 60 percent or more; if there are two or more, one must be 40 percent or more, and the combined rating must be 70 percent or more.[6] According to 38 CFR 3.321, the under secretary for benefits or the director of the C&P Service may grant higher

[3]38 CFR § 4.16b.

[4]Originally, the veteran had to have a single 70 percent evaluation or a combined evaluation of 80 percent, with one disability rated at 60 percent or higher. The standard was changed to the current 60 or 70 percent with one 40 percent disability in 1941.

[5]38 CFR 4.16(b).

[6]38 CFR 4.16(a).

compensation, including total disability (100 percent), than the Rating Schedule allows in "exceptional" cases. "The governing norm in these exceptional ["extraschedular"] cases is: A finding that the case presents such an exceptional or unusual disability picture with such related factors as marked interference with employment or frequent periods of hospitalization as to render impractical the application of the regular schedular standards."[7]

When deciding an IU claim, the rater is supposed to take into account the veteran's current physical and mental condition and his or her employment status, including the nature of employment, and the reason employment was terminated.[8]

The claim must contain sufficient medical evidence to evaluate the veteran's current physical and mental condition. This evidence includes (but is not limited to) the results of VA examinations, hospital reports, and/or outpatient records. RVSRs are instructed to schedule a medical examination if the veteran's medical evidence is incomplete or inconsistent.

Regarding the nature of the veteran's previous employment and the reason for termination, RVSRs are instructed to review employment and work history for the five-year period preceding the date on which the claimant reports that he or she has become too disabled to work, as well as any work performed after this date.[9] Each employer for whom the veteran worked during the 12-month period prior to the date the veteran last worked must complete a form as well.[10] If an employer's form is incomplete (e.g., only states that the veteran retired), raters must request additional information about the nature of the retirement (e.g., whether retirement was due to disability and, if so, the nature of the disability). Instructions to the raters about determining the cause of unemployment and the circumstances surrounding a veteran's retirement imply that IU should not be granted if the veteran retired from the workforce for reasons other than disability, but this is not clearly stated in the regulations, adjudication manual, or training materials.

Social Security Administration reports are supposed to be obtained and considered if the veteran's evidence is insufficient to award compensation and shows that he or she receives Social Security disability benefits. Vocational rehabilitation records may be obtained and considered whenever

---

[7]38 CFR 3.321.

[8]VA's *Compensation and Pension Adjudication Procedure Manual*, M21-1MR, Part IV, Subpart ii, Ch. 2. http://www.warms.vba.va.gov/admin21/m21_1/mr/part4/subptii/ch02/ch02_secf.doc (accessed March 15, 2007).

[9]VA Form 21-8940, "Veteran's Application for Increased Compensation Based on Unemployability."

[10]VA Form 21-4192, "Request for Employment Information in Connection with Claim for Disability Benefits."

there is an indication that training was not found to be medically feasible or a veteran's attempt to be trained was unsuccessful.

RVSRs are instructed *not* to apply the concept of average impairment used in other compensation decisions to IU decisions.

"Extraneous" factors, such as age, nonservice-connected disabilities, injuries occurring after military service, availability of work, or voluntary withdrawal from the market are supposed to be identified and isolated to determine the severity of the service-connected conditions. The severity of service-connected disabilities alone must be enough to preclude the veteran from obtaining or retaining substantially gainful employment.

Certain multiple disabilities may be considered as one disability for the purpose of meeting the 38 CFR 4.16(a) requirements of a 60 percent rating of one condition or 70 percent combined rating with one condition rated at 40 percent or higher. These include (1) disabilities of one or both upper extremities, including the bilateral factor, if applicable; (2) disabilities resulting from common etiology or a single accident; (3) disabilities affecting a single body system, such as orthopedic, digestive, respiratory, cardiovascular-renal, or neuropsychiatric; (4) multiple injuries incurred in action; or (5) multiple disabilities incurred as a prisoner of war.

Marginal employment, defined by VA as earned annual income below the poverty level (or if above the poverty level, employment in a protected environment, such as a sheltered workshop or family business), is not to be considered substantially gainful employment.

The focus of an IU claim record is on the accumulation of medical information, and raters are not required to have vocational records. However, if a veteran's records indicate that he or she is participating in VA's Vocational Rehabilitation and Employment (VR&E) program, the rater is required to obtain the VR&E records and use them in the IU evaluation.[11] Whether vocational records from other sources may be considered is not indicated.

Reevaluation of IU Entitlement

To verify continued eligibility for IU benefits, all IU recipients must complete annual employment certification forms describing work performed in the preceding year for each year they are receiving IU benefits. A veteran is permitted to work and engage in substantially gainful employment for up to 12 months. If a veteran engages in substantially gainful employment beyond 12 months or if a veteran fails to return his or her employment

[11] "Regional Office Handling of Individual Unemployability Claims," VBA Training Letter 07-01, February 21, 2007.

certification form, monthly payments are reduced to amounts corresponding with the schedular rating.

VA'S PROPOSAL TO REVISE AND CODIFY THE INDIVIDUAL UNEMPLOYABILITY REGULATIONS

In October 2001, VA published a Notice of Proposed Rulemaking (NPRM), which was a draft of a totally rewritten set of regulations governing IU. According to the NPRM, the draft regulations would "revise and clarify the procedures and substantive standards for determining whether a veteran's disabilities . . . prevent him or her from engaging in substantially gainful employment."[12] The goal of the revision was to address the "scattered and confusing" set of current regulations by creating better-defined and more clearly stated specific requirements for this entitlement along with clearer standards.

The revision proposed a number of changes throughout sections 4.15–4.18 of the regulations. These included streamlined terminology, elimination of redundancy and unnecessary material, definition of terms, and outlining of specific requirements. Proposed changes included the following:

- Reorganize and rewrite to specify the factors that would trigger consideration of IU rating and total "extraschedular" ratings
- Reduce the percentage threshold for combined ratings from 70 to 60 percent and eliminate the requirement that one of the disabilities must be rated at least 40 percent
- Create a uniform standard to determine an individual's inability to engage in "substantially gainful employment," instead of using as a basis for the determination a presumption of helplessness or bedridden status
- Define "substantially gainful employment" as any work that is generally done for pay or profit that the veteran is able to perform with sufficient regularity and duration to provide a reliable source of income
- Clarify that an assessment of the veteran's ability to perform activities generally considered necessary for "substantially gainful employment" would be the determining factor in assigning a total rating
- In response to *Moore* v. *Derwinski*, require raters to consider medical evidence describing the veteran's service-connected disabilities and the extent to which they limit his or her ability to perform "activities normally required for substantially gainful employment," meaning both exertional

[12]66 FR 49886, October 1, 2001, "Total Disability Ratings Based on Inability of the Individual to Engage in Substantially Gainful Employment (Proposed Rule)," withdrawn December 23, 2005.

and nonexertional activities that as a group affect the ability to engage in any form of employment[13]

- Clarify that if a veteran is employed, earned income that exceeds an amount that is more than twice the maximum annual pension rate for a veteran without dependents will be considered conclusive evidence that the veteran is engaged in substantially gainful employment
- Eliminate the concept of "marginal employment," an individual unemployability eligibility criterion defined by VA as earned annual income below the poverty level, or if above the poverty level, employment in a protected environment such as a sheltered workshop or family business
- Provide a list of specific factors that the rater must address in every claim for a total rating for compensation purposes
- Require the rater to consider evidence of any other unusual limitations imposed by the service-connected disability (e.g., uncharacteristically frequent periods of hospitalization)
- Include a list of factors that VA would disregard in determining entitlement, including age, nonservice-connected disabilities, the veteran's training or lack thereof unless service-connected disabilities would impede further training, the state of the economy in the veteran's community, and the fact that prior employment may have been terminated because of such factors as employer relocation or technological advances that make a prior job obsolete
- VA should state that it will consider age, occupational background, training, and education only to the extent that they limit further training and adaptation

A number of external and VA internal comments were received during the open comment period. Common themes were the questioning of VA's approach to making determinations based solely on "medical evidence" (excluding "lay evidence"); the inclusive and exclusive nature of percentage ratings and related extraschedular issues; the discussion of vocational rehabilitation issues relative to the consideration of benefits granted or denied based on age; the quality and appropriateness of evaluations; training or lack thereof; availability and types of work allowed and disallowed; regularity and duration of periods of work; alternate employment following surgery and during and after convalescence; and the ability or inability to continue working faced with the exigencies of managing disability.

The NPRM was rescinded on December 23, 2005. The reason given in the *Federal Register* was

---

[13]*Moore* v. *Derwinski*, 1 Vet. App. 356, 359 (1991).

> The VA has carefully considered the issues relating to the payment of benefits under the proposed rule and determined that it does not accomplish the stated purpose or intended effect. Accordingly, VA is withdrawing the proposal and is developing a new proposal, which it intends to publish at a later date.[14]

CURRENT STATUS OF INDIVIDUAL UNEMPLOYABILITY: GROWTH AND CONTROVERSY

In May 2005, the VA Office of Inspector General issued a report on state variances in VA disability compensation payments (VA, 2005). This report was in response to congressional interest in the reason for differences in VA's average monthly disability compensation payments from state to state. VA's inspector general selected two clusters of states, one representing the six states with the highest average compensation payments and the other representing the six states with the lowest payments. Among other data methods used, the office issued a questionnaire to 1,992 VA regional office rating specialists, evaluated 2,100 PTSD claims folders, and reviewed the quality and consistency of medical examinations used to support disability rating decisions.

PTSD constitutes the second largest percentage of compensation grants after musculoskeletal conditions and the largest for any specific diagnosis. It is also one of the fastest growing disability conditions. The data showed that the variance in the number of PTSD cases rated at 100 percent is a primary factor contributing to the variance in average annual compensation payments by state. Another factor was the percentage of veterans with disabilities rated for IU. From FY 1999 to FY 2004, the number of veterans receiving IU benefits had more than doubled, from 95,052 to 196,916. One quarter (53,390) of the IU cases in FY 2004 were PTSD cases. The high-state cluster averaged 14.3 percent of veterans with IU compared with 5.4 percent in the low-state cluster.

In October 2005, the Senate Committee on Veterans' Affairs held a hearing on individual unemployability (U.S. Congress, Committee on Veterans' Affairs, 2005). Senator Craig, the chairman, requested the hearing to determine what was being done to ensure that today's veterans with disabilities are able to become productive members of society. He indicated a concern about the 107 percent increase in IU beneficiaries between 1999 and 2004, which in his view is an undesirable life circumstance, one of last resort for all except those for whom it is clearly appropriate.

According to the senator, the purpose of the congressional inquiry was to establish an understanding of the purpose of IU and the standard VA

[14]70 FR 76221, December 23, 2005.

uses in determining a veteran's eligibility. He mentioned a particular concern about the age of IU beneficiaries, based on the fact that a fair number of IU recipients are well beyond traditional retirement ages. He posed the following question:

> Why is a benefit based on unemployability being paid to individuals who, on account of age, would likely not be looking for work anyway? In other words, they are at retirement age by even today's modern terms (U.S. Congress, Senate, Committee on Veterans' Affairs, 2005).

Admiral Daniel Cooper, VA undersecretary for benefits, testified that there is no clear reason for the doubling of IU beneficiaries. However, he pointed out concurrent significant changes:

- From the end of FY 1999 to the end of FY 2005, the number of veterans receiving compensation had increased by 17 percent from 2,252,980 to 2,636,979 at the end of fiscal year 2005
- There was an increase in the average combined disability over the same period
- At the end of 2005, 29 percent of veterans receiving compensation had combined ratings of 60 percent or greater, which makes them eligible to apply for IU, compared with 17 percent in 1999
- Recent court decisions had also increased IU ratings[15]
- Advancing age, diabetes, and various presumptions of service connection for cancers associated with herbicide and radiation, as well as a significant increase in the number of veterans awarded service connection for PTSD, accounted for a substantial portion of the increase

Richard Surratt, deputy national legislative director of the Disabled American Veterans, testified that the increase of veterans rated for IU over the past several years was somewhat consistent with the higher numbers of veterans in the population who are more seriously disabled. From FY 2000 to FY 2004, the number of veterans with 60 percent ratings increased by 31 percent; veterans rated 70 percent increased by 60 percent; veterans rated 80 percent increased by 75 percent; and veterans rated 90 percent increased by 91 percent. During the same period, there was an increase of 78 percent of veterans rated totally disabled due to IU. He added that an aging veteran population also may contribute to increased numbers of unemployable veterans, including those with progressive or degenerative conditions worsening with age and Vietnam veterans with disabilities whose disabilities are on average rated higher than their counterparts from other periods of service, and who had an estimated median age of

[15]*Norris* v. *West*, 12 Vet. App. 304, March 30, 1999.

57.4 years at the end of FY 2004. Mr. Surratt also cited the contribution of PTSD prevalence among Vietnam veterans (the second most prevalent disability for this group) and the availability of judicial review of VA decisions as contributing factors to the expanding number of IU beneficiaries.

Mr. Surratt expressed the view that VA should look at the medical and employment evidence and any available relevant records from the VR&E Service and the Social Security Administration to create an adequately developed record in evaluating individual unemployability.

Admiral Cooper was asked a number of questions about apparently controversial issues: vocational rehabilitation (in its many aspects, including follow-up health care), the ages of beneficiaries and related matters, and PTSD (including VA's decision to conduct a review of PTSD decisions and the attendant workload). For example, he was asked whether trained vocational counselors should be performing IU assessments rather than medical examiners, whether advanced age (31 percent of the recipients of the IU benefits were over the age of 71) should not preclude the receipt of IU benefits, and why periodic future examinations are not requested if an IU recipient is over age 55. Senator Craig stated a general sense that the system to help veterans return to productivity is less emphasized than the granting of benefits. Admiral Cooper indicated that he did not completely agree with this view, stating that both younger and older veterans at retirement age are encouraged to participate in vocational rehabilitation.

In May 2006, GAO issued an IU report that found that VA's process for ensuring ongoing eligibility of beneficiaries is inefficient and ineffective, and relies on old data, has outdated and time-consuming manual procedures, offers insufficient guidance, and provides weak eligibility criteria (GAO, 2006). Further, enforcement activities are not tracked and reviewed to better ensure their effectiveness. GAO found VA to be among the high-risk federal disability programs in need of modernization, including the compensation program, because it had not kept up with trends in science, technology, and medicine, and in the labor market.

CONSISTENCY IN INDIVIDUAL UNEMPLOYABILITY DECISION MAKING

The 2005 report of VA's Office of Inspector General focused on the variation in average disability compensation payments from state to state in FY 2004 (they ranged from a low of $6,961 to a high of $12,004), but data tables in the report's appendix include the number of IU beneficiaries in each state. An analysis of these data shows that the percentage of veterans receiving compensation in FY 2004 who were rated for IU ranged from a low of 3.3 percent in Maryland to a high of 20.1 percent in New Mexico (median state 7.6 percent) (Figure 7-2). In terms of all resident veterans, not

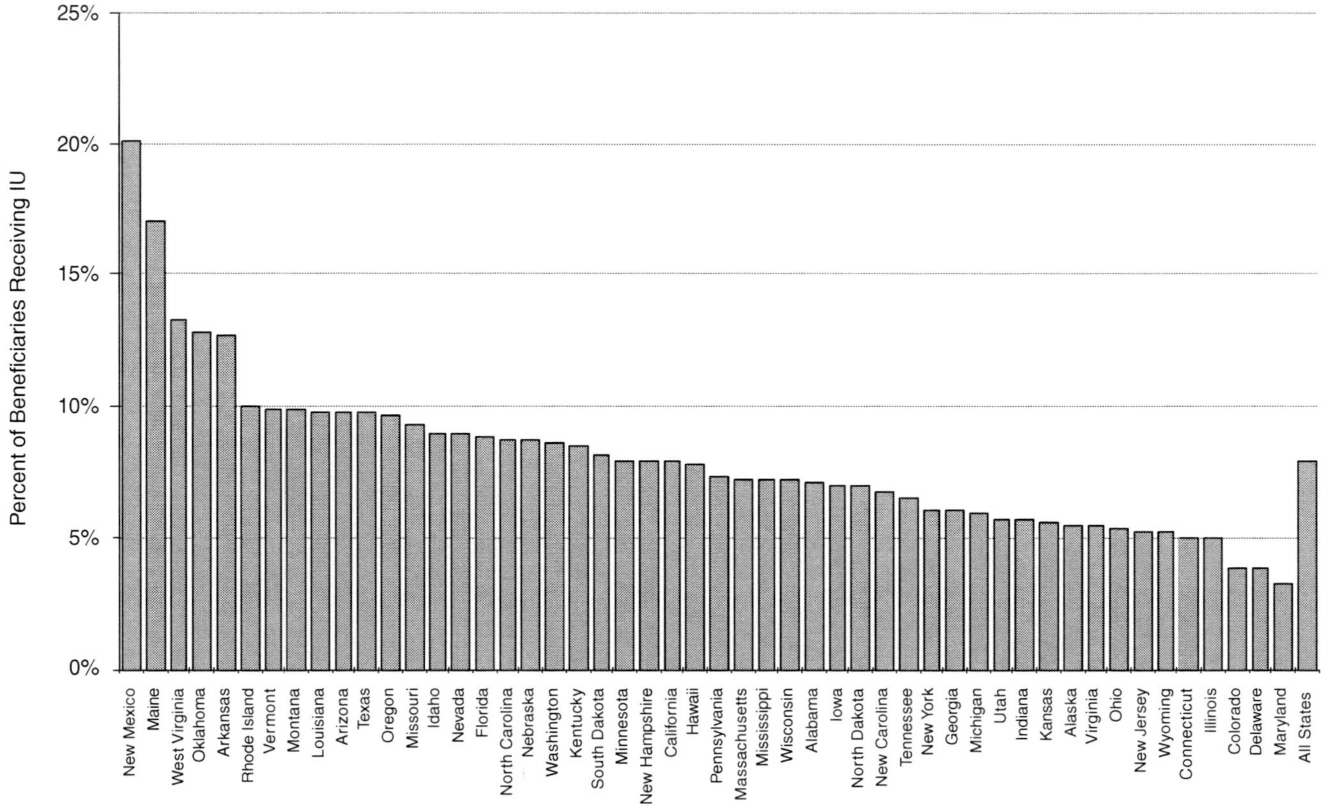

FIGURE 7-2 Number of IU beneficiaries as percentage of veterans receiving disability compensation, by state, FY 2004.
SOURCE: VA (2005:Appendix D, Table 21).

just veterans with disabilities, IU beneficiaries ranged from 2.5 per thousand veterans in Maryland to 28.2 per thousand in New Mexico (median state 7.8 per thousand) (Figure 7-3).

VA RESPONSES

There is evidence that VA is taking steps to address concerns regarding inconsistencies in IU claims processing and the large number of IU recipients of advanced age. On February 21, 2007, the director of the C&P Service issued a training letter to all regional offices and centers handling IU claims. According to the cover memo, the purpose of the letter was to "promote consistency and accuracy in the identification, development, and evaluation of claims for individual unemployability by regional offices." The letter states in its introductory paragraph:

> Benefits granted under the VA Rating Schedule are intended to compensate veterans for the average impairment in earning capacity that results from service-connected disease or injury. IU is a special additional benefit to address the truly unique disability picture of a veteran who is unemployable due to service-connected disability, but for whom the application of the Rating Schedule does not fully reflect the veteran's level of impairment. An award of IU allows the veteran to receive compensation at a rate equivalent to that of a 100 percent schedular award. However, this benefit is not intended, by regulation or policy, to be a quasi-automatic benefit granted whenever a veteran has met a qualifying schedular evaluation or reached an advanced age.[16]

Raters are reminded to consider IU *only in exceptional cases* (emphasis added), and to first determine whether a veteran's disabilities warrant a 100 percent schedular evaluation before considering entitlement to IU.

Regarding age as a factor in IU decision making, the letter states that advanced age (not defined) may relate to voluntary retirement, rather than disability, and that voluntary retirement does not necessarily equate with unemployability. Because of this fact, for IU claims submitted by veterans of advanced age, raters are instructed to take care in distinguishing worsened disability that would have caused unemployability from unemployment due to voluntary retirement. Raters are also instructed to discuss age in their explanation of how the available evidence was evaluated to arrive at the decision to grant or deny IU.

The training letter also elaborates on several of the procedures for identifying and evaluating IU claims (e.g., passive versus active application,

[16]"Regional Office Handling of Individual Unemployability Claims," VBA Training Letter 07-01, February 21, 2007.

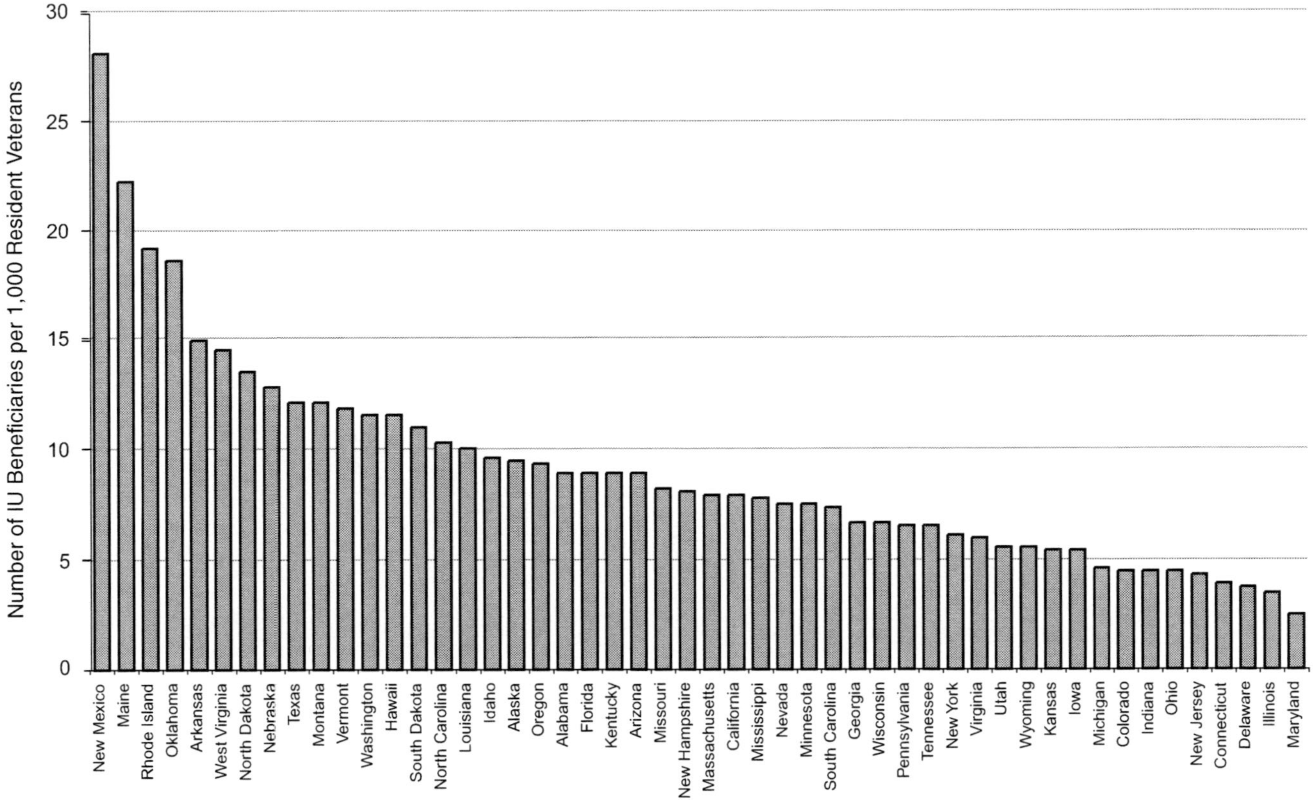

FIGURE 7-3 Number of IU beneficiaries per 1,000 resident veterans, by state, FY 2004.
SOURCE: VA (2005:Appendix D, Table 21).

requirements for continued eligibility), only tersely described in the VBA rating training manual and the *Code of Federal Regulations*.

Perhaps in response to concerns highlighted in the May 2006 GAO report on the number of IU recipients of advanced age, VBA data show that the number of decisions (meaning both grants and denials) on IU claims for veterans ages 70 and older fell from 14,554 in 2004 to 8,897 in 2006. Meanwhile, for all other age groups, the number of IU decisions increased (Figure 7-4).

With the exception of veterans ages 50 and younger, the percentage of IU claims granted fell for all age groups between 2004 and 2006 (Figure 7-5). The largest drop in grants was among applicants ages 70 and older; the percentage granted IU fell from 68.6 percent in 2004 to 42.6 percent in 2006.

FINDINGS AND RECOMMENDATIONS

Vocational Assessment in IU Evaluation

Raters use disability evaluation reports from medical professionals and other medical records to analyze IU claims, but they do not have comparable functional capacity or vocational evaluations from vocational experts

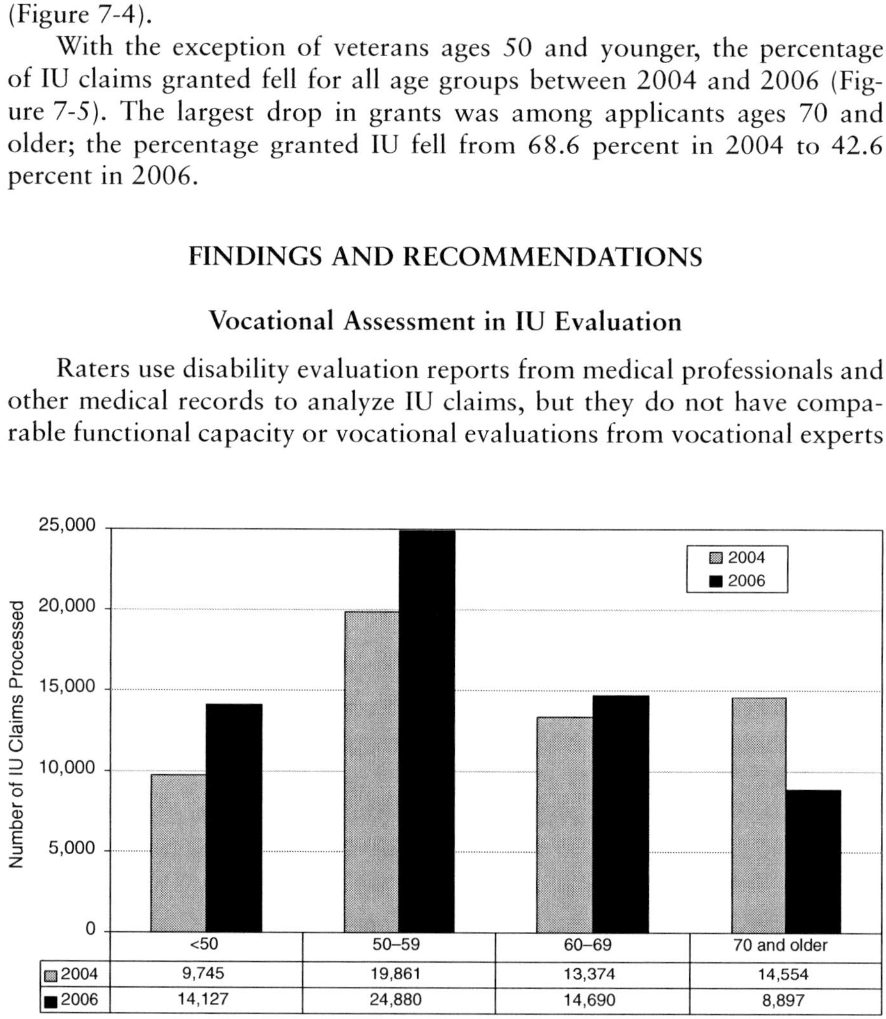

	<50	50–59	60–69	70 and older
2004	9,745	19,861	13,374	14,554
2006	14,127	24,880	14,690	8,897

FIGURE 7-4 Number of IU claims processed by age group, CY 2004–CY 2006.
SOURCE: IOM staff analysis of data provided by VA Office of Performance Analysis and Integrity.

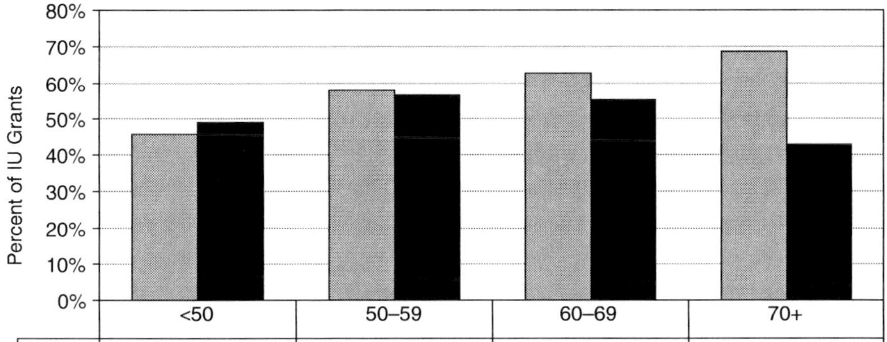

	<50	50–59	60–69	70+
2004	45.5	58.1	62.6	68.6
2006	49.1	56.6	55.2	42.6

FIGURE 7-5 Percentage of IU claims granted by age group, CY 2004–CY 2006.
SOURCE: IOM staff analysis of data provided by VA Office of Performance Analysis and Integrity.

except in cases in which the veteran applicant is participating in VA's VR&E program. Raters must determine the veteran's ability to engage in normal work activities from medical reports and from information in the two-page application for IU and the one-page report from employers, neither of which asks about functional limitations. Raters do not receive training in vocational assessment, nor does VBA have vocational experts whom raters may consult when evaluating IU applications.

The VR&E program has vocational counselors with appropriate education and training to assess employability, but not all veterans claiming IU receive such an evaluation and, if they do, it is usually after they are granted IU. VA could use the vocational portion of a multidisciplinary disability assessment (described in Chapter 3) of veterans separating from service in determining both VR&E needs and IU. In instances in which veterans are applying for IU after separating from service, the multidisciplinary assessment could be done at the time of application.

> **Recommendation 7-1. In addition to medical evaluations by medical professionals, VA should require vocational assessment in the determination of eligibility for individual unemployability benefits. Raters should receive training on how to interpret findings from vocational assessments for the evaluation of individual unemployability claims.**

IU Eligibility Thresholds

The basis for the current thresholds—60 percent for one impairment or 70 percent for more than one, as long as one of them is rated 40 percent—is not known. It was adopted in 1941, replacing the original and stricter 1934 thresholds of 70 and 80 percent. VA's 2001 proposed revised regulations would have changed the threshold to 60 percent for both single and multiple impairments. VA said, "In our view, multiple service-connected disabilities combining to a 60 percent evaluation are no less likely to result in total disability based on individual unemployability than single service-connected disabilities evaluated as 60 percent or higher," but gave no evidence for this conclusion.

Having a threshold makes obvious administrative sense, as long as it is not so high that many people with lower ratings who are legitimately unemployable are excluded. What that threshold should be and the extent to which the current threshold requirements reflect unemployability are not known.

VA regulations allow individuals with lower than current threshold ratings to apply for and receive IU, if approved by the director of the C&P Service.

Recommendation 7-2. VA should monitor and evaluate trends in its disability program and conduct research on employment among veterans with disabilities.

For example, VA could survey a sample of veterans to determine how many of them with lower schedular ratings are unemployed or have earnings low enough to qualify for individual unemployability, and consider appropriate changes in the rating criteria based on survey results. Employment and earnings trends of veterans who do meet individual unemployability eligibility criteria should be followed over time. Further, as a way of checking if the rating criteria for a total schedular rating are too stringent, VA should monitor claims and awards for individual unemployability by condition to discern whether veterans in a particular diagnostic category are disproportionately represented among IU recipients.

Age of IU Recipients

The purpose of IU benefits is to provide full benefits to veterans who do not meet a schedule 100 percent disability rating and who cannot work because of service-connected disability. IU is not meant to provide benefits to every veteran with disabilities without earnings, such as veterans who voluntarily withdraw from the labor market because of retirement or for other reasons. However, GAO statistics indicate that a number of new awards for IU benefits are to veterans who are well beyond the normal retirement age for other government programs, such as Social Security. The committee did not have data indicating whether these veterans were active in the labor market until they applied for IU benefits or whether they had not been active in the labor market for many years prior to their application for IU benefits.

Recommendation 7-3. VA should conduct research on the earnings histories of veterans who initially applied for individual unemployability benefits past the normal age of retirement for benefits under the Old Age, Survivors, and Disability Insurance Program under the Social Security Act.

Factors Considered in IU Evaluation

The labor market has undergone a substantial shift from one largely based on manufacturing for the first three-quarters of the 20th century to today's primarily service-based market. The reduction in the physical demands of many jobs may make employment easier for older workers who have the appropriate education and training. However, for workers whose skills are limited to manufacturing or a particular trade (e.g., construction, mining), finding work may be difficult in the current job market.

In the current system, raters do not consider factors such as education and work experience in IU eligibility determination; service-connected conditions alone must be enough to prevent the veteran from retaining substantially gainful employment.

Recommendation 7-4. Eligibility for individual unemployability should be based on the impacts of an individual's service-connected disabilities, in combination with education, employment history, and the medical effects of that individual's age on his or her potential employability.

Employment of IU Recipients

Under the current system, a veteran on IU is permitted to engage in substantially gainful employment for up to 12 months before IU benefits are terminated. After this grace period the veteran's payments are based on his or her schedular rating of 60, 70, 80, or 90 percent.

Disability compensation amounts do not increase in direct proportion to disability rating percentages. The largest dollar increase in payment is between the 90 percent ($1,483 per month in 2007) and 100 percent ($2,471 per month in 2007) ratings. A veteran receiving IU who engages in substantially gainful employment for more than 12 months will have his or her monthly payments drop by at least 40 percent, or $988 (the difference between a 100 and a 90 percent rating), and by as much as 64 percent, or $1,570 (the difference between a 100 and a 60 percent rating). This poses a sudden "cash cliff" that may deter some veterans from trying to reenter the workforce. Most cash support programs try to provide incentives to work by using some sort of sliding scale to ease the transition from being a beneficiary to being ineligible. The Social Security Administration, for example, is conducting a demonstration to test the impact of reducing disability insurance benefits by $1 for every $2 earned for a period of time after a beneficiary earns more than the amount allowed for eligibility, rather than ending benefits suddenly. Social Security Income recipients already may keep half of their earned income exceeding the first $65 of monthly earnings and $20 in general monthly income. Under the Temporary Assistance to Needy Families (TANF) block grant, California allows a family to keep the first $225 it earns a month and reduces the TANF benefit by $1 for every $2 for every additional dollar earned (Coe, 1998).

Recommendation 7-5. VA should implement a gradual reduction in compensation to individual unemployability recipients who are able to return to substantial gainful employment rather than abruptly terminate their disability payments at an arbitrary level of earnings.

Given the substantial difference in payment at the 100 percent and lower rating levels, the committee believes that implementing a gradual reduction may provide a positive incentive for veterans to find and keep employment. Before adopting this recommendation, VA should study whether incentive effects exist and, if so, experiment with alternative ways to encourage veterans to seek and sustain employment.

REFERENCES

Coe, N. B., G. Acs, R. I. Lerman, and K. Watson. 1998. *Does work pay? A summary of the work incentives under TANF.* Washington, DC: Urban Institute. http://www.urban.org/publications/308019.html (accessed December 4, 2006).

Flohr, B. 2006. *Total disability individual unemployability.* Presentation to the IOM Committee on Medical Evaluation of Veterans for Disability Compensation, Washington, DC, July 7.

GAO (Government Accountability Office). 2006. *Veterans' disability benefits: VA should improve its management of individual unemployability benefits by strengthening criteria, guidance, and procedures.* GAO-06-309. Washington, DC: GAO. http://www.gao.gov/new.items/d06309.pdf (accessed May 30, 2007).

Griffith, C. M. 1945. The Veterans Administration. In *Doctors at war*, edited by M. Fishbein. New York: EP Dutton. Pp. 321–335.

U.S. Congress, Senate, Committee on Veterans' Affairs. 2005. *The rising number of disabled veterans deemed unemployable: Is the system failing? A closer look at VA's individual unemployability benefit.* http://www.access.gpo.gov/congress/senate/ (accessed October 27, 2006).

VA (Department of Veterans Affairs). 2005. *Department of Veterans Affairs Office of Inspector General review of state variances in VA disability compensation payments.* Report No. 05-00765-137. http://www.va.gov/oig/52/reports/2005/VAOIG-05-00765-137.pdf (accessed March 4, 2007).

8

Other Diagnostic Classification Systems and Rating Schedules

The Veterans' Disability Benefits Commission asked the committee about (1) the advantages and disadvantages of adopting universal medical diagnostic codes rather than using a unique system, and (2) the advantages and disadvantages of using the American Medical Association (AMA) *Guides to the Evaluation of Permanent Impairment* (*Guides*) instead of the Department of Veterans Affairs' (VA's) Schedule for Rating Disabilities (Rating Schedule).

ALTERNATIVE DIAGNOSTIC CLASSIFICATION CODES

As a practical matter, the question is whether the Department of Veterans Affairs (VA) should drop or supplement its set of unique diagnostic codes and adopt the diagnostic classifications used by all health-care providers, including the Veterans Health Administration (VHA). These are the *International Classification of Diseases* (ICD), which is maintained by the World Health Organization (WHO), and the *Diagnostic and Statistical Manual of Mental Disorders* (DSM), which is promulgated by the American Psychiatric Association (APA).

International Classification of Diseases

The ICD was originally developed as a consistent way for nations to report mortality statistics. In 1948, the sixth revision of the ICD added causes of morbidity for the first time, based on a proposed statistical classification of diseases, injuries, and causes of death drafted by a U.S.

committee.[1] The 10th and most recent revision of the ICD was published in 1992 and is used by the United States to report mortality statistics. The 9th revision (published in 1977) is still used for clinical and reimbursement purposes.

Use of the ICD

The original purpose of the ICD was to provide internationally consistent statistics that would allow epidemiologic comparisons within populations over time and between populations at a given point in time. In addition, it has come to be the basis for classifying diagnostic information for clinical purposes and for health insurance billing. Several countries, including the United States, have developed clinical modifications of the ICD to make it more useful in primary care settings and for reimbursement and related purposes. In the United States, this is the ICD-9-CM, which was developed by the National Center for Health Statistics (NCHS) and adopted by the federal government for Medicare and Medicaid claims in 1988 (an ICD-10-CM has been developed but has not yet been phased into use).

The ICD has a nested structure allowing users to decide on the level of detail to which they want to code diagnoses. There are four-digit and, in some cases, optional five-digit subdivisions, but users not needing such detail can use the three-digit categories. For example, the three-digit code for diabetes mellitus is 250 (Table 8-1). That three-digit code is subdivided into 10 four-digit codes. Fifth-digit subclassifications can be used with each of the four-digit codes:

0—type II controlled
1—type I controlled
2—type II uncontrolled
3—type I uncontrolled

Thus, for example, the diagnostic code 250.42 indicates type II diabetes with nephropathy or other renal manifestation.

To take another example, the code for chronic bronchitis is 491 (Table 8-1). At the next level of detail, there are four-digit codes for simple chronic bronchitis (491.0), mucopurulent chronic bronchitis (491.1), obstructive chronic bronchitis (491.2), other chronic bronchitis (491.8), and unspecified chronic bronchitis (491.9). Obstructive chronic bronchitis

[1]This account is based on a history of the development of the ICD on the WHO website. http://www.who.int/classifications/icd/en/HistoryOfICD.pdf (accessed March 26, 2007).

TABLE 8-1 Examples of ICD Classifications

250 Diabetes mellitus
- 250.0 Diabetes mellitus without mention of complication
- 250.1 Diabetes with ketoacidosis
- 250.2 Diabetes with hyperosmolarity
- 250.3 Diabetes with other coma
- 250.4 Diabetes with renal manifestations
- 250.5 Diabetes with ophthalmic manifestations
- 250.6 Diabetes with neurological manifestations
- 250.7 Diabetes with peripheral circulatory disorders
- 250.8 Diabetes with other specified manifestations
- 250.9 Diabetes with unspecified complications

491 Chronic bronchitis
- 491.0 Simple chronic bronchitis
- 491.1 Mucopurulent bronchitis
- 491.2 Obstructive chronic bronchitis
  - 491.20 Without mention of acute exacerbation
  - 491.21 With acute exacerbation
- 491.8 Other chronic bronchitis
- 491.9 Unspecified chronic bronchitis

717 Internal derangement of knee
- 717.0 Old bucket handle tear of medial meniscus
- 717.1 Derangement of anterior horn of medial meniscus
- 717.2 Derangement of posterior horn of medial meniscus
- 717.3 Other and unspecified derangement of medial meniscus
- 717.4 Derangement of lateral meniscus
  - 717.40 Derangement of lateral meniscus, unspecified
  - 717.41 Bucket handle tear of lateral meniscus
  - 717.42 Derangement of anterior horn of lateral meniscus
  - 717.43 Derangement of posterior horn of lateral meniscus
  - 717.49 Other
- 717.5 Derangement of meniscus, not elsewhere classified
- 717.6 Loose body in knee
- 717.7 Chondromalacia of patella
- 717.8 Other internal derangement of knee
  - 717.81 Old disruption of lateral collateral ligament
  - 717.82 Old disruption of medial collateral ligament
  - 717.83 Old disruption of anterior cruciate ligament
  - 717.84 Old disruption of posterior cruciate ligament
  - 717.85 Old disruption of other ligaments of knee
  - 717.89 Other
- 717.9 Unspecified internal derangement of knee

SOURCE: St. Anthony's Publishing (2003).

can be classified at the five-digit level as "without mention of acute exacerbation" (491.20) or "with acute exacerbation" (491.21).

Internal derangement of knee, whose three-digit code is 717, has 10 four-digit codes, and 2 of the four-digit codes each can be subdivided into several five-digit codes (Table 8-1).

In 2000, WHO adopted a formal process for updating the ICD between periodic comprehensive revisions. The international collaborating centers, of which one is NCHS, propose revisions and additions to an updating and revision committee, which considers whether to include them in annual updates of the ICD. Annual revisions have been made since 1995.

WHO is currently in the process of developing the ICD-11, which is due to be completed and released in 2011.

International Classification of Functioning, Disability and Health

The ICD is a classification of diagnoses, not of health states. It does not indicate the severity of disease or injury or the patient's level of functioning or quality of life. Another WHO classification, the *International Classification of Functioning, Disability and Health* (ICF), was developed to assess the consequences of disease and injury in terms of an individual's ability to function in his or her environment (WHO, 2001):

> ICF is a multipurpose classification intended for a wide range of uses in different sectors. It is a classification of health and health-related domains—domains that help us to describe changes in body function and structure, what a person with a health condition can do in a standard environment (their level of capacity), as well as what they actually do in their usual environment (their level of performance). These domains are classified from body, individual, and societal perspectives by means of two lists: a list of body functions and structure, and a list of domains of activity and participation. In ICF, the term *functioning* refers to all body functions, activities, and participation, while *disability* is similarly an umbrella term for impairments, activity limitations, and participation restrictions. ICF also lists environmental factors that interact with all these components (WHO, 2002:2).

The ICF is sophisticated conceptually but is difficult to operationalize because of its complexity (see Chapter 3). Researchers in the disability and rehabilitation fields are studying how to measure the functional domains in the ICF. At this point, it has not been adopted for use by any disability benefit programs.

Classification Systems of Other Disability Programs

The Social Security Administration (SSA) has the largest program of cash benefits for persons with disabilities. To receive disability benefits from SSA, a person must be unable to engage in any substantial gainful activity for at least a year because of a physical or mental impairment. The substantial gainful activity concept, currently defined as earning no more than $900 a month, originally derived from the War Risk Insurance Act of 1914, which defined total disability as mental or physical impairment making it impossible for the individual "to follow any substantial gainful occupations" (Berkowitz, 1987:44).

SSA uses a classification system for its disability benefits program based loosely on the ICD-9-CM. Before 1985, SSA used four-digit ICD codes. In 1985, SSA modified the classification to use three digits followed by a zero. The three digits are mostly identical with the three-digit codes in the ICD-9-CM, but SSA does not use all the ICD three-digit codes. In total, the SSA system has about 240 codes. The code for diabetes mellitus (2500) is equivalent to the one in the ICD-9-CM (250), but there are separate codes for diabetic acidosis (2760), diabetic neuropathy (3570), and diabetic retinopathy (3620). The code for chronic bronchitis (4910) is equivalent to the ICD code for simple chronic bronchitis (4910) (Table 8-1). The code for knee impairments is not the same, however. SSA uses 7160 for all dysfunctional joints (e.g., shoulder, elbow, hip) regardless of cause, equivalent to the ICD-9 CM code for other and unspecified arthropathies.

SSA can manage with less than a third of the approximately 800 codes used by VA to specify the impairment in adequate detail. This is because SSA is more concerned with assessment of the functional consequences on ability to work than with specifying the impairment in great detail. SSA must by law establish that a "medically determinable" impairment exists, that is, a well-supported diagnosis, but a diagnosis or the existence of an impairment by itself (with rare exceptions such as amyotrophic lateral sclerosis [ALS] is not a determining factor in making the disability decision. If the medical findings of severity meet or equal the listings, the claimant is allowed; if not, residual functional capacity is evaluated along with occupational factors such as age, education, and work history.

SSA also does not have separate codes for different severities of the same impairment, partly because it is making an all-or-nothing decision—the person is disabled or is not disabled. VA, on the other hand, is concerned with determining degree of impairment. For example, SSA has one diagnostic code for all amputations, while VA has many, depending on which limb or digit is involved and how much loss has occurred. Thus, there are five codes for loss of an arm, depending on if it was severed at the shoulder, above or below the insertion of the deltoid muscle in the upper arm, or above or below the insertion of the pronator teres muscle in the forearm, and the percentage ratings for each differs depending on whether it is the dominant arm.

Diagnostic and Statistical Manual of Mental Disorders

The DSM is a widely used classification of mental disorders. It uses the same numbering system as the ICD, although there are minor differences in what is classified under the same code. The DSM has five axes:

- Axis I includes clinical disorders in 14 categories, such as anxiety, childhood, cognitive, dissociative, eating, factitious, impulse control, mood, psychotic, sexual and gender identity, sleep, somatoform, and substance-related disorders.
- Axis II includes mental retardation and personality disorders, such as antisocial, avoidant, borderline, dependent, histrionic, narcissistic, obsessive-compulsive, paranoid, schizoid, and schizotypal personality disorders.
- Axis III consists of medical conditions that may be relevant to the understanding and treatment of the mental disorder.
- Axis IV includes psychosocial and environmental factors contributing to a disorder, such as housing problems, problems with work, bereavement, and legal problems.
- Axis V is the Global Assessment of Functioning (GAF), which measures psychological, social, and occupational functioning on a 100-point scale.

A psychiatrist uses the DSM to choose the disorder or disorders that most closely match the symptoms and signs of the patient. Each disorder has a classification number, or diagnostic code. Each disorder has diagnostic criteria that must be present. For example, the diagnostic criteria for generalized anxiety disorder (Axis I) are

A. Excessive anxiety and worry (apprehensive expectation), occurring more days than not for at least 6 months, about a number of events or activities (such as work or school performance)

B. The person finds it difficult to control the worry.

C. The anxiety and worry are associated with three (or more) of the following six symptoms (with at least some symptoms present for more days than not for the past 6 months; only one item is required in children):

   1. restlessness or feeling keyed up or on edge,
   2. being easily fatigued,
   3. difficulty concentrating or the mind going blank,

4. irritability,
5. muscle tension, and
6. sleep disturbance (difficulty falling or staying asleep, or restless, unsatisfying sleep).

D. The focus of the anxiety and worry is not confined to features of an Axis I disorder, such as the anxiety or worry is not about having a panic attack (as in panic disorder), being embarrassed in public (as in social phobia), being contaminated (as in obsessive-compulsive disorder), being away from home or close relatives (as in separation anxiety disorder), gaining weight (as in anorexia nervosa), having multiple physical complaints (as in somatization disorder), or having a serious illness (as in hypochondriasis), and the anxiety and worry do not occur exclusively during posttraumatic stress disorder (PTSD).

E. The anxiety, worry, or physical symptoms cause clinically significant distress or impairment in social, occupational, or other important areas of functioning.

F. The disturbance is not due to the direct physiological effects of a substance (e.g., a drug of abuse, a medication) or a general medical condition (e.g., hyperthyroidism) and does not occur exclusively during a mood disorder, a psychotic disorder, or a pervasive developmental disorder.

The DSM also contains three-and-a-half pages of narrative discussion of the diagnostic features of generalized anxiety disorder; associated features and disorders; specific culture, age, and gender features; prevalence; course; familial pattern; and differential diagnosis (APA, 2000).

The DSM was developed by APA in 1952 and has been revised several times. The last major revision, DSM-IV, was published in 1994. A text revision of the DSM-IV, called DSM-IV-TR, was published in 2000. The fifth edition, DSM-V, is scheduled to be released in 2011.

William Narrow, research director for APA's DSM-V task force, briefed the committee on its development. APA is conducting a series of conferences and empirical research on criteria with longitudinal and epidemiologic datasets. Some of the suggestions from the conferences are that DSM-V should include "dimensional" assessments of mental disorders, although not abandoning the categorical system, and that there should be regrouping of disorders based on advances in understanding of mental disorders. Dimensional assessments would include the degree of severity and functional limitations of a diagnosed disorder. A possible candidate for a new diagnostic grouping—based on better understanding of causes of mental disorders—would be "stress-related and fear circuitry disorders" (Narrow, 2006).

VA already uses the DSM, but not the current DSM-IV-TR version, because the mental disorders section of the Rating Schedule was last updated in 1996 before the DSM-IV-TR was published. For example, according to the Rating Schedule:

> The nomenclature employed in this portion of the rating schedule is based upon the *Diagnostic and Statistical Manual of Mental Disorders*, Fourth Edition, of the American Psychiatric Association (DSM-IV). Rating agencies [i.e., raters] must be thoroughly familiar with this manual to properly implement the directives in §4.125 through §4.129 and to apply the general rating formula for mental disorders in §4.130 (38 CFR 4.130).

VA also organizes the schedule of ratings for mental disorders under eight broad categories that correspond to DSM categories, such as schizophrenia and other psychotic behaviors, mood disorders, and somatoform disorders. Some major DSM categories are not used, for example, disorders usually first diagnosed in infancy, childhood, or adolescence (e.g., mental retardation, attention deficit/hyperactivity disorder [ADHD]), substance-related disorders, and personality disorders. Individuals with disabling childhood disorders presumably are not accepted for military service. For policy reasons, substance abuse and personality disorders are expressly barred from being the basis for disability compensation.

Within major categories of mental disorders, VA does not use all the specific disorders that have DSM codes. For example, instead of listing the six specific adjustment disorders (e.g., with depressed mood, with anxiety) in the DSM and allowing each to be acute or chronic, VA uses a single code, called chronic adjustment disorder. In other cases, VA uses some of the specific disorders but not others. Under mood disorders, for example, VA combines seven bipolar diagnoses into one and does not include substance-induced mood disorder, and there is one category for "mood disorder, not otherwise specified (NOS)," instead of separate NOS diagnoses for depressive disorders and for bipolar disorders.

In sum, VA has adapted the DSM classification system to its needs by choosing a three-digit disorder (i.e., adjustment disorders), using some but not all other disorders at the four- and five-digit level, and/or combining diagnoses (e.g., making three DSM diagnoses for dissociative disorders into one—"dissociative amnesia, dissociative fugue, and dissociative identity disorder"). The effect is to simplify categories (VA uses 36 diagnostic codes whereas the DSM uses more than 300), focus the Rating Schedule on diagnoses more common among veterans (e.g., depression, PTSD, schizophrenia), and exclude diagnoses that do not apply (e.g., mental retardation).

VA also uses the GAF, Axis V of the DSM. It is not mentioned in the Rating Schedule, but VA materials for training rating veterans service representatives say that Compensation and Pension (C&P) Services mental examinations must include the DSM-IV multiaxial format, including the GAF. Raters are instructed to use the GAF score as one, although not the sole or main, basis for evaluating mental disability. The C&P examination worksheet calls for the current GAF score, and VHA examiners conducting mental examinations must be trained in use of the GAF.

THE AMA *GUIDES*: AN ALTERNATIVE RATING SCHEDULE?

In the 1950s, AMA began to issue a series of guides to the evaluation of permanent impairment for use by physicians asked to assess patients seeking disability insurance or workers' compensation benefits. In 1971, they were combined in one volume, called *Guides to the Evaluation of Permanent Impairment*. The current fifth edition of the *Guides* was issued in 2000. It defines impairment to be "a loss, loss of use, or derangement of any body part, organ system, or organ function" (AMA, 2001:2). A permanent impairment is one that has reached "maximal medical improvement," meaning it is unlikely to improve substantially for the next year. Disability is defined by the *Guides* as "an alteration of an individual's capacity to meet personal, social, or occupational demands because of an impairment," and it notes that "an impaired individual may or may not have a disability" (AMA, 2001:3). The role of the physician, the *Guides* makes clear, is limited only to determining degree of medical impairment and individual-level functional limitations on activities, and to providing supporting medical information to those making disability determinations, not deciding if someone is disabled for purposes of disability benefits.

The *Guides* is organized into chapters on body systems. Some chapters focus on anatomic loss, and others on functional loss, "depending upon common practice in that specialty" (AMA, 2001:4). The example given of anatomic loss is an enlarged heart. The corresponding functional loss is the loss in the heart's ability to pump blood, as measured by the ejection fraction.[2]

The criteria for evaluating degree of impairment are based on the degree to which the impairment reduces the individual's ability to engage in activities of daily living, "*excluding* work" (emphasis in the original). The ratings are designed to reflect functional limitations, not degree of disability (AMA, 2001:4). This is because the determination of disability involves more than evaluation of impairment. It also involves information about the individual's education, skills, job history, age, and environmental circumstances, which are not matters that physicians are trained or equipped to

[2]The ejection fraction is the percentage of blood that is pumped from a filled heart ventricle with each heartbeat.

assess (AMA, 2001). Although the *Guides* says that activities of daily living (ADLs) are part of the impairment rating process, most of the chapters in the fifth edition are based on anatomic losses and limitations.

Robert Rondinelli, lead medical editor of the sixth edition of the *Guides*, which is due to be completed in late 2007, briefed the committee on plans for the sixth edition (Rondinelli, 2006). He told the committee that this next edition will

- be revised in accordance with the concepts and nomenclature of the ICF, meaning distinguish between impairment of body functions and structures, activity limitations, and participation restrictions;
- clarify that an impairment rating based on the *Guides* is "a consensus-derived percentage estimate of loss of activity, which reflects severity of impairment for a given health condition, and the degree of associated loss of activities of daily living," but not a direct estimate of work disability;
- be as evidence-based as possible, but otherwise be based on expert consensus;
- incorporate as much functional assessment as possible, including assessment of ADLs, to supplement anatomic measures; and
- adopt, if possible, an ADL scale for use in applying the *Guides* (in the absence of an agreed-on scale appropriate for a working population, the fifth edition listed commonly used validated scales and left it to the physician to choose the most appropriate one).

FINDINGS AND CONCLUSIONS

Diagnostic Classification Systems

The Rating Schedule has been in use since 1945. It includes almost 800 unique diagnostic codes categorized by body system. Raters match the medical conditions of veterans applying for disability compensation with one or more of the codes and then use the criteria associated with each code to assign a percentage rating. Therefore, it is important that the diagnostic categories represented by the diagnostic codes in the Rating Schedule be as medically correct as possible or else the criteria used for determining the rating will not be appropriate.

Numerical codes first appeared in the 1933 Rating Schedule and were continued in 1945, when the current Rating Schedule was promulgated. They are unique to VA. According to VA, the codes "are arbitrary numbers for the purpose of showing the basis of the evaluation assigned and for statistical analysis in the VA" (38 CFR § 4.27).

VA has periodically updated diagnostic codes within the Rating Schedule to reflect changes in medical nomenclature and to add new diseases (e.g., HIV and chronic fatigue syndrome). Many of the body systems were comprehensively revised in the early to mid 1990s, when many, if not all, diagnostic codes were revised, including infectious diseases/immune disorders/nutritional deficiencies, respiratory, cardiovascular, genitourinary, gynecological, hemic/lymphatic, endocrine, mental, dental/oral, and the muscles part of cardiovascular. The skin system was overhauled in 2001. In most of these cases, 90 to 100 percent of the diagnostic codes were changed in some way, ranging from updating the name to redefining what the code covers to changing the rating criteria. Some body systems have not been comprehensively revised, namely, the orthopedic part of musculoskeletal, neurological, and digestive systems. In all, as shown in Table 4-1 in Chapter 4, 35 percent (281 of 798) of the codes have not changed since 1945, most of them in the musculoskeletal (105), neurological (105), and digestive systems (20). As a result, there are areas in which conditions are misclassified in comparison with current medical standards. For example, multiple sclerosis and myasthenia gravis are categorized as neurodegenerative diseases in the Rating Schedule, but are currently thought of as autoimmune diseases. Multiple sclerosis is not necessarily degenerative; it is known to have several forms, including a relapsing-remitting, secondary progressive, and primary progressive type, each with a different course and impact on function. The subcategorization of epilepsy is out of date.

There are pros and cons to changing the diagnostic classification system to the ICD. The strongest arguments for adopting the ICD are that it would (1) use the categories of diagnoses, definitions of what fits those categories, and nomenclature used in current medical practice and make the exchange of information between the examiners and raters more effective in identifying a veteran's medical problems, and (2) facilitate better understanding of trends in the health of the veteran population. The strongest arguments against adopting the ICD are (1) the costs involved and (2) loss of the role the current diagnostic criteria play in identifying the location and degree of injury in great detail for rating purposes.

Veterans are diagnosed, treated, and rehabilitated in a health-care system in which the ICD and the DSM are the bases of common language and understanding. The VA disability compensation system relies heavily on medical records, which are expressed in terms of ICD and DSM categories and terms. Raters use these records, whether from private providers or the VHA health-care system, as part of establishing the diagnosis or diagnoses pertinent to a veteran's claim. C&P examinations, whether by VHA clinicians or contract clinicians, play a prominent role in the disability compensation system, probably in part because the examiner provides the service of interpreting the medical information and translating it into Rating Schedule terms for raters to use. This may mean that more prominence than warranted is given to the C&P examiner's snapshot evaluation of a veteran than to the longitudinal information found in the treating physician's records.

Having the same diagnostic categories for the disability compensation program as VHA and other health-care providers would facilitate communication and understanding of a veteran's health problems. The rater would be better able to relate information in medical records to the Rating Schedule if the diagnostic categories corresponded. It would also help the program keep up with advances in medical understanding, because the ICD and the DSM undergo regular revision and periodic comprehensive revisions. This would help avoid situations in which some currently identified conditions are not found in the Rating Schedule. Raters probably realize that paralysis agitans is called Parkinson's disease and that dementia of the Alzheimer's type is called Alzheimer's disease, but they would have to determine which codes to use for veterans who are diagnosed with multiple system atrophy, corticobasal degeneration, or progressive supranuclear palsy. Also, closely-related diseases such as progressive muscular atrophy, bulbar palsy, and ALS are grouped together in the ICD as motor neuron disease (although they have different five-digit codes), but they are separated in the Rating Schedule, and one, bulbar palsy, has different rating criteria than the other two.

The Rating Schedule contains a number of instances of outdated terms and names, especially in the orthopedic section of the musculoskeletal and neurological systems, which have not been comprehensively updated since 1945. Raters must match conditions in the medical records to the proper diagnostic code in the Rating Schedule. Knowing that Parkinson's disease should be rated under paralysis agitans has already been mentioned. Similarly, raters have to know that veterans presenting with an unstable shoulder or elbow should be evaluated under one of the codes in the Rating Schedule for "flail joint," because it is an obsolete term unlikely to appear in their medical treatment records.

As noted in Chapter 2, traumatic brain injury is the signature injury of the war in Iraq. The Rating Schedule has a diagnostic code for brain disease due to trauma (8045), which was last revised in 1961 (VA, 2006). The rater is directed to evaluate the condition according to its various neurological consequences, "such as hemiplegia, epileptiform seizures, facial nerve paralysis, etc." There is no other guidance in the Rating Schedule on the likely sequelae of brain injury for the rater to consider. In recent years, for example, with better measures and definitions, medical researchers have discovered significant neurobehavioral impacts of mild to moderate brain trauma. Each condition that is service connected and rated is given a hyphenated code with 8045 as a prefix (before the hyphen) and the diagnostic code for the related condition as the suffix (after the hyphen). This permits tracking the number of veterans being compensated for traumatic brain injury; however, this is not possible for spinal cord injury, which has no diagnostic code, but is rated only on the basis of the nerves that no longer work and on the impact on organ function.

Another advantage of using ICD codes would be the reduction in the rate of analogous codes. No classification system can identify every possible diagnosis ahead of time, not even one with 800 codes such as those found in the VA Rating Schedule. VA provides flexibility by allowing the rater to use an analogous condition as a guide for determining the rating percentage. The first two numbers are those of the relevant body system, the second two numbers are 99, and the four-digit number following the hyphen is for the analogous condition being used for rating purposes. At the end of FY 2005, 9 percent (370,000) of the 7.7 million service-connected disabilities had analogous codes (Figure 8-1). These percentages were higher for some body systems, especially dental/oral (25 percent), genitourinary (18 percent), and hemic/lymphatic (16 percent). The rate of use for musculoskeletal conditions is 12 percent, but analogous codes are concentrated in the orthopedic part of musculoskeletal, where they constituted 15 percent of the codes.

Analogous codes could be analyzed to identify impairments that occur often enough to deserve their own code or for which the criteria in existing codes are not adequate. The Army has cited Crohn's disease as an example of the latter (U.S. Army, 2007). There is no diagnostic code for Crohn's, so it must be rated by analogy. Raters may choose to use the criteria for ulcerative colitis (7323) or irritable colon syndrome (7319) to rate the claimed condition, depending on the symptomatology. Code 7319 allows ratings for abdominal distress up to 30 percent, while 7323 allows ratings up to 100 percent in more severe cases. The use of multiple codes makes it difficult to track the number of Crohn's disease claims, compare the incidence of Crohn's with other populations, or recognize when the number of cases of Crohn's would justify establishment of a diagnostic code to make rating more uniform and efficient.

Use of DSM categories illustrates the potential effect of using a universal code. The categories are designed to be comprehensive and mutually exclusive. This is probably the reason that the rate of analogous codes for mental ratings was less than 1 percent, the lowest rate of all the body systems.

Use of common diagnostic categories would also allow VA managers and researchers to compare populations and trends that would help in program planning and in epidemiologic and health services research. VA's diagnostic codes are unique and do not allow comparisons of trends in disabilities in populations served by VHA or the Department of Defense (DoD) or research normed to the veteran population. Lack of ICD codes makes it difficult to project actuarial trends or to identify emerging trends, such as Gulf War illnesses. Tracking trends in the ailments of veterans who served

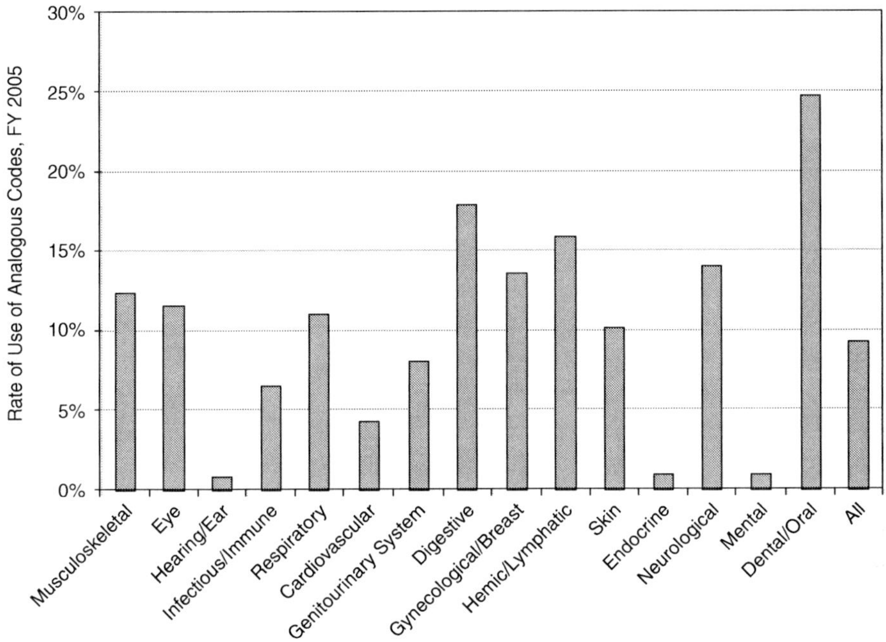

FIGURE 8-1 Rate of use of analogous codes by body system, FY 2005.
NOTE: Rate is the number of service-connected disabilities coded as analogous (XX99) divided by the number of all service-connected disabilities in each body system.
SOURCE: IOM (2007).

in a particular war and comparing them with other veterans or the general population would help VA identify health-care needs and be part of the surveillance system for recognizing conditions that should be presumptively service connected. Tracking trends in the disabling conditions of veterans in particular military occupational specialties could help VA identify occupational health problems for DoD to address.

Switching to ICD codes would have some downsides. The short-term direct costs would be significant in terms of changing computer systems and retraining raters. These costs would already be incurred, however, if the Rating Schedule undergoes a comprehensive revision in which most of the codes would be changed anyway. The costs of switching to a different set of codes would also be offset by the benefits for veterans of having a system aligned with modern medical practice and record keeping. In addition, the switch does not have to be sudden. Raters could continue to use the current codes while phasing in ICD codes.

Another downside would be changing the way the current codes are used to specify the degree of loss of a particular body structure or system. For example, there are different codes for different degrees of amputation of an arm or leg or various combinations of amputated fingers and toes. However, there is nothing inherent to the ICD that prevents achieving this purpose because of the way the numbering can be nested. The ICD-9-CM code for traumatic amputation of leg(s) is 897, but there are fourth-digit modifiers for the height of the amputation on the leg. ICD users may pick their own set of codes, perhaps at the three-digit level for some conditions, and at the four- or five-digit level for others, as VA has done with the DSM-IV. VA could add modifiers when subcategories not needed in regular medical practice are desired for its own purposes.

Recommendation 8-1. VA should adopt a new classification system using the *International Classification of Diseases* (ICD) and the *Diagnostic and Statistical Manual of Mental Disorders* (DSM) codes. This system should apply to all applications, including those that are denied. During the transition to ICD and DSM codes, VA can continue to use its own diagnostic codes, and subsequently track and analyze them comparatively for trends affecting veterans and for program planning purposes. Knowledge of an applicant's ICD or DSM codes should help raters, especially with the task of properly categorizing conditions.

VA should use the most recent versions of the ICD and the DSM in the disability determination process. When the Rating Schedule is revised, it should include the conditions most prevalent in the veteran population, classified according to current medical concepts and terminology. Then each should be given the relevant ICD or DSM code, probably at the three-digit level, which would be a relatively small subset of ICD codes.

AMA *Guides* Impairment Rating System

Use of the AMA *Guides* would have some advantages. As with the ICD and the DSM, it undergoes comprehensive updating on a periodic basis and, at this point, it is medically more up to date than the Rating Schedule. If VA is going to revamp the Rating Schedule to align with current medical knowledge, as recommended in Chapter 4, it might consider adopting the already proven, more up-to-date *Guides*, or adopt it for certain body systems. It should be noted, however, that the *Guides* was designed for use in a different disability decision system than VA's (that is, workers' compensation), which has a different division of labor between the medical examiner and the disability decision maker. In workers' compensation, the physician is asked to evaluate the claimant and determine a percentage rating of total impairment. The *Guides* leaves it to the adjudicator in the workers' compensation program or other disability program to determine degree of disability, which involves considerations of functioning that the *Guides* does not address. The *Guides* was designed for use by a licensed physician and limited to a physician's areas of competence, meaning evaluation of impairment of body structures and functions and of the ability of the individual to carry out basic daily activities of self-care, such as bathing, dressing, toileting, getting in or out of a chair or bed, and eating, and to live independently, such as making meals, managing money, shopping for groceries or personal items, performing light or heavy housework, and using a telephone.[3]

According to the *Guides*, physicians have the discretion to provide an assessment of an individual's work-related disability only if they are knowledgeable about the essential requirements of a specific job and work environment. Evaluation of an individual's ability to return to work in general, such as to any job in the person's field, is a different matter:

> A decision of this scope usually requires input from medical and non-medical experts, such as vocational specialists, and the evaluation of both stable and changing factors, such as the person's education, skills, and motivation, the state of the job market, and local economic considerations (AMA, 2001:14).

The *Guides* includes an example of individuals with the same degree of clinical impairment (e.g., 30 percent because of pericardial heart disease) but very different degrees of disability, depending on whether their job is sedentary or involves manual labor (AMA, 2001).

The *Guides* is organized by body system but uses a broad numbering system. The cardiovascular system, for example, has four categories: 4.1, hypertensive cardiovascular disease; 4.2, diseases of the aorta; 4.3, vascular disease affecting the extremities; and 4.4, diseases of the pulmonary arteries. The neurological system has more categories—eight—and some are subdivided. The criteria for rating cranial nerves (13.4), for example, are discussed under subheadings for the olfactory nerve, 13.4a; optic nerve, 13.4b; oculomotor, trochlear, and abducens nerves, 13.4c; and so on, through the hypoglossal nerve, 13.4i. Diagnostic codes are not used in the *Guides*. It is left to the physician examiner to know which criteria to use for which diagnosis. For instance, the section on criteria for rating cerebral impairments mentions some conditions in examples, such as traumatic brain injury, Parkinson's disease, uremic encephalopathy, epilepsy,

[3]These correspond to activities of daily living (ADLs) and instrumental activities of daily living (IADLs) (AMA, 2001). For definitions of ADLs and IADLs, see NCHS (2007a,b).

and dysphasia, but many others, such as multiple sclerosis and ALS, are not mentioned.

The *Guides*, designed to measure degree of permanent impairment and not degree of ability to work (which is to be determined by government agencies or insurance companies), tends to have lower ratings than the Rating Schedule. An example in the *Guides* is upper extremity amputation (Table 8-2). The AMA *Guides* rates amputation of a leg at the hip at 40 percent (whole person) and the Rating Schedule rates it at 90 percent[4].

Similarly, an individual with severe loss of hearing in both ears would receive a rating of 50 percent from the Rating Schedule and 34 percent from the *Guides*.[5] Total loss of hearing is rated 100 percent in the Rating Schedule and 35 percent in the *Guides*. For diabetes mellitus, the AMA *Guides* allows ratings of 0 to 5 percent and 6 to 10 percent for type 2 diabetes, the higher rating if control of plasma glucose requires both a restricted diet and medication (oral agent or insulin) and there is evidence of microangiopathy (retinopathy or albuminaria of greater than 30 mg/dL). The *Guides* allows 11 to 20 percent for type 1 diabetes and 21 to 40 percent if there is frequent hyper- or hypoglycemia despite conscientious efforts to control plasma glucose levels by the individual and his or her physician. Secondary manifestations of type 1 or 2 diabetes (e.g., retinopathy, nephropathy, neuropathy, atherosclerosis) are rated separately. The Rating Schedule provides percentages from 10 to 100 percent for diabetes mellitus, with the 100 percent rating requiring: (1) more than one daily injection of insulin, (2) restricted diet, and (3) activity restrictions with (4) episodes of ketoacidosis or hypoglycemic reactions requiring (a) at least three hospitalizations annually or (b) weekly visits to a diabetic care provider, plus (5) either progressive loss of weight and strength or complications that would be compensable if separately evaluated. As in the *Guides*, secondary manifestations are rated separately.

The *Guides* does not determine percentage of impairment from mental disorders. According to the fifth edition:

> Unlike cases with some organ systems, there are no precise measures of impairment in mental disorders. The use of percentages implies a certainty

[4]The AMA *Guides* rates impairment for specific body parts and then translates that rating into a whole person rating. For example, a 100 percent amputation of the leg at the hip translates into a 40 percent whole person rating.

[5]This assumes a pure-tone average (PTA) of 90 decibels hearing loss at the four frequencies used to calculate the PTA. In the VA Rating Schedule, the four frequencies are 1,000, 2,000, 3,000, and 4,000 Hertz. For the *Guides*, the four frequencies are 500, 1,000, 2,000, and 3,000 Hertz. Because noise-induced hearing loss primarily affects the frequencies of 3,000, 4,000, and 6,000 Hertz, both of these methods underestimate the extent of the acquired hearing loss, although the Rating Schedule more accurately reflects the effects of noise-induced hearing loss than the *Guides*.

TABLE 8-2 Comparative Impairment Ratings for Upper Limb Amputation

	VA Rating Schedule		AMA *Guides*	
Amputation Level	Dominant Hand	Nondominant Hand	Upper Extremity	Whole Person
Shoulder disarticulation	90	90	100	60
Arm above deltoid insertion	90	80	100	60
Arm below deltoid insertion	80	70	95	57
Forearm above pronator teres (VA)/bicipital insertion (AMA)	80	70	95	57
Forearm below pronator teres (VA)/bicipital insertion (AMA)	70	60	94–90	56–54
Wrist	70	60		
All digits	70	60	90	54

NOTE: The insertion points for the pronator teres and bicipital muscles are at slightly different points on the upper forearm, so it is possible for someone to have an amputation above the pronator teres and below the bicipital insertion, which is just below the elbow.
SOURCES: VA Schedule for Rating Disabilities (diagnostic codes 5120–5125) and AMA *Guides* (Table 16–4).

> that does not exist. Percentages are likely to be used inflexibly by adjudicators, who then are less likely to take into account the many factors that influence mental and behavioral impairment. In addition, the authors are unaware of data that show the reliability of the impairment percentages (AMA, 2001:361).

Instead, the *Guides* asks examiners to rate four domains of behavior using a five-category scale ranging from 1 (no impairment noted) to 5 (extreme impairment). The dimensions are

- ADLs;
- social functioning;
- concentration, persistence, and pace; and
- adaptation to stressful situations in complex or worklike settings (tendency to decompensate).

Thus an individual might be assigned a 3 on social function, a 5 on concentration, a 1 on ADLs, and a 4–5 on adaptation (as was done in an example of an individual with a major depressive episode and associated anxiety after recovering from a heart attack). It would then be up to the adjudicator to determine a percentage of disability based on all the information in the veteran's medical record, including the four mental assessments with supporting rationales.

In sum, there are both advantages and disadvantages to adopting the AMA *Guides*. The advantages are that it is more up to date medically, and (or because) it is updated on a regular basis. The disadvantages are that it is designed to be used by licensed physicians; measures and rates impairment and, to some extent, daily functioning, but not disability or quality of life; and does not provide mental ratings. The sixth edition is expected to improve the evidence base for impairment evaluation and include more assessment of ADLs, but it still will not be intended for use as a tool for evaluating ability to work.

Recommendation 8-2. Considering some of the unique conditions relevant for disability following military activities, it would be preferable for VA to update and improve the Rating Schedule on a regular basis rather than adopt an impairment schedule developed for other purposes.

VA should update its Rating Schedule and improve it to the extent possible by including validated functional limitations measures. The evaluation procedures and severity criteria found in the AMA *Guides*, but not in the Rating Schedule, could be adopted for certain conditions, as does Social Security, for example, by requiring use of the techniques in the AMA *Guides* for measuring joint motion.

REFERENCES

AMA (American Medical Association). 2001. *Guides to the evaluation of permanent impairment*, 5th Edition. Chicago, IL: AMA.

APA (American Psychiatric Association). 2000. *Diagnostic and statistical manual of mental disorders*, 4th Edition. Text Revision (DSM-IV-TR). Washington, DC: APA.

Berkowitz, M. 1987. *Disabled policy–America's programs for the handicapped*. New York: Cambridge University Press.

IOM. 2007. IOM staff analysis of data in VA statistical report, RCS 20-0227, "Diagnoses counts grouped by percentage, service-connected compensaton only, all periods [of service], as of September 30, 2005." Report prepared by VBA/D&IS, December 27, 2005, and provided to IOM.

Narrow, W. E. 2006. *APA's work toward DSM-V*. Presentation to the IOM Committee on Medical Evaluation of Veterans for Disability Compensation, Washington, DC, September 21.

NCHS (National Center for Health Statistics). 2007a. *Instrumental activities of daily living (IADLs)*. http://www.cdc.gov/nchs/datawh/nchsdefs/iadl.htm (accessed March 26, 2007).

NCHS. 2007b. *Activities of daily living (ADLs)*. http://www.cdc.gov/nchs/datawh/nchsdefs/ADL.htm (accessed March 26, 2007).

Rondinelli, R. D. 2006. *AMA guides 6th ed: Applications to compensation and pensioning within the Veterans Benefits Administration.* Presentation to the IOM Committee on Medical Evaluation of Veterans for Disability Compensation, Washington, DC, September 21.

St. Anthony's Publishing. 2003. *Professional ICD-9-CM Code Book 2001*, 6th Edition, Vols.1, 2, and 3. Reston, VA: St. Anthony's Publishing.

U.S. Army. 2007. *Department of the Army Inspector General inspection of the physical disability evaluation system.* Washington, DC: Office of the Inspector General, Department of the Army, March 6. http://www.army.mil/institution/operations/reports/IGReport-APDESI/IG%20Report%20-%20Army%20Physical%20Disability%20Evaluation%20System%20Inspection.pdf (accessed March 15, 2007).

VA. 2006. *Veterans Benefits Administration program guide 21.2, Part II, index to transmittal sheets for compensation and pension regulations, 38 CFR Part 4.* Washington, DC: Veterans Benefits Administration, VA. http://www.warms.vba.va.gov/admin21/guide/pg21_2/part4.doc (accessed August 7, 2006).

WHO (World Health Organization). 2001. *International classification of functioning, disability and health: ICF.* Geneva: WHO.

WHO. 2002. *Towards a common language for functioning, disability and health: ICF.* Geneva: WHO. http://www3.who.int/icf/beginners/bg.pdf (accessed March 25, 2007).

9

Service Connection on Aggravation and Secondary Bases

The Veterans' Disability Benefits Commission asked the committee to

> *From a medical perspective, analyze the current Department of Veterans Affairs (VA) practice of assigning service connection on "secondary" and "aggravation" bases. In secondary claims, determine what medical principles and practices should be applied in determining whether a causal relationship exists between two conditions. In aggravation claims, determine what medical principles and practices should be applied in determining whether a preexisting disease was increased due to military service or was increased due to the natural process of the disease.*

This chapter summarizes what is known about how aggravation of preservice disability and secondary claims are evaluated and rated, and provides recommendations on how the current process can be enhanced for each.

COMPENSATION FOR AGGRAVATION OF PRESERVICE DISABILITY CLAIMS

According to VA regulations, *aggravation* is defined as occurring under the following conditions:[1]

> A preexisting injury or disease will be considered to have been aggravated by active military, naval, or air service, where there is an increase

[1]38 CFR § 3.306.

> in disability during such service, unless there is a specific finding that the increase in disability is due to the natural progress of the disease.

In the two-year period ending September 30, 2006, more than 21,000 veterans were service connected on the basis of aggravation of a preservice disability by military service, constituting less than two percent of disabilities that were service connected during that time period. The ten most common aggravated conditions (Table 9-1) accounted for nearly half of the total number of cases service connected on the basis of aggravation. Five percent were rated 50 percent or higher, while 87 percent were rated 20 percent or lower (Figure 9-1).

Establishing Preservice Disability

VA begins its evaluation of claims for aggravation of preservice disabilities under a "presumption of soundness" whereby, unless the evidence indicates otherwise, it is to be presumed that veterans were in sound condition on enlistment into service:

> 38 CFR §3.304(b), "Presumption of soundness."
>
> The veteran will be considered to have been in sound condition when examined, accepted, and enrolled for service, except as to defects, infirmities, or disorders noted at entrance into service, or where clear and unmistakable (obvious or manifest) evidence demonstrates that an injury or disease existed prior thereto and was not aggravated by such service. Only such conditions as are recorded in examination reports are to be considered as noted.

VA can note preservice illness or injury during a veteran's service.[2] For example, if the presence of disease residuals (e.g., scars, healed fractures) is discovered during service, and there is no evidence of the antecedent disease or injury during service, the conclusion is that the antecedent disease or injury preexisted service. Where this information is noted, and the evidentiary weight that is given to this information should the veteran file an aggravation claim in the future, are not clear.

Rating specialists consult medical records from before, during, and after a claimant's enlistment date to evaluate claims involving preservice disability. Likely to be included in these records are findings from a general medical examination that rating specialists request for almost all new claims. According to the medical history section of the compensation and pension (C&P) examination worksheet for general medical exams, the physician should include in the report a discussion of "whether an injury

[2] 38 CFR 3.303(c).

TABLE 9-1 10 Most Common Conditions Service Connected on the Basis of Aggravation, FY 2005–FY 2006

Diagnostic Code	Disability	Number of Cases
6100	Hearing loss	3,066
5276	Flat feet	1,737
5260	Leg, limitation of flexion of	1,043
5010	Traumatic arthritis	832
5237	Lumbrosacral/cervical strain	772
7101	Hypertensive vascular disease	586
5242	Major depression	572
5257	Knee, other impairment of	538
6602	Bronchial asthma	493
5271	Ankle, limited motion of	485

SOURCE: Communication from Bradley G. Mayes, director, C&P Service, Department of Veterans Affairs, December 14, 2006.

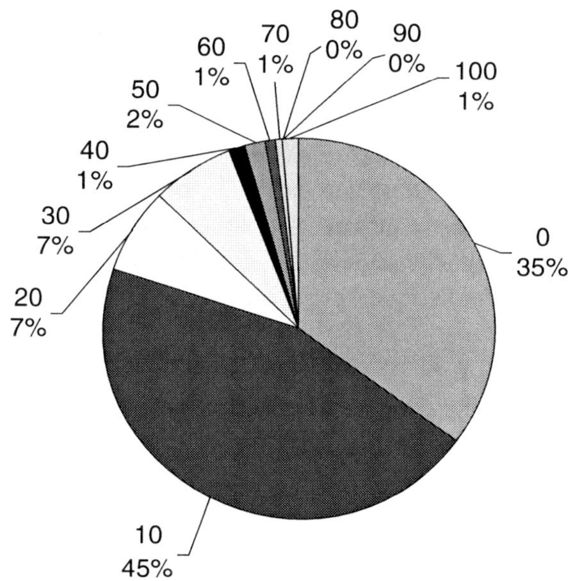

FIGURE 9-1 Distribution of grants for aggravation of preservice disability by rating degree from 0 to 100 percent, FY 2005–FY 2006.
SOURCE: Communication from Bradley G. Mayes, director, C&P Service, Department of Veterans Affairs, December 14, 2006.

or disease that is found *occurred during active service, before active service, or after active service.* To the extent possible, describe the circumstances, dates, specific injury or disease that occurred, treatment, follow-up, and residuals. If the injury or disease occurred *before active service*, describe any worsening of residuals due to being in military service."[3]

If medical records indicate that the claimant had an illness or injury prior to enlistment, this will not confirm that the condition existed, but will be used as one piece of evidence in an overall evaluation "with due regard to accepted medical principles pertaining to the history, manifestations, clinical course, and character of the particular injury or disease or residuals thereof."[4]

Under the presumption of soundness principle, if a preservice disability is not noted in the veteran's medical records, VA has the burden of showing by clear and unmistakable evidence that the disease or injury existed prior to service, and was not aggravated by service.[5]

Aggravation vs. Natural Process of Disease

According to VA rating policy instructions, "Where the advancement in severity is beyond that to be expected by natural progress of the condition, service connection is warranted.[6] This will require analysis of the facts in the individual case and knowledge of the particular condition concerned" (VA, 2005). In practice, when the presence of a preservice disability and an increase in that disability is established, rating specialists assume that the increase is due to aggravation by service, unless there is specific evidence indicating that the increase is due to the natural progress of the disease.

For veterans whose service was during wartime or peacetime after December 31, 1946, clear and unmistakable evidence (defined as "medical facts and principles that may be considered to determine whether the increase is due to the natural progress of the condition") is required to rebut the presumption of aggravation.[7]

For veterans who served during peacetime prior to December 7, 1941, disease or injury will be found to be due to the natural progress of the condition when "available evidence of a nature generally acceptable as competent shows that the increase in severity of a disease or injury or

---

[3]http://www.vba.va.gov/bln/21/Benefits/exams/disexm23.htm (accessed December 20, 2006).

[4]38 CFR 3.304(b)(1).

[5]VA's *Compensation and Pension Adjudication Procedures Manual* (M21-1MR) is the Veterans Benefits Administration's (VBA's) manual for the disability determination process. The section on aggravation is attached as Appendix A of the manual.

[6]Phrases "natural *process* of disease" and "natural *progress* of disease" are used interchangeably throughout VA regulations and training materials.

[7]38 CFR 3.306(b).

acceleration in progress was that normally to be expected by reason of the inherent character of the condition, aside from any extraneous or contributing cause or influence peculiar to military service."[8]

The places, types, and circumstances of service are also taken into consideration for veterans who served during wartime. For example, if there are found to be manifestations of a preservice disease or injury during or soon after combat, or following status as a prisoner of war, aggravation of a preservice condition will be established.[9] Hardships of service may also be considered in claims for veterans who served during peacetime.

Rating Aggravation of Preservice Disability Claims

The final rating of an aggravation claim takes into account the degree of disability over and above that which existed on entry into service. For instance, if a veteran has an overall rating of 90 percent and it can be ascertained from medical evidence that the degree of disability at entry into service was 10 percent, he or she will receive a final rating of 80 percent. If, however, the degree of disability at time of enlistment is not ascertainable, such a deduction will not be made and the veteran will receive the overall rating of 90 percent. When the overall rating at evaluation is 100 percent, the degree of preservice disability is never deducted.[10]

How rating specialists go about determining a veteran's degree of disability prior to service compared with his or her current degree of disability is not clear. The physician performing the general medical examination is not responsible for assigning these percentages. The rater, therefore, through his or her own review of the medical records, most likely makes these determinations to make the deduction.

Temporary and intermittent flare-ups of illnesses or injuries that existed prior to service cannot be considered as aggravation due to service. A veteran is eligible for compensation only when his or her underlying condition (as opposed to symptoms) has been worsened by service. Also, should a veteran seek compensation for side effects (e.g., scars, absent or poorly functioning body parts) of medical or surgical treatment received during service for an illness or injury that existed preservice, his or her application will not be granted unless the preservice condition has otherwise been aggravated by service.[11]

---

[8]38 CFR § 3.306(c) "Peacetime service prior to December 7, 1941."
[9]38 CFR § 3.306(b)(2).
[10]38 CFR § 3.322, "Ratings of disabilities aggravated by service."
[11]38 CFR § 3.306(b)(1).

Chronic and Hereditary Disease

Splane v. *West* (Fed. Cir. 2000) led to the November 7, 2002, publication of a final rule (67 FR 67792) amending VA's adjudication regulations concerning presumptive service connection. Under the new rule, chronic illnesses that preexisted a veteran's entry into service that manifest themselves to a degree of disability of at least 10 percent within a specified period after service are to be considered aggravated by service, unless there is evidence to the contrary. The specified period is within one year (except for leprosy and tuberculosis within three years, and multiple sclerosis within seven years) from the date of separation from service.[12]

The presumption may be rebutted by evidence showing that the chronic illness has not manifested itself to a degree of at least 10 percent within the specified period or, if it has, that the disability is due to a disease or injury acquired after separation from service.[13]

Despite their hereditary origin, diseases such as sickle cell anemia, polycystic kidney disease, and retinitis pigmentosa, are included in the Rating Schedule and can be service connected if symptoms of these diseases first manifest themselves after entry into service. Such diseases can also be found to have been aggravated by service when there is evidence that there were symptoms of disease prior to entry into service and evidence that there was progression during service at a rate greater than normally expected according to the accepted medical authority.[14]

Role of C&P Medical Examiners in Evaluating Aggravation of Preservice Disability Claims

As already noted, the general medical examination worksheet directs the examiner in the Veterans Health Administration (VHA) to determine whether an injury or disease occurred before, during, or after active military service and, if before active service, to describe any worsening of the preexisting condition due to being in active service.

When ordering the examination of someone claiming aggravation of a preservice condition, the rater could ask for the examiner's opinion of whether it is more likely than not that a veteran's condition existed preservice and was worsened by being on active duty rather than by the natural progression of the condition. Whether and how often this is done is not known.

---

[12]38 CFR § 3.307(a)(3).

[13]38 CRF § 3.307(d).

[14]VA's *Compensaton and Pension Adjudication Procedures Manual* M21-1MR, Part IV, Subpart ii, Ch. 2, Sec. B.

In addition, according to VHA policy,

> Veteran patients may request descriptive statements regarding their medical conditions and/or opinions concerning the "possible cause(s)" of an existing medical condition for VA disability claims purposes. VHA health-care providers shall provide a statement or opinion describing a patient's medical condition. If the health-care provider is the veteran's treating physician, and is unable, or deems it inappropriate, to provide an opinion or statement, such physician shall refer the veteran's request to another health-care provider for the opinion or statement (VHA, 2000).

COMPENSATION FOR SECONDARY SERVICE CONNECTION AND FOR SECONDARY SERVICE CONNECTION BY AGGRAVATION

As the title of the regulation suggests, there are two categories of claims that can be granted secondary service connection under VA regulation 3.310, "Disabilities that are proximately due to, or aggravated by, service-connected disease or injury."

The first category includes claims for which there is an initial service-connected disability, and then a subsequent disability or disabilities found to be proximately due to (caused by) the service-connected disability. One example of this type of claim would be loss of limb due to amputation occurring subsequent to a service-connected diabetes diagnosis.[15] The loss of a limb, it might be argued, should be service connected in addition to the diabetes because the amputation may not have been needed had the veteran not developed diabetes.

In the two-year period from October 2004 through September 2006, nearly 260,000 veterans were service connected for conditions proximately due to service-connected disabilities. This accounted for approximately 19 percent of the more than 1.3 million disabilities that were service connected during that period. Most of the disabilities were rated at 10 or 20 percent (Figure 9-2). Less than 10 percent were rated at 50 percent or higher.

Ten conditions (Table 9-2) accounted for 55 percent of the disabilities compensated as secondary to service-connected disabilities in 2005–2006.

In accord with a 1995 court decision (*Allen* v. *Brown*, 7 Vet. App. 439), VA will also grant service connection under this regulation in claims where there is an increase in the severity of nonservice-connected disability that is found to be due to aggravation by a service-connected disability. These are called *secondary service connection by aggravation* claims or, after the

---

[15]In people with diabetes, an increased risk of amputation comes from damage to nerves and blood vessels through decreased circulation efficiency and diabetic neuropathy. According to the American Diabetes Association, more than 60 percent of nontraumatic lower-limb amputations occur in people with diabetes and the rate of amputation for people with diabetes is 10 times higher than for people without diabetes (ADA, 2007).

TABLE 9-2 10 Most Common Diagnoses Service Connected as a Secondary Condition, FY 2005–FY 2006

Diagnostic Code	Disability	Number of Cases
8520	Sciatic nerve, paralysis	40,761
7522	Erectile dysfunction	24,406
8515	Median nerve, paralysis	17,790
8521	External popliteal nerve	13,685
7005	Arteriosclerotic heart disease	10,188
7114	Arteriosclerosis obliterans	8,538
7101	Hypertensive vascular disease	7,103
7541	Renal involvement in systemic diseases	7,008
8620	Sciatic nerve, neuritis	6,476
9434	Degenerative arthritis of the spine	5,371

SOURCE: Communication from Bradley G. Mayes, director, C&P Service, Department of Veterans Affairs, December 14, 2006.

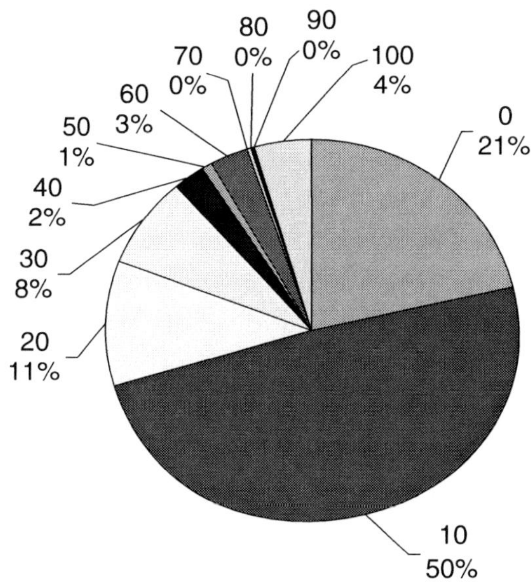

FIGURE 9-2 Distribution of grants for secondary service connection by rating degree from 0 to 100 percent, FY 2005–FY 2006.
SOURCE: Communication from Bradley G. Mayes, director, C&P Service, Department of Veterans Affairs, December 14, 2006.

name of the court case, *Allen aggravation* claims. One example of this type of claim would be a veteran with a service-connected left knee injury who, after service, goes on to develop arthritis in his or her right hip. It could be argued that, through the effects of the knee injury on gait, the hip arthritis is exacerbated to a level beyond what would have been had there not been a service-connected knee injury.

For the period October 2004 through September 2006, approximately 41,000 claims were granted service connection based on aggravation of a nonservice-connected condition by a service-connected condition.[16]

What Is a Secondary Condition?

Secondary condition is a relatively new term in the disability and public health arenas. It began to be accepted around 1990 as an expansion of the concept of comorbidity, which is used to refer to conditions that exist in a single person simultaneously, but that are not known to be related in any manner (CDC, 2004a). A person having coexisting skin malignancy and hearing loss would be said to have comorbidities, because there is no known relationship between these two conditions.

From a strictly medical perspective, a secondary condition is a condition with its own pathophysiology that is due to, or caused by, the presence of a preceding primary condition. Secondary conditions can be distinguished from secondary *manifestations*, the latter referring to sequelae or subsequent complications arising from the same underlying pathophysiologic process as the primary condition.

Diabetes is a good example of a condition with many secondary manifestations. Diabetes itself is an abnormal metabolism of glucose (that can be induced in several ways, including trauma), which has an associated abnormality in lipid metabolism, which leads to an accelerated process of arteriosclerosis. This combination leads to a higher frequency and earlier onset of, among other things, peripheral vascular disease, coronary arteriosclerosis, peripheral neuropathy, and premature cataracts of the eyes. These can be considered secondary manifestations because they are expressions of the person's underlying diabetes and share the same underlying pathophysiology.

At times the Rating Schedule treats what are in fact secondary manifestations as secondary conditions. The instructions on rating diabetes mellitus (diagnostic code 7913 under CFR 4.119 Schedule of ratings—endocrine system), for example, tell raters to evaluate compensable complications of diabetes separately, except in cases where they are a part of a 100 percent

---

[16]Communication from Bradley G. Mayes, director, C&P Service, Department of Veterans Affairs, December 14, 2006.

evaluation (diabetes ratings below 100 percent do not take into account compensable complications).

Rating Secondary Service Connection Claims

In a presentation before the committee, C&P Service staff stated that decisions on secondary claims are based on the facts of the individual case and the medical opinion solicited from the VHA examiner on the general medical examination form. Using this evidence, the rater determines whether it is at least as likely as not that each claimed secondary condition was caused by the primary service-connected condition.

The process of assigning ratings in secondary claims is the same as in claims involving multiple individually service-connected conditions. Each condition is first evaluated separately and assigned a percentage rating. Starting with the condition with the highest percentage rating, the rater then uses VA's combined ratings table to calculate an overall percentage rating for the primary condition and all conditions found to be proximately due to the primary condition.

Cardiovascular Disease

Ischemic or other cardiovascular disease that develops in a veteran with a service-connected amputation of a lower extremity at or above the knee, or service-connected amputations of both lower extremities at or above the ankles, is presumptively secondary to the amputation or amputations.[17]

Alcohol and Drug Abuse

In some cases there are nonmedical considerations in allowing service connection for secondary conditions. Examples in training materials include alcohol or drug abuse resulting secondarily from a service-connected disorder, such as posttraumatic stress disorder (PTSD). Federal law (38 U.S.C. § 1110) permits a veteran to receive compensation for an alcohol abuse or drug abuse disability acquired as secondary to, or as a symptom of, a veteran's service-connected disability, although according to the Federal Circuit Court of Appeals, it precludes compensation for secondary disabilities, such as cirrhosis of the liver, that result from primary alcohol abuse (i.e., voluntary and willful drinking to excess during the time of service).[18]

---

[17]38 U.S.C. 501, 1110–1131, and 38 CFR § 3.320(b).

[18]*Allen* v. *Principi*, 237 F.3d 1368 (Fed. Cir. 2001), rehearing en banc denied, 268 F.3d 1340 (2001). The Federal Circuit Court of Appeals defined *primary* as meaning an alcohol abuse disability arising during service from voluntary and willful drinking to excess.

Rating Secondary Service Connection by Aggravation Claims

Regulation 3.310(b), or aggravation of nonservice-connected disabilities (referred to in our report as Allen aggravation claims) reads as follows:

> Any increase in severity of a nonservice-connected disease or injury that is proximately due to or the result of a service-connected disease or injury, and not due to the natural progress of the nonservice-connected disease, will be service connected. However, VA will not concede that a nonservice-connected disease or injury was aggravated by a service-connected disease or injury unless the baseline level of severity of the nonservice-connected disease or injury is established by medical evidence created before the onset of aggravation or by the earliest medical evidence created at any time between the onset of aggravation and the receipt of medical evidence establishing the current level of severity of the nonservice-connected disease or injury. The rating activity will determine the baseline and current levels of severity under the Schedule for Rating Disabilities and determine the extent of aggravation by deducting the baseline level of severity as well as any increase in severity due to the natural progress of the disease from the current level.

According to the Veterans Benefits Administration (VBA) rating manual, the first step in rating Allen aggravation claims is to collect all "potentially relevant" medical records from the veteran's providers. Once this is complete, the rater requests a medical examination.

The examination is conducted by a VHA physician and includes a review of all records in the claims folder to establish the baseline level of nonservice-connected disability, and the additional level of disability that occurred due to the service-connected disability.

To be considered adequate for rating purposes, the examiner's report must separately address the following:[19]

- the baseline manifestations that are due to the effects of nonservice-connected disease or injury;
- the increased manifestations that, in the examiner's opinion, are proximately due to a service-connected disability based on medical considerations; and
- the medical considerations supporting an opinion that increased manifestations of a nonservice-connected disease or injury are proximately due to a service-connected disability.

[19]VA's *Compensation and Pension Adjudication Procedures Manual,* M21-1MR, Part IV, Subpart ii, Ch. 2, Sec. B.

An examination that fails to identify baseline findings, or the increment of increased disability due to service-connected causes, should not be considered adequate for rating purposes. In the event that the report does not meet these requirements and also fails to explain why it would be mere speculation to comment on these matters, the rater is instructed to send the report back to the examiner. When the examination report is complete, the rater uses the findings to assign a rating to the claimed conditions.

There are no instructions on how the rater is to use the findings from the examination to adjudicate the claim. However, as is the case in aggravation of preservice disability claims, in Allen aggravation claims there is assessment of whether disability is the result of the service-connected disability (military service, in aggravation of preservice disability claims) or the natural progress of disease, and in both types of claims the veteran is compensated for the degree of disability over and above that existing prior to aggravation. Because of these similarities, the rating process in Allen aggravation claims may be similar to that outlined in the earlier sections of this chapter on aggravation versus natural progress of disease and rating aggravation of preservice disability claims. However, there is one important distinction. In aggravation of preservice disability claims, when the evidence of degree of preservice disability is not available, there is no penalty to the veteran; the veteran receives the overall rating for his or her condition at the time of application with no deduction of the percent of disability existing preservice. In Allen aggravation claims, if there is no medical evidence of the baseline level of severity of the nonservice-connected disability before the onset of aggravation by the service-connected disability, VBA will not consider the claim.

FINDINGS AND RECOMMENDATIONS

Aggravation of Preservice Disability and Allen Aggravation Claims

Aggravation of preservice disability claims involve an assessment of the worsening of a condition existing preservice due to service. Allen aggravation claims involve an assessment of the worsening, due to a service-connected condition, of a nonservice-connected condition that could have developed either before or after service. Regarding aggravation, the statement of task asks the committee to "determine what medical principles and practices should be applied in determining whether a preexisting disease was increased due to military service or was increased due to the natural process of the disease." The committee interprets this task as referring to aggravation of preservice disability claims and not Allen aggravation claims, and assumes its sponsor either intended for Allen aggravation to be addressed with secondary conditions (since these claims are categorized under secondary conditions in VA regulations), or omitted it unintentionally from the statement of task. However, insofar as both aggravation of preservice disability and Allen aggravation claims involve an assessment of worsening of disability over and above some previous level, both can be addressed by the committee simultaneously.

When a veteran files an aggravation of preservice disability claim, VA has the burden of proving the veteran was in sound condition on enlistment. If, in this process, it is discovered from medical evidence that there was a condition existing preservice, and that the condition has since increased in severity, VBA must proceed with adjudication of the claim. Raters weigh medical evidence, which may include the opinion of a VHA medical examiner, to determine whether it is at least as likely as not that the preservice disability was aggravated by service rather than increased in severity due to the natural process of the disease.

The adjudication process in Allen aggravation claims is similar. The rater collects medical records and requests a medical examination by a VHA physician, the findings of which are used to document the baseline level of the nonservice-connected disability when it began, and the presence and degree of worsening of the nonservice-connected disability since. If the condition has worsened, the rater must then determine whether the worsening of the nonservice-connected disability is due to the service-connected disability or the natural process of disease.

As is the case in all disability claims, raters who often have no medical training are responsible for reviewing medical evidence and assigning ratings. In aggravation claims, raters have the additional task of deciding whether a condition has worsened and, if it has, whether the worsening is due to the natural process of disease or military service (or, in Allen aggravation claims, whether the worsening is due to the natural process of disease or a nonservice-connected disability).

The committee has learned that, when ordering the examination of someone claiming aggravation of a preservice condition, the rater could ask for the physician's opinion of whether it is more likely than not that the condition existed preservice and was worsened by being on active duty rather than by the natural progression of the condition. For all types of claims, VHA policy also allows veterans to request descriptive statements regarding the possible causes of their conditions from VHA examiners. However, how often either is done is not known.

Recommendation 9-1. VA should seek the judgment of qualified experts, supported by findings from current peer-reviewed literature, as guidance for adjudicating both aggravation of preservice disability and Allen aggravation claims. Judgment could be provided by VHA examiners, perhaps from VA centers of excellence, who have the appro-

priate expertise for evaluating the condition(s) in question in individual claims.

Secondary Service Connection

The statement of task asks the committee to "determine what medical principles and practices should be applied in determining whether a causal relationship exists between two conditions." Currently, raters consult medical records to determine whether it is at least as likely as not that a claimed secondary condition was caused by a service-connected condition.

Causation

In epidemiology, well-established criteria are used to aid in judging the strength of the relationship between two variables at the population level. Perhaps the best known are those that were set forth in the U.S. Surgeon General's 1964 report on the relationship between smoking and health (CDC, 1964). These include the following:

1. Temporal relationship—relationship in time between two variables; an exposure cannot be considered a cause of an outcome unless it can be shown to have preceded the outcome in time
2. Consistency—replication of research findings on the relationship between a given exposure and an outcome, especially across study designs and populations
3. Strength of association—degree of association between two variables as measured statistically; the greater the association, the more likely the causal role of the exposure
4. Specificity—degree to which the occurrence of the outcome depends on the presence of the exposure; if the outcome is known to occur in relation to exposures other than the one in question, then the relationship is considered less specific
5. Biological plausibility—known biological mechanism by which a certain exposure might increase or decrease likelihood of the outcome

Using such criteria, evidence classification schemes can be developed. In the U.S. Surgeon General's 2004 report (CDC, 2004b) on the health consequences of smoking, for example, conclusions concerning the evidence that smoking causes health outcomes such as cancer and cardiovascular disease were placed into one of the following four categories:

1. sufficient to infer a causal relationship
2. suggestive but not sufficient to infer a causal relationship

3. inadequate to infer the presence or absence of a causal relationship
4. suggestive of no causal relationship

In VA's case, raters and examiners are dealing with determining causation at the individual level, where the primary service-connected condition is the exposure and the claimed secondary condition is the outcome. Where research is available, VA could use epidemiologic criteria for causation and evidence classification schemes to inform decision-making on secondary claims. The committee is aware that this might require regulatory action to implement.

Recommendation 9-2. VA should guide clinical evaluation and rating of claims for secondary service connection by adopting specific criteria for determining causation, such as those cited above (e.g., temporal relationship, consistency of research findings, strength of association, specificity, plausible biological mechanism). VA should also provide and regularly update information to compensation and pension examiners about the findings of epidemiological, biostatistical, and disease mechanism research concerning the secondary consequences of disabilities prevalent among veterans.

REFERENCES

ADA (American Diabetes Association). 2007. *Complications of diabetes in the United States.* http://www.diabetes.org/diabetes-statistics/complications.jsp (accessed May 23, 2007).

CDC (Centers for Disease Control). 1964. *Smoking and health: Report of the Advisory Committee to the Surgeon General of the Public Health Service.* PHS Publication No. 1103. Washington, DC: CDC.

CDC (Centers for Disease Control and Prevention). 2004a. *Children and adults with disabilities: Secondary conditions.* http://0-www.cdc.gov.mill1.sjlibrary.org/NCBDDD/factsheets/DH_sec_cond.pdf (accessed December 5, 2006).

CDC. 2004b. *The health consequences of smoking: A report of the Surgeon General.* Atlanta, GA: CDC. http://www.cdc.gov/tobacco/data_statistics/sgr/sgr_2004/chapters.htm (accessed April 3, 2007).

VHA (Veterans Health Administration). 2000. *VHA Directive 2000-029, provision of medical opinions by VA health care practitioners.* http://www.va.gov/vhapublications/ViewPublication.asp?pub_ID=74 (accessed December 20, 2006).

VA (Department of Veterans Affairs). 2005. *Instructor guide: General policy in rating.* Washington, DC: VA.

10

Conclusion: Into the 21st Century

In the course of responding to the specific tasks assigned by the Veterans' Disability Benefits Commission, the committee encountered some themes that underlie the somewhat disparate topics. First, the Veterans Benefits Administration (VBA) is so focused on serving veterans applying for the various services it provides that there do not appear to be adequate resources for systematic analysis of how well it is providing those services (process analysis) or the impact of the services on the lives of veterans (outcome analysis), which in turn would enable the Department of Veterans Affairs (VA) to be more responsive to changes affecting its programs. Second, VBA does not have adequate resources for a systematic program of research oriented toward understanding and improving the effectiveness of its benefits programs. Third, VA is missing the opportunity to take a more veteran-centered approach to service provision across its benefits programs. Veterans with severe disabilities need coordinated care that is able to integrate their needs for medical rehabilitation, vocational rehabilitation, assistive technologies, accessible transportation and housing, education and training services, and compensation to make up for loss of earning capacity that may remain after rehabilitation. VA provides some of these services, but they are not readily accessible nor well coordinated. Addressing these issues is beyond the scope of the committee's assignment, but we think it is worthwhile to discuss them and point to the need for them to be addressed.

NEED FOR ANALYSIS AND PLANNING

It is instructive that much of the information about the operations of the disability compensation program came from external sources or, if internal, from ad hoc panels and task forces. The effort to update the Rating Schedule in the 1990s was triggered by a 1988 report of the General Accounting Office (GAO), which found that ten of the body systems had not been updated for 10 years or more and the rest had been updated, but not comprehensively.[1] Internal ad hoc reviews formed in response to perceived problems include the 1993 Blue Ribbon Panel on Claims Processing and the 2001 Claims Processing Task Force. Congress established the Veterans' Claims Adjudication Commission of 1996, initiated the study of the management of compensation and pension (C&P) benefits claim processes for veterans by the National Academy of Public Administration in 1997, and created the current Veterans' Disability Benefits Commission. GAO and the VA Office of the Inspector General have issued a number of reports on the operation and results of the C&P process.

Another indicator of limited planning is the insufficient capacity of VBA's management information systems to provide data needed for planning and evaluation. Until recently, the information system on C&P disability cases—the Benefits Delivery Network (BDN)—could not provide information on the characteristics of disabilities that were not allowed and could not detect changes in aggregate grant rates or differences in these rates across regional offices. The BDN could only list up to seven diagnostic codes at a time and their rating levels, and if a veteran was granted an increase or a new service-connected disability, the historical information was overwritten. This limits analysis of trends in reopened cases, such as the impact of the progression of diabetes and the manifestation of its complications over time, which will have an unknown but large impact on program capacity and costs.

VBA is aware of the problems and has made some progress. An Office of Performance Analysis and Integrity (PA&I) was established in 2001 to consolidate data quality and analysis functions of the various VBA programs, and a data warehouse was established. VA now has an Office of Planning, Evaluation, and Preparedness, which has sponsored evaluations of some VBA programs. A 2000 evaluation of VA's education benefit programs found that the benefit level had lagged significantly behind the rising cost of education. In 2001, an evaluation of the program for survivors of veterans with service-connected disabilities was performed, which looked at the Dependency and Indemnity Compensation program and four insurance programs.

[1] GAO was renamed the Government Accountability Office in 2004.

Following a recommendation of the 1996 Veterans' Claims Adjudication Commission, VA established an Office of the Actuary in 1999, but it does not yet produce the kinds of actuarial forecasts of the number of veterans with service-connected disabilities receiving Department of Defense (DoD) disability benefits done by the DoD Office of the Actuary.

VBA now has an information system for the C&P Service that provides much better information beginning with calendar year 2004 for planning and evaluation purposes as well as program management. The new system—Rating Board Automation (RBA 2000)—provides a more complete range of information and can produce historical data for trend analyses and forecasts. RBA 2000 can also produce information on inconsistencies in decision making.

The policy analysis group in PA&I is small, however, in relation to the analysis and planning needs of VBA.

PROGRAM-ORIENTED RESEARCH

This report also recommends a greater research effort to improve the Rating Schedule and keep it up to date (Recommendations 4-2, 4-3, 4-6, 5-3, 6-2, and 7-3). The recommended research program focuses on the evaluation and rating processes and on program outcomes. VBA does not have a large research capacity, however, nor are there adequate resources and staff to conduct policy research and to contract for research and evaluation studies relating to the adequacy of the process and outcomes of veterans benefit programs and services. Examples of the research that might be performed are described below.

Process Research

Process research would focus on continuous improvement of the VBA rating system and process, including ways of increasing accuracy and reducing variability in outcomes. Examples of areas to be examined would include decision-making studies, in which the same patients are examined by several C&P examiners to understand the range and sources of variability in results, and cases would be rated by different examiners to understand the range and sources of variability in those results. Currently, most C&P examinations are performed by generalists, including those involving the worksheets for the heart, the various musculoskeletal impairments, HIV infection, and so forth, because VA believes that generalists can produce adequate reports for rating.[2] This hypothesis could be tested. The use

[2]Certain conditions require specialists, such as hearing (audiologist) and initial posttraumatic stress disorder (PTSD) (psychiatrist).

of nurses and physician assistants under physician supervision, which is allowed, could also be tested.

Clinical Outcomes Research

Clinical outcomes research would help identify and validate the use of severity scores and disease-staging protocols used in clinical settings for rating purposes. Research on the effectiveness of using measures of individual functioning, such as activities of daily living, instrumental activities of daily living, and specific functional tests, recommended in Chapter 4, falls in this category of research, as does research on the utility of health-related quality-of-life (QOL) measures in quantifying loss in QOL not accounted for in the current Rating Schedule.

Economic Outcomes Research

Economic outcomes research is recommended in Chapter 4 to provide information on how well the criteria in the Rating Schedule can measure loss of earnings. The same research could also provide information on the adequacy of benefits in compensating for lost earning capacity. The results of this research would be a factor in revising the criteria, because it is the closest measure to loss of earning capacity available. This would not necessarily limit adjustment of the criteria to account for other losses, such as loss of QOL, but it would provide a benchmark in assessing the income security impact of disability compensation.

VETERAN-CENTERED SERVICES

The committee's scope of work was centered on the disability compensation program, but it also included consideration of the medical criteria for eligibility for ancillary services (Chapter 6). It became apparent that while VA has the collective body of services needed to maximize the potential of veterans with disabilities, the separate services are not actively coordinated, which ultimately makes them less effective. It is up to the veteran to apply for each benefit, and he or she must apply and be granted service connection to become eligible for other services. Ideally, there would be a comprehensive initial evaluation of a veteran's needs and a case worker to assist in obtaining the applicable services. This approach would treat the veteran as a client. This would create tension with the veteran's role as a claimant ("we would like to help you, but first you have prove you are eligible"), but this would be minimized if there were a more coordinated intake process.

In Chapter 3, we laid out a model of a rating process in which there would be rating of impairment severity, degree of disability, and loss of

QOL. Some research and analysis must be done to understand how best to determine the nonwork disability and QOL ratings and whether they can be combined—whether, for example, work disability and nonwork disability measures could be included in one Rating Schedule or would have to be rated separately, or whether it is feasible to operationalize QOL measures as a basis for compensation. Impairment ratings are based on medical findings and expert judgment, but disability evaluation requires additional information and expertise to judge what a person can do in daily life. The disability evaluation process provides the opportunity to evaluate the veteran with disabilities for the other services VA provides, such as vocational rehabilitation, employment services, education benefits, and specialized medical services (e.g., centers for spinal cord injury, traumatic brain injury, and vision impairment rehabilitation). This process would coordinate VA's programs for each veteran and make it a more veteran-centered agency.

Appendix A

Biographical Sketches of Committee Members, Consultants, and Staff

Lonnie R. Bristow, M.D., M.A.C.P., (*chair*) is a former president of the American Medical Association (AMA), after earlier serving as vice-chair and chair of AMA's Board of Trustees. Dr. Bristow has written and lectured extensively on medical science as well as socioeconomic and ethical issues related to medicine. He is a board-certified internist and has practiced medicine for more than 40 years. He received his M.D. from New York University College of Medicine. He is a member of the Institute of Medicine (IOM) and was appointed to its Quality of Health Care in America committee, which in 1999 and 2001, respectively, authored the widely-read reports *To Err Is Human* and *Crossing the Quality Chasm*. He chaired the IOM Committee on Strategies for Increasing the Diversity of the U.S. Health-Care Workforce, which issued its report, *In the Nation's Compelling Interest—Ensuring Diversity in the Health-Care Workforce*, in 2004. Dr. Bristow's research interests and expertise are broad and, over the decades, his writings have included papers on medical ethics, socialized medicine as practiced in Great Britain and Canada, health-care financing in America, professional liability insurance problems, sickle cell anemia, and coronary care unit utilization. Dr. Bristow recently served as vice-chair for the Physician Leadership for a New Drug Policy and also, by presidential appointment, he served for six years as chair of the board of regents of the Uniformed Services University of Health Sciences. He continues as an active member of both groups. In addition, Dr. Bristow is a reviewer for the *Journal of the American Medical Association*. He recently retired from private practice but continues his other activities as a professional consultant. Dr. Bristow is a Navy veteran.

Gunnar B. J. Andersson, M.D., Ph.D., is professor and chairman of the Department of Orthopedic Surgery, and vice-dean, Surgical Sciences and Services, Rush University Medical Center, and senior attending vice-president of Medical Affairs, and president, Medical Staff, Rush-Presbyterian-St. Luke's Medical Center, Chicago. His areas of expertise include disorders of the spine, lower back pain, surgery for herniated disk, and evaluation of the lumbar spine following surgery. He is an editor of the *Guides to the Evaluation of Permanent Impairments*, 5th edition (2000), and *Disability Evaluation*, 2nd edition (2003), both published by AMA. Dr. Andersson is also a member of numerous medical societies and committees, including chairman of the Research Planning Committee of the North American Spine Society, member of the Council of the American Academy of Orthopaedic Surgeons, and member of the U.S. National Safety Council. He was president of the U.S. Orthopaedic Research Society in 2000. He received his M.D. from the University of Goteborg, Sweden, and did his residency at Sahlgren Hospital, University of Goteborg. He also holds a Ph.D. in medical science.

John F. Burton, Jr., Ph.D., LL.B., is professor emeritus in the School of Management and Labor Relations at Rutgers University. Dr. Burton is an authority in workers' compensation and occupational safety and health law, as well as other types of social insurance programs. He has published many articles on workers' compensation programs, has edited and coauthored several books, and was president of the Labor and Employment Relations Association. In 1971–1972, he chaired the National Commission on State Workmen's Compensation Laws, which led to changes in many states. Dr. Burton served as dean of the School of Management and Labor Relations (1994–2000) and director of the Institute of Management and Labor Relations (1991–1994) at Rutgers University. He was a founding member of the National Academy of Social Insurance (NASI) and is currently a member of the NASI board of directors. He received his law degree and his Ph.D. in economics from the University of Michigan.

Lynn H. Gerber, M.D., is a graduate of Tufts University School of Medicine, and a diplomate of the American Board of Internal Medicine, subspecialty rheumatology, and the American Board of Physical Medicine and Rehabilitation. She is currently the director of the Center for Chronic Illness and Disability, and professor of Rehabilitation Science at George Mason University in Fairfax, Virginia. In this capacity, she is responsible for developing a research program to help describe the mechanisms by which chronic illness produces disability, determine how disability may accelerate illness, and explore treatments that can prevent or reduce disabilities and restore function. Dr. Gerber retired from the Clinical Center, National Institutes of Health (NIH), in 2005, after 30 years, where she served as the founding chief of the Rehabilitation Medicine Department, and coordinated care for patients with disabilities and collaborated in clinical research. Much of her clinical research interest has centered on measuring and treating impairments and disability in patients with musculoskeletal deficits, particularly children with osteogenesis imperfecta and persons with rheumatoid arthritis and cancer. Dr. Gerber has authored and coauthored 90 peer-reviewed, published manuscripts and 45 chapters in major textbooks.

Sid Gilman, M.D., F.R.C.P., is William J. Herdman Distinguished University Professor of Neurology in the Department of Neurology at the University of Michigan. He is also director of the Michigan Alzheimer's Disease Research Center, which is funded by NIH. Dr. Gilman is an expert on the neurochemical bases of human diseases causing cognitive and movement disorders and has published more than 350 research articles on the diagnosis, treatment, imaging characteristics, and neurophysiological changes underlying neurodegenerative disorders, including Parkinson's and Alzheimer's diseases. He is editor-in-chief of *Experimental Neurology*, *Neurobiology of Disease*, *MedLink Neurology*, and the *Contemporary Neurology Series*, and a member of the editorial boards of several other neurological and neuroscience journals. He is a consultant for the U.S. Food and Drug Administration, chair of the safety monitoring committees for two ongoing clinical trials, and a member of the scientific advisory boards of several companies. Gilman was elected a member of IOM in 1995. He received his M.D. from the University of California, Los Angeles, in 1957, and his F.R.C.P. from the Royal College of Physicians (London) in 2001.

Howard H. Goldman, M.D., M.P.H., Ph.D., is a professor of psychiatry and director of Mental Health Policy Studies at the University of Maryland, Baltimore School of Medicine. Between 1983 and 1985, Dr. Goldman was assistant director at the National Institute of Mental Health (NIMH), where he was responsible for mental health-care financing and policy research. He was also part of a working group to revise the Social Security Administration's listings of mental impairments during this period. Dr. Goldman has since continued as a consultant to the federal government on health-care financing, including the *President's Task Force on Health Care Reform* (1993) and the *President's New Freedom Commission on Mental Health* (2002–2003). He has authored more than 275 articles in the areas of mental health services research and economics and is current editor of the journal *Psychiatric Services*. He also serves on the editorial boards of several other journals, including the *American Journal of Psychiatry* and the *Journal of Mental Health Policy and Economics*. In 1999, he served as the senior scientific editor of the Surgeon General's report on mental health. Well regarded in his field, Dr. Goldman is the recipient of numerous awards, including the American Psychiatric Association's Senior Award for Research Development in Mental Health Services (1991). He is a member of the National Academy of Social Insurance (1996) and IOM (2002).

Sandra Gordon-Salant, Ph.D., is a professor in the Department of Hearing and Speech Sciences at the University of Maryland, College Park, and director of the Doctoral Program in Clinical Audiology. She has published more than 50 articles and book chapters pertaining to age-related hearing loss, speech perception, auditory temporal processing, and hearing aids. Her articles have appeared in the *Journal of the Acoustical Society of America; Journal of Speech, Language, and Hearing Research; Ear and Hearing;* and the *Journal of the American Academy of Audiology.* Dr. Gordon-Salant's research program has been supported by NIH for the past 20 years. She was the editor of the hearing section of the *Journal of Speech, Language, and Hearing Research,* and recently served as a member of the National Research Council's Committee on Disability Determination for Individuals with Hearing Impairment.

Jay S. Himmelstein, M.D., M.P.H., is a professor of Family Medicine and Community Health and director of the Center for Health Policy and Research (CHPR) at the University of Massachusetts (UMass) Medical School. He is board certified in both internal and occupational medicine and serves as assistant chancellor for Health Policy at UMass. His health policy research interests include Medicaid policy, health-care quality, workers' compensation medical care, and general health services research. As director of CHPR, Dr. Himmelstein oversees a wide range of applied policy research aimed at improving health outcomes for those served by public agencies, focusing on improving the evidence base for making policy decisions. As a Robert Wood Johnson health policy fellow in 1991, Dr. Himmelstein worked with a Senate Labor and Human Resources Committee on issues of national health reform and integration of workers' compensation with other health and disability benefit systems. He recently directed a national Robert Wood Johnson Foundation grant program called the Workers' Compensation Health Initiative aimed at supporting demonstration and evaluation projects testing innovations in the delivery and financing of the medical care portion of workers' compensation. Dr. Himmelstein received his M.D. from the University of Maryland and his M.P.H from the Harvard School of Public Health.

Ana E. Núñez, M.D., is an associate professor of medicine, director of the Center of Excellence in Women's Health, and director of the Women's Health Education Program at Drexel University College of Medicine. She received her M.D. training at Hahnemann University. She has additional fellowship training in medical education, health policy, and health services research. Dr. Núñez is a nationally recognized medical educator in women's health, primary care, cultural competency, and health disparities. She has served on numerous expert panels on women's health and cultural competency. She was principal investigator on a number of educationally focused health services research studies funded by the Department of Health and Human Services and the National Heart, Lung, and Blood Institute. Dr. Núñez has presented nationally at conferences addressing women's health, curricular reform, women and minorities in medicine, and cultural issues in health-care delivery and practice. Her research interests are in girls' and women's health, minority women's health, and culturally effective care. She has been an advocate on eliminating health disparities along gender and ethnic lines. She is a member of several professional societies including the American College of Physicians, American Medical Association, Association of Academic Women's Health Professionals, and National Academy of Women's Health Educators.

James W. Reed, M.D., M.A.C.P., is a professor of medicine and associate chair of Medicine for Research at Morehouse School of Medicine, and chief of endocrinology at Grady Memorial Hospital in Atlanta, Georgia. Dr. Reed is also a medical consultant at the Tuskegee Veterans Affairs Hospital in Alabama. He began his career as an Army physician, holding distinguished positions in medicine and clinical investigation at the Madigan and Eisenhower Army Medical Centers. He has lectured extensively on issues relating to the diagnosis and management of diabetes mellitus and hypertension, and is author of many articles, chapters, and books on diabetes and high blood pressure management. He is president of the International Society of Hypertension in Blacks, and a master (M.A.C.P.) of the American College of Physicians and fellow of the American College of Clinical Endocrinology. Dr. Reed received his M.D. from the Howard University College of Medicine.

Denise G. Tate, Ph.D., A.B.P.P., F.A.C.R.M., is a professor of rehabilitation psychology and neuropsychology in the Department of Physical Medicine and Rehabilitation at the University of Michigan. She is an expert on cognitive and emotional dysfunction among patients with chronic illness and physical impairment. Dr. Tate is particularly interested in adjustment following spinal cord injury, and she has published several articles on quality of life, return to work, and substance abuse among people with spinal cord injuries. Dr. Tate is also director of the Advanced Rehabilitation Research Training Project, a training program for professionals interested in pursuing research in rehabilitation of individuals with traumatic brain and spinal cord injury, at the University of Michigan. She received her M.A.

in experimental psychology from the Getulio Vargas University in Rio de Janeiro, Brazil, and her Ph.D. in rehabilitation psychology from Michigan State University.

Brian M. Thacker is a U.S. Army veteran and in 1973 received the Congressional Medal of Honor for extraordinary courage displayed while serving in Vietnam. Before retiring in 2002, Mr. Thacker had worked for the Department of Veterans Affairs (VA) for more than 25 years in various program evaluation and administration capacities. He began his career at VA's Long Beach Medical Center evaluating the efficacy of counseling services for veterans and the quality of continuing medical education programs for health-care providers. In the next phase of his career, he worked as director of the Management Services Division at the VA headquarters in Washington, D.C. Mr. Thacker is an active member and regional director of the Congressional Medal of Honor Society. He lives in Wheaton, Maryland.

Dennis C. Turk, Ph.D., is the John and Emma Bonica Professor of Anesthesiology and Pain Research and director of the Fibromyalgia Research Center at the University of Washington. He has published more than 400 articles on pain assessment, management, and treatment, as well as on the psychological characteristics of pain sufferers. Dr. Turk is co-coordinator of the Initiative on the Methods, Measurement, and Pain Assessment in Clinical Trials. He was formerly the editor-in-chief of the *Annals of Behavioral Medicine* and *Pain Management Today* and is currently editor-in-chief of the *Clinical Journal of Pain*. An international survey conducted by the University of Regina (Canada), published in the *Pain Clinic* (2001), identified Dr. Turk as one of the top ten leaders in pain research and treatment development. Dr. Turk received his Ph.D. in clinical psychology from the University of Waterloo in Ontario, Canada.

Raymond John Vogel, M.S., is a U.S. Army veteran with direct knowledge of veterans services and benefit programs. Mr. Vogel has held several executive positions with the VA, including three years as under secretary for veterans benefits, six years as director of VA regional benefits offices in Pennsylvania and Oregon, and seven years as director and CEO of VA medical centers in Florida and South Carolina. Mr. Vogel has also been involved with several veterans service organizations, including the Disabled American Veterans, Vietnam Veterans of America, and AMVETS. Mr. Vogel received his M.S. degree in government administration from George Washington University.

Rebecca A. Wassem, R.N., D.N.Sc., is a tenured associate professor with the University of Utah College of Nursing. Dr. Wassem began her nursing career in acute care (emergency room, triage, intensive care unit, anesthesia) but has concentrated since 1980 on the study of adjustment and rehabilitation for people who have a chronic physical illness or disability. Her research has focused on people with multiple sclerosis, arthritis, cardiac disease, fibromyalgia, and chronic fatigue. Recently, she began designing assistive technology for the disabled. Dr. Wassem is committed to helping individuals with disabilities have more productive lives and a better quality of life. Currently, she serves on the Utah State Independent Living Council (vice-chair), Utah State Rehabilitation Council, and the advisory council for a national grant for a rehabilitation engineering center on accessible medical instrumentation. Dr. Wassem is a veteran who served in Vietnam in the Army Nurse Corps.

Edward H. Yelin, Ph.D., is professor of medicine and health policy at the University of California, San Francisco Medical School. He is also director of the Arthritis Research Group within the Division of Rheumatology, director of the Multidisciplinary Clinical Research Center in the Rheumatic Diseases, and director of Medical Effectiveness Review for the California Health Benefits Review Program, an effort on the part of the University of California to provide assessments for the state legislature of the impact of proposed health insurance mandates. Dr. Yelin's research interests include the intersection of work and health, quality of life, and the social and economic impact of chronic disability. He has over 160 publications in these areas, and over 50 concern work disability issues. Dr. Yelin received his Ph.D. from the University of California, Berkeley.

Consultants

David K. Barnes operates Advanced Policy Solutions (APS), a private consulting firm that provides expert advice to individuals, organizations, and government agencies on disability program policy and administration, claim adjudication, program analysis, rulemaking, and procurement. Prior to founding APS, Mr. Barnes completed a 27-year career with the Social Security Administration (SSA). After beginning as a claims representative in an SSA field office, he advanced to a variety of staff and management positions within the agency, eventually becoming the director of SSA's Office of Disability Evaluation Policy, where he oversaw development, implementation, and analysis of disability decision-making policy for both the Social Security Disability Insurance and Supplemental Security Income disability programs. While at SSA, Mr. Barnes became known as a leading authority on disability policy and decision making, and a respected expert in research and development, personnel management, teambuilding, procurement, rulemaking, and litigation. He was also the recipient of more than 30 awards and citations for service, including the Commissioner's Citation, the Deputy

Commissioner's Citation (three times), and the Associate Commissioner's Citation (twice).

Robert J. Epley is an independent consultant working in the areas of strategic planning, training, performance management, and the operations of federal entitlement programs. Mr. Epley served with the Department of Veterans Affairs for 31 years, dividing his tenure between positions in headquarters and in the field. In VA field offices, he progressed through positions as benefits counselor and claims examiner to director of two regional offices in Detroit and St. Louis. At VA headquarters, Mr. Epley was chief of field operations for the education program, and later he served as deputy director and director of the Compensation & Pension Service. His final position with VA was associate deputy under secretary for policy and program management, where he was responsible for administration and oversight of the Veterans Benefits Administration's business lines: compensation, pension, housing, insurance, vocational rehabilitation, and education. During his tenure with VA, Mr. Epley received two Vice President Al Gore Hammer Awards for reinventing government and two Presidential Rank Awards.

IOM Staff

Michael McGeary (study director) is a political scientist specializing in science, health, and technology policy analysis and program evaluation. Between 1995 and 2004, he was an independent consultant to government agencies, foundations, and nonprofit organizations in issues of science and technology. Between 1981 and 1995, Mr. McGeary was at IOM and the National Academy of Sciences, where he was staff director of more than a dozen major reports on such topics as federal funding of research and development; graduate education and employment of scientists and engineers; priority setting, funding, and management of the National Institues of Health; merit review at the National Science Foundation; and regulation of nursing homes. Before this report on evaluating veterans for disability compensation, he was staff director for a committee that recommended improvements in Social Security disability decision-making process. Mr. McGeary is a graduate of Harvard College and completed all requirements for a doctorate in political science from MIT except the dissertation.

Morgan A. Ford (program officer) has been on staff at IOM since October 2005. During this time she has supported the work of two committees evaluating the disability compensation policies of government agencies. Prior to joining the IOM staff, Ms. Ford spent three years at Georgetown University's Lombardi Cancer Center coordinating cancer research. Between 1998 and 2002, she worked with Harvard nutrition and cancer epidemiologists on several projects, including a longitudinal study of risk factors for overweight and obesity among adolescents and a study of the impact of a cancer risk assessment on perceived cancer risk. Ms. Ford has a B.A. in psychology from Seattle University and an M.S. in health and social behavior from the Harvard School of Public Health.

Susan R. McCutchen (research associate) has been on staff at the National Academies for 26 years and has worked in several institutional divisions and with many different boards, committees, and panels within those units. The studies in which she has participated have addressed a broad range of subjects and focused on a variety of issues related to science and technology for international development, technology transfer, aeronautics and the U.S. space program, natural disaster mitigation, U.S. education policy and science curricula, needle exchange for the prevention of HIV transmission, the scientific merit of the polygraph, human factors/engineering, research ethics, and disability compensation programs. She has assisted in the production of more than 50 publications. Ms. McCutchen has a B.A. in French, with a minor in Italian and Spanish, from Ohio's Miami University, and an M.A. in French, with a minor in English, from Kent State University.

Reine Y. Homawoo (senior program assistant) is a staff member of IOM's Board on Military and Veterans Health. She has an associate degree in computer programming from the National Center for Computer Studies (CENETI) in Togo. She plans to pursue a bachelor's degree in information systems management at University of Maryland University College starting in September 2007.

Frederick (Rick) Erdtmann, M.D., M.P.H., is director of IOM's Board on Military and Veterans Health and its Medical Follow-up Agency. He attended medical school in Philadelphia where he earned his M.D. degree from the Temple University School of Medicine, and he also holds an M.P.H. from the University of California, Berkeley. He completed a residency program in general preventive medicine at Walter Reed Army Institute of Research in 1975 and is board certified in that specialty. Dr. Erdtmann's assignments with the Army Medical Department included chief of the preventive medicine services at Fitzsimons Army Medical Center, Frankfurt Army Medical Center in Germany, and Madigan Army Medical Center. He also served as division surgeon for the Second Infantry Division in Tongduchon, Korea. He later served as deputy chief of staff for clinical operations within the Department of Defense's TRICARE Region 1, prior to assuming hospital command at Walter Reed Army Medical Center in March 1998. Following that he was assigned to the Office of the Surgeon General as the deputy assistant surgeon general for force development. In 2001, following 30 years of commissioned military service, Dr. Erdtmann joined The National Academies and assumed his present responsibilities.

Appendix B

Committee Charge

STATEMENT OF TASKS

1. How well do the medical criteria in the Department of Veterans Affairs (VA) Rating Schedule and VA rating regulations enable assessment and adjudication of the proper levels of disability to compensate both for the impact on quality of life and impairment in earnings capacity? Provide an analysis of the descriptions associated with each condition's rating level that considers progression of severity of condition as it relates to quality-of-life impairment and impairment in average earnings capacity.

2. Certain criteria and/or levels of disability are required for entitlement to ancillary and special-purpose benefits. To what extent, if any, do the required thresholds need to change? Determine from a medical perspective at what disability rating level a veteran's medical or vocational impairment caused by disability could be improved by various special benefits such as adapted housing, automobile grants, clothing allowance, and vocational rehabilitation. Consideration should be given to existing and additional benefits.

3. Analyze the current application of the individual unemployability (IU) extraschedular benefit to determine whether the Rating Schedule descriptions need to more accurately reflect a veteran's ability to participate in the economic marketplace. Propose alternative medical approaches, if any, to IU that would more appropriately reflect individual circumstances in the determination of benefits. For the population of disabled veterans, analyze

the cohort of IU recipients. Examine the base rating level to identify patterns. Determine if the Rating Schedule descriptions of conditions provide a barrier to assigning the base disability rating level commensurate with the veteran's vocational impairment.

4. What are the advantages and disadvantages of adopting universal medical diagnostic codes rather than using a unique system? Compare and contrast the advantages and disadvantages of the VA Schedule for Rating Disabilities and the American Medical Association *Guides to the Evaluation of Permanent Impairment.*

5. From a medical perspective, analyze the current VA practice of assigning service connection on "secondary" and "aggravation" bases. In secondary claims, determine what medical principles and practices should be applied in determining whether a causal relationship exists between two conditions. In aggravation claims, determine what medical principles and practices should be applied in determining whether a preexisting disease was increased due to military service or was increased due to the natural process of the disease.

6. Compare and contrast the role of health-care professionals in the claims and appeals processes in VA and the Department of Defense (DoD), the Social Security Administration, and federal employee disability benefits programs. What skills, knowledge, training, and certification are required of the persons performing the examinations and assigning the ratings?

Appendix C

The Relationship Between Impairments and Earnings Losses in Multicondition Studies

John F. Burton, Jr., Seth Seabury, Michael McGeary, and Robert T. Reville

The purpose of this study is to provide assistance to the Institute of Medicine (IOM) Committee on Medical Evaluation of Veterans for Disability Compensation, and, in particular, to help address portions of the committee's first task:

> *How well do the medical criteria in the VA Rating Schedule and VA rating regulations enable assessment and adjudication of the proper levels of disability to compensate both for the impact on quality of life and impairment in earnings capacity? Provide an analysis of the descriptions associated with each condition's rating level that considers progression of severity of condition as it relates to quality-of-life impairment and impairment in average earnings capacity.*

This study focuses on the aspect of task 1 concerned with the relationship between the medical criteria used to determine the level of disability and the impairment (or limitation) in earning capacity associated with that level of disability. More specifically, this study examines the relationship between impairments (the medical consequences of injuries or diseases) and the actual loss of earnings (the economic consequences of the impairments). We also discuss the intermediate consequences between impairments and actual earnings losses, such as the loss of earning capacity. The relationships will be examined with evidence from multicondition studies (that is, studies involving two or more medical conditions). The study will not examine the relationship between impairments (the medical consequences of injuries and diseases) and quality-of-life impairment (sometimes referred to as "noneconomic losses" or "nonwork disability"). The study will rely

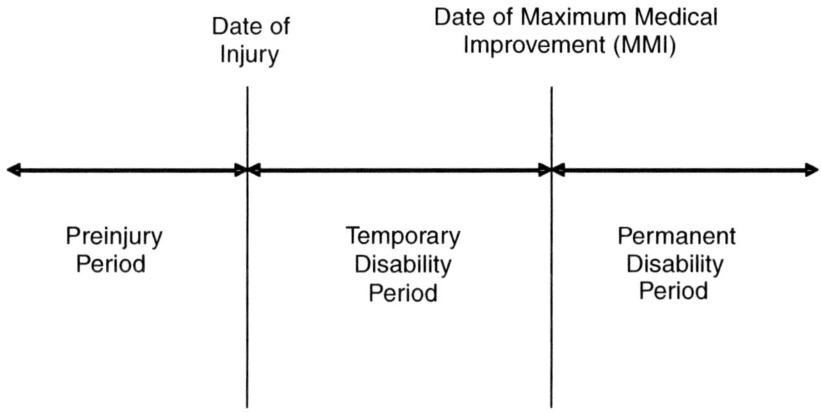

FIGURE C-1 Three time periods in a workers' compensation case where the injury has permanent consequences.

on selected previous studies from workers' compensation, on new data from the Californian workers' compensation program, and on the 1971 Economic Validation of the [Veterans Administration] Rating Schedule (ECVARS) study.

CONCEPTUAL FRAMEWORK[1]

Three Time Periods

As shown in Figure C-1, three time periods are pertinent in compensating a worker with an injury serious enough to result in permanent disability benefits. The *preinjury period* is relevant because *inter alia* the employee's average weekly wage is used to calculate the cash benefits after the worker is injured. The *temporary disability period* refers to the time from the onset of the injury or disease until the date of maximum medical improvement (MMI) has been reached; and the *permanent disability period* refers to the period following MMI. The distinction between the temporary and disability periods is important because workers' compensation programs provide different types of cash benefits in the two periods.

The permanent disability period is the crucial period for our study of the veterans disability compensation program because we are examining the benefits provided to veterans with permanent consequences of their injuries or diseases.

[1]This section is based in part on Burton (2005).

The Permanent Consequences of an Injury or Disease

The study will rely on the conceptual relationship shown in Figure C-2 because this provides a useful framework for presenting the evidence on the relationship between impairment ratings and earnings losses. Figure C-2 differs from the model of disability presented in Chapter 3 of this report in two ways. First, Figure C-2 is only concerned with work disability, while the report also considers losses in quality of life, which are defined as "the consequences of an injury or disease other than work disability." Second, Figure C-2 divides both impairment and work disability into subcomponents in order to facilitate the analysis in this study.

The concepts in Figure C-2 described below correspond to the operational measures currently used to determine the amount of cash benefits provided by workers' compensation programs and to the outcome measure used in the research on disability programs examined in this study.

IA. Medical impairment: Anatomical loss—The American Medical Association's (AMA's) *Guides to the Evaluation of Permanent Impairment, Fifth Edition* (Cocchiarella and Andersson, 2001, hereafter referred to as the *Guides*) provides impairment ratings for certain medical conditions based on the anatomical loss. For example, Table 17-32 at page 545 of the *Guides* indicates that amputation of the leg above the knee at the midthigh is rated at 90 percent of the loss of the leg and 36 percent impairment of the whole person.

IB. Medical impairment: Functional loss—The *Guides* provides impairment ratings for certain medical conditions based on the extent of the functional loss. Example 16-78 at page 514 explains how to determine the rating for a person who sustained a Colles' fracture of the right distal radius: "The factors to be rated are the loss of motion of the wrist and forearm rotation."

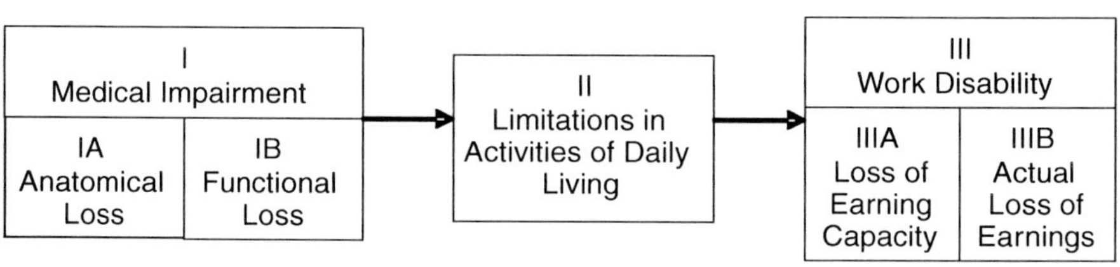

FIGURE C-2 The consequences of an injury or disease resulting in work disability.

II. Limitations in activities of daily living—These are the limitations in the activities of daily living resulting from the impairment. These can be measured by some of the questions in the SF-36. (For example, Question 8 asks if the person's health now limits bending, kneeling, or stooping.)

IIIA. Work disability: Loss of earning capacity—This is the presumed loss of earning capacity resulting from the functional limitations. This can be measured by some of the questions in the SF-36. (For example, Question 13 asks if during the past four weeks the person cut down the amount of time spent on work or other activities as a result of his or her physical health.) The loss of earning capacity approach is used in a number of workers' compensation programs for certain types of injuries.

IIIB. Work disability: Actual loss of earnings—This is the actual loss of earnings resulting from the injury or disease and its consequences (e.g., impairment).

The actual loss of earnings is measured by the difference between the worker's actual earnings and the earnings the individual could have been expected to earn if he or she had not been injured (potential earnings) as shown in Figure C-3. In this example, prior to the date of injury, wages increased through time from A to B, reflecting the worker's increasing productivity and other factors that caused wages to increase, such as inflation. At point B, the worker experiences a work-related injury that permanently reduces his or her earnings. Had the worker not been injured, his or her

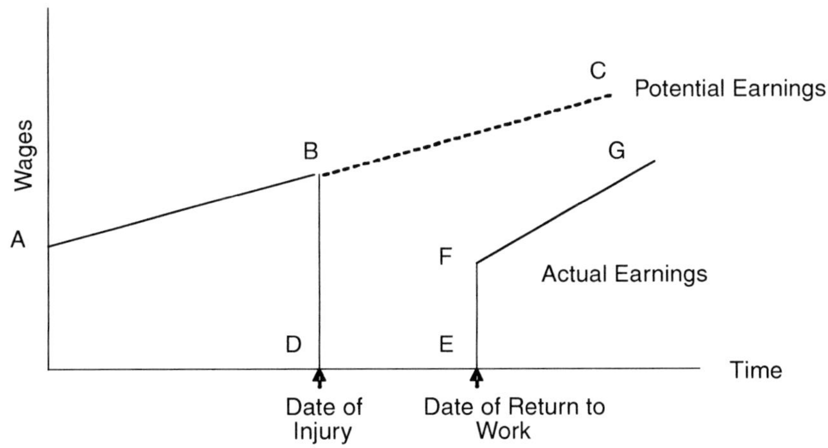

FIGURE C-3 Actual losses of earnings for a worker with a permanent disability.

earnings would have continued to grow along the line BC. The worker's actual earnings in this example dropped from B to D and continued at this zero earnings level until point E, when the worker returned to work at wage level F. Thereafter, actual earnings grew along the line F to G. In this example, it is assumed the worker's actual earnings never returned to the potential earnings (line BC) that he or she would have earned if the injury had not occurred. The worker's *"true" wage loss* due to the injury is equal to his or her potential earnings after the date of injury (BC) minus the actual earnings after the date of injury (BDEFG).

The calculation of potential earnings (line BC) is a crucial step in the analysis. Different researchers have used different methods to estimate potential earnings. We will describe these methods in connection with the research on the two workers' compensation programs and the veterans disability compensation program examined in this study.

The Causes of the Injury or Disease

Both workers' compensation programs and the veterans disability compensation program provide benefits only when specified causation requirements are satisfied. For workers' compensation, the injury or disease must be work-related, which in most states requires several legal tests to be met.[2] For veterans benefits, the injury or disease must be incurred or aggravated during active military service. We assume for this study that the injuries and diseases and the resulting impairment and disability meet the causation requirements of the programs we are examining.

The distinction between causes and consequences of injuries and diseases is important. For example, work disability is a consequence of an injury or disease, but the cause may or may not be work-related. Indeed, one of our central inquiries is the relationship between injuries and diseases caused by military service and the consequences of those injuries and diseases on the loss of earnings (i.e., work disability).

The Purpose of Cash Benefits

A fundamental issue is which of the consequences of injuries and diseases shown in Figure C-2 provide the reasons or purpose of the cash benefits provided by workers' compensation programs and by the veterans disability program.

[2]Most workers' compensation statutes require a worker to satisfy four legal tests: there must be (1) an injury (2) resulting from an accident that (3) arose out of employment and (4) in the course of employment (Willborn et al., 2007: 894-937).

Workers' Compensation

The possible reasons for workers' compensation program cash benefits were examined by Burton:

> To the extent that the rationale for benefits is discernable . . . two schools of thought can be identified. One view considers lost wages due to the injury (work disability) as the sole justification for workers' compensation benefits. . . .
>
> An alternative view of the rationale for benefits workers with permanent consequences of their injuries accepts work disability as the primary basis for benefits, but argues there is a secondary role for benefits paid for nonwork disability. Arguments for these "impairment benefits" indicate that the purpose is not only to compensate impairment per se but to also use permanent impairment as a convenient proxy for the functional limitations and nonwork disability that result from the impairment. A variant of this alternative view is to argue that nonwork disability merits compensation, and that the degree of permanent impairment serves as a proxy for the extent of nonwork disability.
>
> The dominant view probably is that the only permanent consequences that warrant benefits in a workers' compensation program are medical care, rehabilitation, and work disability (Burton, 2005:80).

The view that the only purpose of workers' compensation cash benefits is to compensate for work disability is explicitly or implicitly adopted in almost all research on the program. Studies of the relationship between earnings losses and cash benefits, for example, use the entire amount of cash benefits to evaluate the performance of the system of cash benefits.[3] We assume for this study that the sole purpose of cash benefits in workers' compensation is to compensate for work disability and not for the other consequences shown in Figure C-2.

Veterans Disability Compensation Program

The statement of tasks for the IOM committee asks for an evaluation of VA's Schedule for Rating Disabilities (Rating Schedule) and rating regulations for both quality-of-life impairment and impairment in average earning capacity. However, the sole purpose of the cash benefits specified by § 4.1 of the *Code of Federal Regulations* dealing with VA's Rating Schedule is limited to work disability (as that term is used in this study):

[3]Examples of studies of the relationship between earnings losses and cash benefits that use the entire amount of the cash benefits for the evaluation—thus implicitly or explicitly assuming that the sole purpose of the cash benefits is to compensate for work disability—are Berkowitz and Burton (1987) and Boden et al. (2005).

> The percentage ratings represent as far as can practicably be determined the average impairment in earning capacity resulting from such diseases and injuries and their residual conditions in civil occupations.

We assume for the purposes of this study that the sole purpose of the cash benefits provided by the VA Rating Schedule and rating regulations is to compensate for work disability and not for the other consequences of injuries and disease shown in Figure C-2.

The Operational Basis for Cash Benefits

The generally accepted view is that the sole or dominant purpose of cash benefits in workers' compensation and in the VA disability compensation program is to compensate for work disability. Ideally, the extent of work disability would be determined by measuring each worker's actual loss of earnings. However, it is impractical and probably inappropriate to directly measure actual loss of earnings for each worker and to determine the amount of cash benefits based on the measure of actual wage loss.[4] As a result, one of the other consequences shown in Figure C-2 is used as a proxy (or predictor) of actual loss of wages.

There are several possible reasons why disability compensation programs use proxies, such as the extent of the applicant's impairment, to provide benefits for which the purpose is actual loss of earnings. The first reason is administrative convenience: It is easier to conduct a medical examination of an applicant than to monitor the worker's actual labor market experience over an extended period of time. The second reason is that linking benefits to actual loss of earnings may result in incentive effects for some beneficiaries, who may limit their extent of participation in the labor force if higher earnings result in reduced benefits. Despite these reasons for the use of proxies, one possible drawback is that they may not provide accurate estimates of the actual loss of earnings. We examine how well proxies predict the amount of actual wage loss in this study.

One possible objection to using the amount of actual wage loss as the test of the accuracy of the predictions of the disability rating systems is that the stated purpose of the veterans disability compensation program is average impairment in earning capacity, not the average loss of actual earnings. However, there is no meaningful test of the accuracy of the current Rating Schedule if a comparison is made between (1) the *ratings* produced by application of the criteria for evaluating medical conditions in the Rating Schedule and (2) the *average reduction in earning capacity*, since in practice

[4]The difficulties of using each worker's own actual earnings as a basis for cash benefits is discussed by Berkowitz and Burton (1987).

they are the same thing. The only meaningful test is whether the ratings produced by the Rating Schedule (which are estimates of the loss of earning capacity) are closely related to the actual losses of earnings.

THE 1987 STUDY OF THE WISCONSIN WORKERS' COMPENSATION PROGRAM

The Wisconsin Workers' Compensation Program

Berkowitz and Burton (1987) conducted a wage-loss study of Wisconsin, Florida, and California workers who were injured in 1968. The results for one of the two samples from Wisconsin are shown in Table C-1. The sample consists of male Wisconsin workers who received permanent partial disability (PPD) benefits without a legal contest.

The system of cash benefits in Wisconsin relied on several distinctions found in most (although not all) state workers' compensation programs.[5] As shown in Figure C-1, three time periods were relevant for determining benefits for workers who received PPD benefits. During the temporary disability period, most Wisconsin workers in the study qualified for temporary total disability (TTD) benefits. In 1968, the TTD benefits were 66-and-two-thirds percent of the workers' preinjury wages, subject to a maximum weekly benefit. Once the worker reached the date of MMI, the TTD benefits stopped and most workers with permanent disabilities qualified for permanent partial disability (PPD) benefits.[6]

Scheduled PPD benefits were paid to workers who had an injury included in a list (or schedule) of body parts included in the Wisconsin workers' compensation statute. The statute also specified the number of weeks of PPD benefits associated with the total loss of each body part. The complete loss of an arm, for example, entitled a worker to 400 weeks of PPD benefits. A 50 percent loss of an arm meant the worker received 200 weeks of PPD benefits.

Nonscheduled PPD benefits were paid to workers who had an injury not included in the list of body parts in the statute. The seriousness of the nonscheduled injury—typically a back condition—was rated "as the nature of the injury bears to one causing permanent total disability." A 40 percent rating for the back was multiplied by 1,000 weeks to determine the duration of the PPD benefits.

---

[5]An extended discussion of the various approaches to cash benefits in workers' compensation programs is included in Burton (2005).

[6]A limited number of Wisconsin workers qualified for permanent total disability (PTD) benefits. However, the number of PTD cases was so small that the workers were not included in the study.

TABLE C-1 Wisconsin Uncontested Permanent Partial Disability Cases for Men with 1968 Injuries

	Classification of Workers	Percent Rating 1–2	3–5	6–10	11–15	16–50	51–100	Mean Ratings	Total
Panel A		Weighted counts of workers and mean disability ratings							
1	Workers ages 20–59	941.0	467.0	177.0	52.0	48.0		3.70	1,685.0
2	Workers ages 20–29	294.0	105.5	36.0	15.0	14.0		3.54	464.5
3	Workers ages 30–39	226.0	122.0	39.5	10.0	14.0		3.69	411.5
4	Workers ages 40–49	219.5	140.5	53.5	11.0	13.0		3.68	437.5
5	Workers ages 50–59	201.5	99.0	48.0	16.0	7.0		3.71	371.5
6	Upper extremities	785.0	192.0	82.0	20.0	20.0		2.80	1,099.0
7	Trunk cases	17.0	93.0	42.0	10.0	0.0		5.83	162.0
8	Lower extremities	120.0	150.0	34.0	9.0	4.0		3.76	317.0
9	All other cases	19.0	32.0	19.0	13.0	24.0		9.62	107.0
Panel B		Mean potential earnings (1968–1973, in dollars)[a]							
1	Workers ages 20–59	42,567	43,938	43,320	42,472	37,960			42,892
2	Workers ages 20–29	40,144	44,412	38,743	41,693	32,671			40,829
3	Workers ages 30–39	43,641	46,232	47,880	52,464	42,605			44,995
4	Workers ages 40–49	45,298	44,383	48,995	48,364	41,628			45,414
5	Workers ages 50–59	41,925	39,973	36,673	32,905	32,434			40,159
6	Upper extremities	42,740	44,084	41,644	39,699	35,516			42,706
7	Trunk cases	37,364	44,193	45,224	44,276				43,748
8	Lower extremities	42,497	43,123	43,355	37,036	37,720			42,670
9	All other cases	40,529	46,136	46,279	49,113	40,036			44,159

Panel C		Mean earnings losses (1968–1973, in dollars)[a]					
1	Workers ages 20–59	1,554	2,759	*4,292	* 7,483	*7,175	*2,519
2	Workers ages 20–29	1,714	1,890	1,337	6,627	8,757	*2,096
3	Workers ages 30–39	3,009	7,595	*6,399	*13,028	*9,611	*5,162
4	Workers ages 40–49	2,822	954	4,647	*4,131	4,241	2,520
5	Workers ages 50–59	–1,694	287	4,379	7,124	*4,586	117
6	Upper extremities	1,535	1,688	2,913	5,098	7,503	*1,838
7	Trunk cases	4,583	5,417	*3,395	8,916		5,022
8	Lower extremities	1,808	2,307	9,349	*11,740	1,984	3,137
9	All other cases	–1,978	3,581	3,178	7,102	*7,766	*3,889
Panel D		Standard deviation of mean earnings losses (1968–1973, in dollars)[a]					
1	Workers ages 20–59	860	1,150	1,138	2,236	2,046	662
2	Workers ages 20–29	1,482	2,057	2,987	4,479	3,398	1,237
3	Workers ages 30–39	2,194	2,449	2,272	6,193	3,059	1,559
4	Workers ages 40–49	1,768	1,951	1,760	5,321	5,055	1,228
5	Workers ages 50–59	1,294	2,596	2,248	2,250	4,129	1,213
6	Upper extremities	875	1,952	1,726	2,754	2,328	809
7	Trunk cases	4,430	1,364	2,132	5,040		1,115
8	Lower extremities	1,639	1,160	2,351	8,283	4,188	935
9	All other cases	2,613	3,354	3,767	3,513	3,436	1,596

continued

TABLE C-1 Continued

	Classification of Workers	Percent Rating 1–2	3–5	6–10	11–15	16–50	51–100	Mean Ratings	Total
Panel E		Proportional earnings losses							
1	Workers ages 20–59	0.036	0.063	0.099	0.176	0.189			0.059
2	Workers ages 20–29	0.043	0.043	0.035	0.159	0.268			0.051
3	Workers ages 30–39	0.069	0.164	0.134	0.248	0.226			0.115
4	Workers ages 40–49	0.062	0.021	0.095	0.085	0.102			0.055
5	Workers ages 50–59	–0.040	0.007	0.119	0.216	0.141			0.003
6	Upper extremities	0.036	0.038	0.070	0.128	0.211			0.043
7	Trunk cases	0.123	0.123	0.075	0.201				0.115
8	Lower extremities	0.043	0.053	0.216	0.317	0.053			0.074
9	All other cases	–0.049	0.078	0.069	0.145	0.194			0.088
Panel F		Mean benefits of legal fees (1968–1973, in dollars)							
1	Workers ages 20–59	696	2,479	4,957	7,807	10,980			2,150
2	Workers ages 20–29	742	2,316	5,078	8,388	12,846			2,047
3	Workers ages 30–39	626	2,509	5,451	7,224	10,286			2,136
4	Workers ages 40–49	706	2,316	4,999	7,360	10,327			2,201
5	Workers ages 50–59	696	2,846	4,412	7,934	9,851			2,234
6	Upper extremities	593	2,057	4,503	6,716	11,641			1,453
7	Trunk cases	1,288	3,141	5,371	8,410				3,850
8	Lower extremities	1,261	2,636	5,803	10,254	13,537			2,809
9	All other cases	842	2,348	4,485	7,326	10,003			4,782

Panel G		Replacement rates: Benefits as proportion of earnings losses						
1	Workers ages 20–59	0.45	0.90	1.15	1.04	1.53		0.85
2	Workers ages 20–29	0.43	1.23	3.80	1.27	1.47		0.98
3	Workers ages 30–39	0.21	0.33	0.85	0.55	1.07		0.41
4	Workers ages 40–49	0.25	2.43	1.08	1.78	2.44		0.87
5	Workers ages 50–59	[b]	9.91	1.01	1.11	2.15		19.11
6	Upper extremities	0.39	1.22	1.55	1.32	1.55		0.79
7	Trunk cases	0.28	0.58	1.58	0.94			0.77
8	Lower extremities	0.70	1.14	0.62	0.87	6.82		0.90
9	All other cases	[b]	0.66	1.41	1.03	1.29		1.23

*Significant at the .05 level.

[a]1968 present value dollars discounted at 6 percent.

[b]The replacement rate is not shown because the mean earnings loss estimate is negative.

Both scheduled and nonscheduled PPD beneficiaries received weekly benefits that were 66-and-two-thirds percent of the workers' preinjury weekly wages, subject to a maximum weekly benefit. As of 1968, the ratings for both the scheduled and nonscheduled PPD benefits were based on an evaluation of medical impairment, corresponding to the extent of anatomical loss (IA) or functional loss (IB) shown in Figure C-2. In short, while the purpose of the Wisconsin PPD benefits was to compensate for work disability, in 1968 the operational approach for the benefits was to measure the extent of medical impairment and to use the rating as a proxy for work disability.

As discussed by Berkowitz and Burton (1987), Wisconsin began to base nonscheduled PPD benefits on the loss of earning capacity (corresponding to consequence IIIA in Figure C-2) beginning in the 1970s. Thus the results in this section probably would not be applicable to workers who receive PPD benefits from the current Wisconsin workers' compensation program.

Summary of the Wisconsin Results

The male Wisconsin workers who were injured in 1968 and received PPD benefits were separated into two categories. Most workers were paid benefits without litigation or use of compromise and release (C&R) agreements. These uncontested cases are shown in Table C-1 (which corresponds to Table 10.1 in Berkowitz and Burton [1987]). Other workers were paid benefits after a contest (litigation or use of C&R agreements). The results for the contested cases are not shown in this report. Table C-1 contains seven panels of information.

Panel A. The Wisconsin uncontested cases were selected using a stratified sampling procedure that selected a higher proportion of cases in cells with fewer workers. The sample represented a total of 1,685 workers from ages 20 to 59 (line 1). The sample was placed into columns based on the permanent disability ratings and into rows corresponding to 10-year age categories (lines 2 to 5) and into rows corresponding to four locations of injury (lines 6 to 9). The numbers of the various types of injuries ranged from upper extremities (1,099) to all other cases (107). The mean disability rating for the entire sample was 3.70 percent. The mean ratings varied by age (from 3.54 percent for workers ages 20–29 to 3.71 percent for workers ages 50–59) and by location of injury (from 2.80 percent for upper extremities to 9.62 percent for all other cases).

Panel B. The potential earnings for each worker were calculated by multiplying the worker's actual earnings in 1966–1967 by his expected earnings growth ratio (EGR). The EGR was derived from the ratio of the actual earnings in 1968–1973 to the actual earnings in 1966–1967 of workers in the control group, as shown in Social Security earnings records.

The control group workers were matched to the injured Wisconsin workers in the sample on the basis of each worker's sex, age in 1968, and level of actual earnings in 1966–1967. The potential earnings in Panel B correspond to the potential earnings in Figure C-3 calculated for the six years between 1968 and 1973, and represent the estimate of what the workers in the sample would have earned if they had not been injured in 1968. The mean potential earnings for all workers in the sample were $42,892. (All dollar figures in Table C-1 are in 1968 dollars.) For workers with injuries to the upper extremity rated at 1–2 percent, the mean potential earnings were $42,740.

Panel C. The actual earnings for each worker from 1968 to 1973 were determined based on Social Security earnings records. The actual earnings used to calculate the results in Panel C correspond to the actual earnings shown in Figure C-3. The actual earnings were subtracted from the potential earnings to determine the earnings losses shown in Panel C. The mean earnings losses for all workers in the sample were $2,519. For workers with injuries to the upper extremity rated at 1–2 percent, the mean earnings losses were $1,535. Of interest, there are two entries in Panel C in which the mean earnings losses are negative: The mean actual earnings exceeded the mean potential earnings for workers in those categories.

Panel D. The earnings losses varied significantly for workers in the sample of Wisconsin workers. The standard deviations (a measure of dispersion) of the mean earnings losses are shown in Panel D. The standard deviation for all workers in the sample was $662. The mean for all workers was $2,519. The ratio of the standard deviation to the mean is low enough that we can be 95 percent certain that the mean earnings losses for all workers in the sample were greater than zero. The significance at the .05 level is shown by the asterisk by the $2,519 entry in Panel C. In contrast, the standard deviation for workers with injuries to the upper extremity rated at 1–2 percent was $875, and so we cannot be 95 percent certain that the mean earnings losses of $1,535 were greater than zero. A perusal of Panel C shows that a number of entries are not significant.

Panel E. The proportional earnings losses are shown in Panel E. These figures represent the mean earnings losses in Panel C divided by the mean potential earnings in Panel B. The proportional earnings loss for all workers in the sample was 0.059 ($2,519 divided by $42,892), which means that all workers had earnings losses that were 5.9 percent of potential earnings. For workers with injuries to the upper extremities rated at 1–2 percent, the proportional earnings loss was 0.036 ($1,535 divided by $42,740), which means that the earnings losses for workers with this type of injury were 3.6 percent of potential earnings.

Panel F. The mean workers' compensation benefits net of legal fees are shown in Panel F. These include all temporary disability benefits as well as PPD benefits received between 1968 and 1973. The mean benefits for all workers in the sample were $2,150. For workers with injuries to the upper extremity rated at 1–2 percent, the mean benefits net of legal fees was $593.

Panel G. The replacement rates are shown in Panel G. The replacement rates are the mean benefits net of legal fees received by the Wisconsin workers between 1968 and 1973 (Panel F) divided by the mean earnings losses for these workers during those six years (Panel C). For all workers in the sample, the replacement rate was 0.85 ($2,150 divided by $2,519), which means these workers received benefits that replaced 85 percent of their earnings losses. For workers with injuries to the upper extremity rated at 1–2 percent, the replacement rate was 0.39 ($875 divided by $1,535), which means these workers received benefits that replaced 39 percent of their earnings losses. A perusal of Panel G indicates there were great variations in replacement rates, ranging from 21 percent for workers ages 30–39 with injuries rated at 1–2 percent to 991 percent for workers ages 50–59 with injuries rated at 3–5 percent. There were also two entries (shown in Panel G with "b") where the workers in the category received workers' compensation benefits but on average had no earnings losses.

The Wisconsin Disability Rating System and Equity

Background on the Equity Criteria

The concepts of horizontal and vertical equity have a long history in the public finance literature. Musgrave provides an example:

> A proper definition of income is important, not only to establish equity in a vertical sense—that is, to plan taxes and transfers so as to adjust relative positions; it is important also to establish equity in a horizontal sense—that is, to give equal treatment to people in equal positions (Musgrave, 1959:20).

The equity criteria were used to evaluate a disability benefits program in *The Report of the National Commission on State Workmen's Compensation Laws*:

equitable: delivering benefits and services fairly as judged by the program's consistency in providing equal benefits or services to workers in identical circumstances and its rationality in providing benefits and services in proportion to the impairment or disability for those with different degrees of loss (The National Commission, 1972:137).

We expand the use of the horizontal and vertical equity criteria to evaluate the performance of the rating system used to provide benefits to people who experience loss of earnings as a result of injuries or diseases.[7] The balance of this section discusses a series of figures derived from the information in Table C-1 pertaining to the Wisconsin workers' compensation program. (The figures transform the proportions in Table C-1 into percentages in order to expedite exposition.)

Vertical Equity for Ratings

The data in Figure C-4 can be used to explain vertical equity. *Vertical equity requires that actual wage losses increase in proportion to the increase in disability ratings.* In this instance, there is reasonably good vertical equity in the ratings of the upper extremity injuries. With the exception of the lowest and highest disability category, the percentage earnings losses are close to the midpoint of the corresponding category of disability ratings. For example, workers with disability ratings of 11–15 percent experienced 12.8 percent earnings losses.[8]

Intra-Injury Horizontal Equity for Ratings

Intra-injury horizontal equity for ratings requires that the actual wage losses for workers with the same disability ratings and the same type of injury should be the same or similar. The data for upper extremities shown in Figure C-5 indicates there are substantial variations in earnings losses for these workers with the same disability ratings. The entries include the mean amount of earnings losses for workers in each rating category, plus the earnings losses associated with plus or minus two times the standard deviation for the earnings losses. As can be seen, the range of earnings losses contains some workers who had negative earnings losses in the six years after their

[7]The adequacy and equity criteria are discussed at greater length in Burton (2005) and Berkowitz and Burton (1987).

[8]The top category (16–50 percent ratings) is very broad because of confidentiality considerations. Most of the observations are likely to involve injuries at the lower end of the category; therefore, the lack of correspondence between the extent of wage loss and the midpoint of the range is understandable.

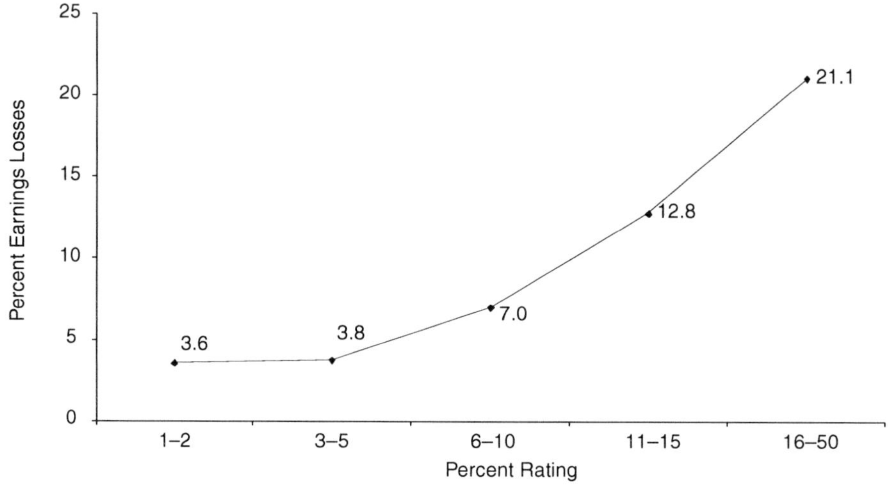

FIGURE C-4 Percentage earnings losses for Wisconsin workers with upper extremity injuries.

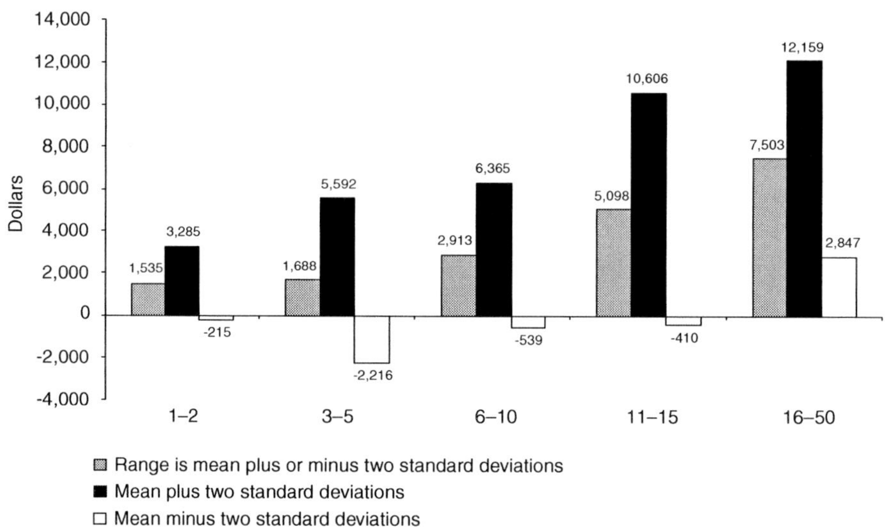

FIGURE C-5 Earnings losses for Wisconsin workers with upper extremity injuries: means and ranges of losses.

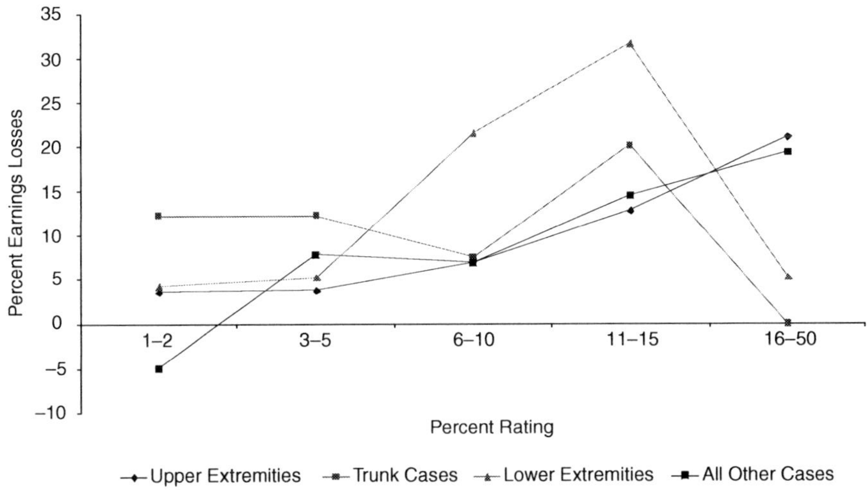

FIGURE C-6 Percentage earnings losses for Wisconsin workers with four types of injuries.

injuries.[9] Indeed, the earnings losses are only statistically significantly different than zero for workers with injuries of the upper extremities with ratings of 16–50 percent.

One "lesson" of Figure C-5 in conjunction with Panels C and D of Table C-1 is that the Wisconsin workers' compensation program did a reasonably good job on vertical equity for upper extremity cases when the emphasis is placed on mean values of losses, but that the program did not do as well on intra-injury horizontal equity, as shown by the considerable variability in lost wages for workers with similar disability ratings.

The relationships between disability ratings and earnings losses for four types of injuries are shown in Figure C-6.

Inter-Injury Horizontal Equity for Ratings

Inter-injury horizontal equity for ratings requires that the actual wage losses for workers with the same disability ratings, but different types of injuries, should be the same or similar. However, the results in Figure C-6 suggest there are significant differences among the types of injuries in the relationships between disability ratings and lost earnings. For example,

[9] "Negative earnings losses" means these workers had actual earnings that exceeded the estimates of their potential earnings.

for workers with disability ratings of 11 to 15 percent, earnings losses ranged from 31.7 percent for lower extremities to 12.8 percent for upper extremities.

Vertical Equity for Ratings—Revisited

Figure C-6 is also useful in illustrating the challenges of achieving vertical equity for particular types of injuries. As shown earlier in Figure C-4, there is a reasonably close relationship between higher ratings for workers with upper extremity injuries and higher earnings losses. However, the data in Figure C-6 "tell" a somewhat different story. For two types of injuries (upper extremities and all other cases), earnings losses generally increase with higher disability ratings. However, for trunk cases and lower extremities, earnings losses are much lower for workers in the most serious rating category than in most of the categories with lower disability ratings.

Vertical Equity for Ratings—Revisited Again!

Shall we look at the trees (represented by Figures C-5 and C-6) or the forest (represented by Figure C-7)? As shown in Figure C-7, for all Wisconsin workers, there is a very close relationship between rating categories and percentage earnings losses. The dashed line represents an exact correspondence between ratings and losses (for example, an 8 percent disability rating equals an 8 percent earnings loss). At this level of aggregation, the Wisconsin rating system does an excellent job of providing vertical equity.

The Wisconsin Replacement Rates and Adequacy

It is useful to separate the analysis of the ability of the rating system to predict earnings losses from the analysis of the ability of the compensation system to replace an appropriate portion of lost earnings with benefits. It is possible, for example, that the rating system does an excellent job in predicting earnings losses, but that the design or implementation of the benefit system results in a poor match between benefits and lost wages. The next set of figures looks at the equity and adequacy of the Wisconsin workers' compensation benefits for workers with PPD benefits.

Background on the Adequacy Criterion

There is also a long history of the use of the adequacy criterion to assess social insurance programs, including those providing benefits to persons with disabilities. One possible standard is the Social Adequacy Model, which requires that benefits provide at least enough income to assume the

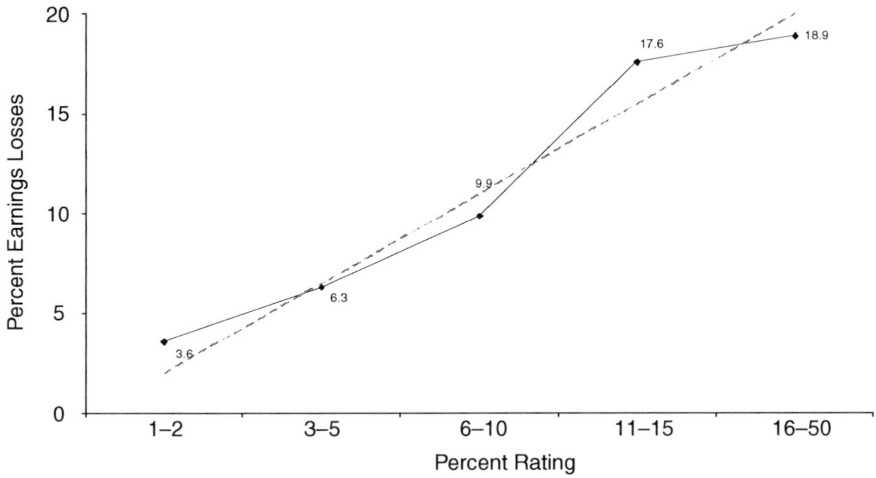

FIGURE C-7 Percentage earnings losses for all Wisconsin workers.

beneficiary is not living in poverty (Hunt, 2004). Other standards rely on replacement rates, which represent the proportion of lost wages replaced by the cash benefits from a program.

The National Commission argued that workers' compensation should replace a substantial proportion of the worker's lost income.

> Replacement of a substantial proportion is justified by a feature of workmen's compensation which distinguishes the program from other forms of social insurance. In exchange for the benefits of workers compensation, workers renounced their right to seek redress for economic damages and pain and suffering under the common law. In no other social insurance program, such as Social Security or unemployment compensation, did workers surrender any right of value in exchange for benefits (The National Commission, 1972:36).

The generally accepted standard of adequacy for workers' compensation is that the benefits should replace two-thirds of lost wages (Hunt, 2004). This replacement rate, which is shown by the horizontal line 66.67 percent in Figures C-8 to C-10, can be used to assess the adequacy of benefits provided by the Wisconsin workers' compensation program for workers receiving permanent partial disability benefits. One meaning of adequacy is to consider the replacement rate for the entire sample of injured workers. In Wisconsin, cash benefits replaced 85 percent of earnings losses for the entire sample, as shown in Panel G of Table C-1, which clearly met the adequacy test.

The Wisconsin Replacement Rates and Equity

Vertical Equity for Benefits

The data in Figures C-8 through C-10 can also be used to examine vertical equity of the PPD benefits. Vertical equity requires that the same proportion of lost wages should be replaced for workers at all disability ratings. (This definition is refined in the next paragraph.) In Figure C-8, there is fairly good vertical equity for the benefits for upper extremity injuries. The least serious category (1–2 percent ratings) has a replacement rate of only 39 percent, but the other categories have replacement rates that are within the range of 122 to 155 percent. The results for the four types of injuries in Figure C-9 suggest that there was a reasonable degree of vertical equity for the four lowest rating categories, but there were serious equity problems for the highest rating category.

Vertical Equity for Benefits—Revisited

Vertical equity has two possible meanings. A narrow view asserts that all levels of severity should have the same proportion of earnings losses replaced by benefits. An alternative view is that more serious injuries should have a higher replacement rate. Those who subscribe to the alternative view can take some comfort from Figure C-10, which indicates the Wisconsin

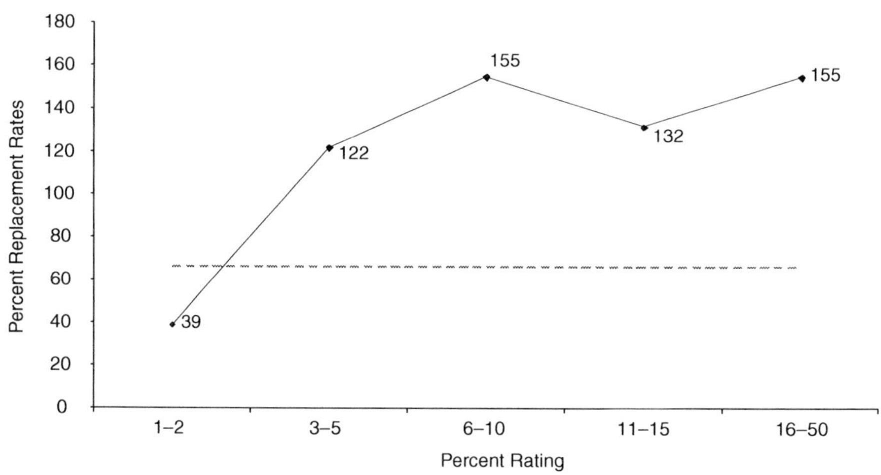

FIGURE C-8 Replacement rates (benefits as a percentage of earnings losses) for Wisconsin workers with upper extremity injuries.

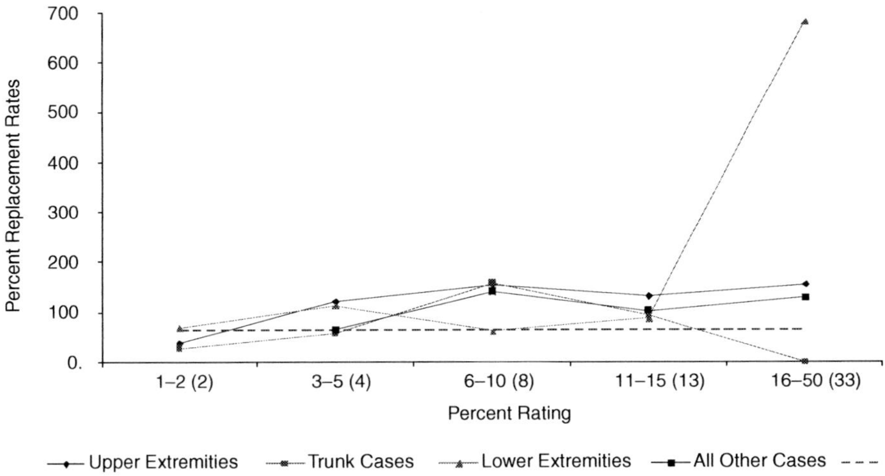

FIGURE C-9 Replacement rates (benefits as a percentage of earnings losses) for Wisconsin workers with four types of injuries.

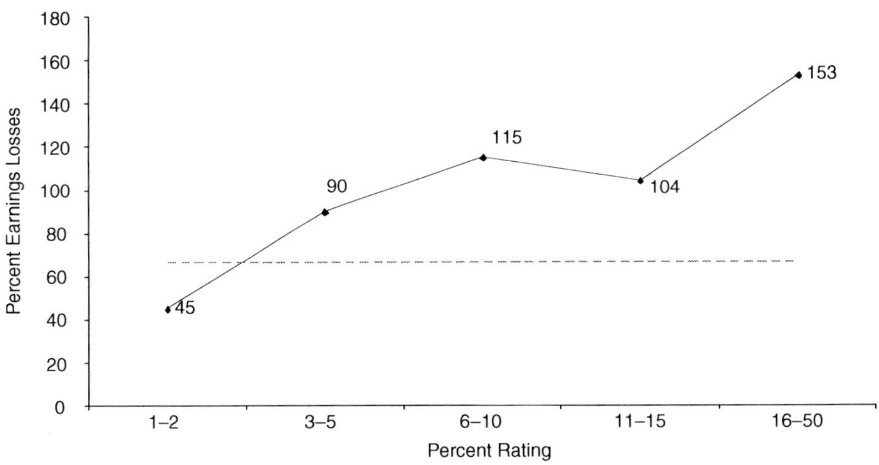

FIGURE C-10 Replacement rates (benefits as a percentage of earnings losses) for all Wisconsin workers.

workers' compensation program was in general replacing a higher proportion of earnings loss for workers with more serious disability ratings.

Inter-Injury Horizontal Equity for Benefits

Inter-injury horizontal equity for benefits requires that the replacement rates for workers with the same disability ratings and different types of injuries should be the same or similar. The results in Figure C-9 suggest there are significant differences among the types of injuries concerning the relationships between benefits and lost earnings.

Observations on the Wisconsin Results

1. It is important to distinguish between the ability of the disability rating system to accurately predict earnings losses (discussed in entries 2 through 5 below) and the ability of the benefit system to match benefits to earnings losses (discussed in entries 6 through 8). These are related, but different, matters. The former is of greater interest for this study because an assessment of the accuracy of the disability ratings produced by the VA Rating Schedule is part of the assignment for the IOM committee for which this study is being prepared.

2. At the most aggregate level—the entire sample of Wisconsin workers—the Wisconsin rating system did an excellent job of providing vertical equity. As shown in Figure C-7, there is a close correspondence between higher disability ratings and greater earnings losses.

3. When the Wisconsin sample is separated into the four injury types, the Wisconsin rating system does not do as well in terms of vertical equity. As shown in Figure C-6, the earnings losses generally increase with higher ratings for two types of injuries, but there are serious problems with vertical equity for two other types of injuries.

4. There are also serious problems with the Wisconsin rating system in terms of inter-injury horizontal equity. As shown in Figure C-6, there are significant differences among the four types of injuries in the relationships between disability ratings and lost earnings.

5. There are also serious problems with the Wisconsin rating system in terms of intra-injury horizontal equity. As shown in Figure C-5 (and in Panels C and D of Table C-1), with cells defined by injury type (or age) and percent rating, there are large variations in earnings losses among different workers.

6. The Wisconsin cash benefits system met the generally accepted test of adequacy, since the average replacement rate for the entire sample was more than 66.67 percent.

7. The Wisconsin rating system did a fairly good job of providing vertical equity for benefits. As shown in Figure C-9, the replacement rates generally were roughly the same for workers with different ratings for the same injury (although there were some important exceptions).

8. Finally, the Wisconsin benefit system had serious problems with inter-injury horizontal equity. As shown in Figure C-9, there were significant differences among the types of injuries concerning the relationships between benefits and lost earnings.

A CURRENT STUDY OF THE CALIFORNIA WORKERS' COMPENSATION PROGRAM

The California Worker's Compensation Program

The workers' compensation programs in California and several other states have been examined in a series of studies conducted by the RAND Corporation in recent years.[10] Boden et al. (2005) provide a summary of the results for California, New Mexico, Oregon, Washington, and Wisconsin. Reville et al. (2005) examined various aspects of the California program for permanent disability rating system; we rely on material from that study. We produced new empirical results for this study involving workers who were injured between January 1, 1991, and December 31, 1993, and who received permanent partial disability benefits in California.[11]

The California workers' compensation benefit system applicable to the workers in this study had some similarities to the Wisconsin workers compensation program described in the previous section. California used different benefit formulae during the temporary disability period and the permanent disability period (Figure C-1). During the temporary disability period, most California workers in the study qualified for TTD benefits, which were 66-and-two-thirds percent of the worker's preinjury wages, subject to a maximum weekly benefit. Once the worker reached the date of MMI, the TTD benefits stopped and most California workers with permanent disabilities qualified for PPD benefits. The weekly benefit for PPD

[10]These studies include Peterson et al. (2001) and Reville et al. (2001).

[11]The RAND data include some injuries in later years, but this study focuses on injuries from 1991 to 1993 in order to include five years of post-injury earnings, which is comparable to the Wisconsin data from Berkowitz and Burton (1987) used in the present study.

was 66-and-two-thirds percent of the worker's preinjury wages, subject to a maximum weekly benefit. These attributes of the California system were basically the same as in Wisconsin.

There were also significant differences between the PPD benefits in California and Wisconsin. In Wisconsin, a distinction was made between scheduled injuries (those involving injuries to body parts listed in the workers' compensation statute) and unscheduled injuries (those involving injuries to other body parts, such as backs), whereas in California all injuries were rated using a rating schedule adopted by the administrative director of the Division of Workers' Compensation.

Another major distinction between the states pertained to the basis for the permanent disability ratings.[12] In Wisconsin, both the scheduled and nonscheduled injuries were rated based on an evaluation of medical impairment, corresponding to the extent of anatomical loss (IA) or functional loss (IB) shown in Figure C-2. In California, there were several sets of criteria that could be used to apply the "standard rating" for permanent disabilities. *Objective factors* roughly corresponded to IA or IB in Figure C-2, and were largely based on information the rating physician could directly observe or measure. *Subjective factors* could be based on the worker's description of the severity or frequency of pain and the resulting limitations on his or her ability to perform various activities. Such subjective factors roughly correspond to IB or limitations in activities of daily living (II) in Figure C-2. *Work-capacity Guidelines* were developed to rate spines and then were extended to other medical conditions. The guidelines in part correspond to II in Figure C-2 ("contemplates the individual has lost approximately half of his pre-injury capacity for performing such activities as bending, stooping, lifting"). The guidelines in part also correspond to loss of earning capacity (IIIA) in Figure C-2 ("disability precluding heavy work").

An additional complication of the California permanent disability rating system is that the objective factors, subjective factors, and work-capacity guidelines were not mutually exclusive categories. Rather, it was quite common for an injury to have rating factors from more than one category, such as an injury to the wrist that causes immobility plus pain. Finally, a distinctive attribute of the California rating system is that the standard rating was modified on the basis of the individual worker's age and occupation. The ultimate basis for the rating was provided in the workers' compensation statute: namely, "the diminished ability of such injured employee to compete in an open labor market." In essence, the California rating system used measurements of a variety of consequences of an injury or disease to

[12]The California permanent disability rating system is described in more detail in Reville et al. (2005).

serve as proxies or predictors of the loss of earning capacity and/or actual loss of earnings.

The California rating system for permanent disabilities was significantly changed in 2004, subsequent to the period when the injuries analyzed in this section occurred. One significant change was the adoption of the *Guides* as the basis for rating permanent impairments. Therefore, the results in this section likely would not be applicable to workers who receive PPD benefits from the current California workers' compensation program.

Summary of the California Results

The California workers who were injured between 1991 and 1993 and who received PPD benefits were classified into 21 impairment categories based on the California permanent disability rating system, which are shown in Table C-2.

There are four panels of data for California, which roughly correspond to four of the seven panels of data presented for Wisconsin. There are no California data on the standard deviation of mean earnings losses corresponding to Panel D in the Wisconsin data in Table C-1. In addition, the only benefits data readily available for California are confined to PPD benefits and do not include temporary disability benefits, as in Wisconsin, and so there are no Panels F and G in Table C-2. Because we lack data on all types of cash benefits, we will not evaluate the adequacy and equity of the California cash benefits.

Panel A. There are 78,696 California PPD cases shown in Table C-2.

Panel B. The potential earnings for each worker were determined by matching the injured worker to a *control group*, which consisted of other workers in the same firm who had similar earnings in the four quarters prior to the date of injury and who did not experience workplace injuries.[13] The uninjured workers' actual earnings in the five years after the date of injury as recorded in the California unemployment insurance database correspond to the potential earnings shown in Figure C-3. For workers with injuries that resulted in general lower extremity impairments rated at 1 to 5 percent, the mean potential earnings for the five years were $222,772. (The figures are in 2003 dollars discounted to the present value of the potential earnings at the date of injury.[14])

---

[13]Reville et al. (2005) provide an extended discussion on the matching procedure used to construct the data used in this study and the tests used to assure the quality of the matches.

[14]Reville (1999) discusses the discounting procedure.

TABLE C-2 California Permanent Partial Disability Cases

		Percent Rating								
	Classification of Workers	1–5	6–10	11–15	16–20	21–25	26–50	51–100	Mean Ratings	Total
Panel A		Counts of workers								
1	General lower extremity impairment	299	134	152	136	117	147	65	18.7	1,050
2	Hip impairment	65	44	44	17	26	42	25	20.6	263
3	Knee impairment	2,549	1,500	1,313	843	690	825	206	14.6	7,926
4	Ankle impairment	988	473	335	253	134	218	100	13.7	2,501
5	Impaired function in toe(s)	196	35	23	23	11	13	10	9.4	311
6	Vision impairment	93	22	12	8	28	7	1	10.2	171
7	Hearing impairment	732	255	227	103	74	62	79	11.0	1,532
8	Hand/fingers	2,322	615	507	233	102	273	17	8.7	4,069
9	Loss of grasping power	1,721	2,421	1,167	771	234	511	85	11.3	6,910
10	Chronic lung impairment	19	68	9	13	4	15	16	20.4	144
11	Heart disease	6	34	26	43	10	64	47	32.0	230
12	General impairment to shoulder or arm	895	886	1,187	621	272	1,003	75	17.9	4,939
13	Impaired function in shoulder	1,808	1,023	930	410	109	106	14	9.8	4,400
14	Impaired function in elbow	760	388	292	107	43	59	1	9.3	1,650
15	Impaired function in wrist	1,244	711	716	334	115	437	18	13.0	3,575

16	Impaired function of neck, spine, or pelvis	3,414	4,664	4,771	3,290	3,534	4,572	687	19.6	24,932
17	General impairment to abdomen	57	77	41	37	16	33	10	17.3	271
18	Psychiatric impairment	135	201	162	108	49	181	77	22.2	913
19	Posttraumatic head syndrome	6	18	9	17	1	17	4	24.4	72
20	Headaches	70	18	8	2	2	3	1	7.7	104
21	Other	155	82	41	17	14	20	13	13.6	342
22	Multiple impairments	478	1,310	1,765	1,679	1,381	4,266	1,512	27.9	12,391
23	Total	18,012	14,979	13,737	9,065	6,966	12,874	3,063	17.6	78,696
Panel B		Mean potential earnings (5 years in dollars)								
1	General lower extremity impairment	222,772	212,342	201,888	191,640	210,192	193,088	173,165		205,757
2	Hip impairment	216,122	222,054	186,194	255,052	202,375	172,636	152,215		200,246
3	Knee impairment	248,030	226,808	219,113	225,184	221,475	206,545	181,574		228,436
4	Ankle impairment	213,040	210,958	225,356	183,737	213,007	183,213	159,130		206,574
5	Impaired function in toe(s)	226,615	171,619	250,608	158,705	165,986	187,296	302,528		215,831
6	Vision impairment	179,462	163,693	182,941	152,001	214,175	173,203	907,883		186,080
7	Hearing impairment	327,325	298,036	286,521	300,473	322,791	263,565	342,879		312,602
8	Hand/fingers	209,404	212,214	192,877	201,203	181,845	188,842	173,162		205,078
9	Loss of grasping power	202,594	197,372	184,260	182,303	171,652	187,648	206,208		193,295
10	Chronic lung impairment	209,446	187,187	172,809	236,983	161,239	199,785	216,351		197,553

continued

TABLE C-2 Continued

		Percent Rating								
	Classification of Workers	1–5	6–10	11–15	16–20	21–25	26–50	51–100	Mean Ratings	Total
11	Heart disease	230,212	321,699	386,182	296,066	441,916	320,496	271,779		316,501
12	General impairment to shoulder or arm	221,518	212,543	192,945	186,673	179,654	186,235	160,057		198,256
13	Impaired function in shoulder	229,916	218,578	224,585	191,834	177,413	201,546	181,857		220,468
14	Impaired function in elbow	244,375	236,635	217,595	217,276	211,776	187,296	25,710		233,035
15	Impaired function in wrist	196,603	204,600	191,931	187,747	173,689	195,437	205,847		195,597
16	Impaired function of neck, spine, or pelvis	211,659	201,228	198,319	193,793	186,691	181,240	185,695		194,965
17	General impairment to abdomen	298,018	283,966	202,290	252,706	351,237	173,110	219,259		258,382
18	Psychiatric impairment	252,582	203,768	209,605	199,731	233,809	215,352	231,894		217,825
19	Posttraumatic head syndrome	109,461	133,884	254,696	199,530	199,818	132,797	215,269		167,631
20	Headaches	171,730	216,163	215,627	66,244	70,903	136,991	221,950		178,310
21	Other	222,476	172,208	268,260	352,335	194,575	211,438	218,442		220,426
22	Multiple impairments	232,058	205,536	191,462	193,938	188,114	184,851	190,298		192,060
23	Total	224,315	209,364	202,352	197,457	192,891	187,224	193,817		204,505

Panel C		Mean earnings losses (5 years in dollars)							
1	General lower extremity impairment	33,533	35,278	37,981	51,788	68,946	85,767	82,942	51,081
2	Hip impairment	39,905	55,351	37,400	114,564	76,527	32,562	76,796	52,850
3	Knee impairment	37,506	33,523	44,222	55,132	75,147	81,495	103,220	49,303
4	Ankle impairment	27,987	29,882	54,860	35,299	67,201	63,883	72,010	39,675
5	Impaired function in toe(s)	32,144	27,913	73,854	–7,694	31,962	90,456	174,570	38,817
6	Vision impairment	1,518	27,353	24,981	–31,339	50,294	81,007	769,050	20,680
7	Hearing impairment	97,275	105,490	106,834	134,188	147,299	112,385	126,603	107,081
8	Hand/fingers	30,674	40,465	47,015	53,352	62,070	76,110	117,422	39,687
9	Loss of grasping power	29,904	35,871	46,702	48,068	49,262	72,625	83,994	41,338
10	Chronic lung impairment	53,569	62,087	14,616	49,687	-41,265	51,094	151,581	62,804
11	Heart disease	54,910	80,954	62,862	135,073	222,307	131,962	191,720	131,322
12	General impairment to shoulder or arm	41,267	47,078	51,570	60,893	58,731	74,778	89,442	55,752
13	Impaired function in shoulder	41,217	56,103	74,430	65,240	64,813	94,681	94,728	55,980
14	Impaired function in elbow	43,771	48,292	59,764	49,634	72,154	54,021	9,145	49,130
15	Impaired function in wrist	30,876	48,626	44,769	51,796	46,014	69,838	107,651	44,779
16	Impaired function of neck, spine, or pelvis	34,857	37,488	46,577	50,187	58,597	67,237	103,985	50,822
17	General impairment to abdomen	106,332	96,965	45,454	121,247	165,557	53,324	120,402	94,057

continued

TABLE C-2 Continued

		Percent Rating								
	Classification of Workers	1–5	6–10	11–15	16–20	21–25	26–50	51–100	Mean Ratings	Total
18	Psychiatric impairment	114,519	107,346	105,382	103,634	136,278	146,619	189,275		123,867
19	Posttraumatic head syndrome	60,075	17,161	86,519	53,981	–75,641	85,629	200,984		63,190
20	Headaches	39,739	66,326	98,959	–32,016	50,423	20,066	–12,946		46,647
21	Other	41,070	13,888	38,994	170,609	61,545	114,093	152,655		50,093
22	Multiple impairments	54,613	41,508	39,885	57,043	57,888	74,409	104,045		64,671
23	Total	38,687	42,198	49,856	55,293	62,038	73,530	106,482		53,623
Panel E		Proportional earnings losses								
1	General lower extremity impairment	0.15	0.17	0.19	0.27	0.33	0.44	0.48		0.25
2	Hip impairment	0.18	0.25	0.20	0.45	0.38	0.19	0.50		0.26
3	Knee impairment	0.15	0.15	0.20	0.24	0.34	0.39	0.57		0.22
4	Ankle impairment	0.13	0.14	0.24	0.19	0.32	0.35	0.45		0.19
5	Impaired function in toe(s)	0.14	0.16	0.29	–0.05	0.19	0.48	0.58		0.18
6	Vision impairment	0.01	0.17	0.14	–0.21	0.23	0.47	0.85		0.11
7	Hearing impairment	0.30	0.35	0.37	0.45	0.46	0.43	0.37		0.34
8	Hand/fingers	0.15	0.19	0.24	0.27	0.34	0.40	0.68		0.19
9	Loss of grasping power	0.15	0.18	0.25	0.26	0.29	0.39	0.41		0.21
10	Chronic lung impairment	0.26	0.33	0.08	0.21	–0.26	0.26	0.70		0.32

11	Heart disease	0.24	0.25	0.16	0.46	0.50	0.41	0.71	0.41
12	General impairment to shoulder or arm	0.19	0.22	0.27	0.33	0.33	0.40	0.56	0.28
13	Impaired function in shoulder	0.18	0.26	0.33	0.34	0.37	0.47	0.52	0.25
14	Impaired function in elbow	0.18	0.20	0.27	0.23	0.34	0.29	0.36	0.21
15	Impaired function in wrist	0.16	0.24	0.23	0.28	0.26	0.36	0.52	0.23
16	Impaired function of neck, spine, or pelvis	0.16	0.19	0.23	0.26	0.31	0.37	0.56	0.26
17	General impairment to abdomen	0.36	0.34	0.22	0.48	0.47	0.31	0.55	0.36
18	Psychiatric impairment	0.45	0.53	0.50	0.52	0.58	0.68	0.82	0.57
19	Posttraumatic head syndrome	0.55	0.13	0.34	0.27	-0.38	0.64	0.93	0.38
20	Headaches	0.23	0.31	0.46	–0.48	0.71	0.15	–0.06	0.26
21	Other	0.18	0.08	0.15	0.48	0.32	0.54	0.70	0.23
22	Multiple impairments	0.24	0.20	0.21	0.29	0.31	0.40	0.55	0.34
23	Total	0.17	0.20	0.25	0.28	0.32	0.39	0.55	0.26

Panel C. The actual earnings for each injured worker in the five years after the date of injury were determined based on California unemployment insurance earnings records. These actual earnings correspond to the actual earnings shown in Figure C-3. The actual earnings were subtracted from the potential earnings to determine the earnings losses shown in Panel C. For workers with injuries that resulted in general lower extremity impairments rated at 1 to 5 percent, the mean earnings losses for the five years were $33,533.[15] Of interest, there were five entries in Panel C in which the mean earnings losses are negative: The mean actual earnings exceeded the mean potential earnings for workers in those categories.

Panel D. There are no data on the standard deviation of the earnings losses for California workers; therefore, this panel is missing in Table C-2.

Panel E. The proportional earnings losses are shown in Panel E. These figures represent the mean earnings losses in Panel C divided by the mean potential earnings in Panel B. For workers with injuries that resulted in general lower extremity impairments rated at 1 to 5 percent, the proportional earnings loss was 0.15 ($33,533 divided by $222,772), which means these workers experienced earnings losses that were 15 percent of potential earnings.

The California Disability Rating System and Equity

The results from the study of California workers can be used to illustrate the use of the equity criterion to evaluate the performance of a system providing benefits to persons experiencing loss of earnings as a result of injuries or diseases. The balance of this section discusses a series of figures derived from the information in Table C-2. (The figures transform the proportions in Table C-2 into percentages in order to expedite exposition.) We have selected eight medical conditions from Table C-2 for this discussion.

Vertical Equity for Ratings

The data in Figures C-11 and C-12 can be used to evaluate vertical equity. *Vertical equity requires that actual wage losses increase in proportion to the increases in disability ratings.* There are some conditions for which earnings losses consistently increase as the permanent disability rating increases. These are condition 1 (general lower extremity impairment) and condition 3 (knee impairment) in Figure C-11, and condition 12

[15]The figures are in 2003 dollars discounted to the present value of the actual earnings at the date of injury.

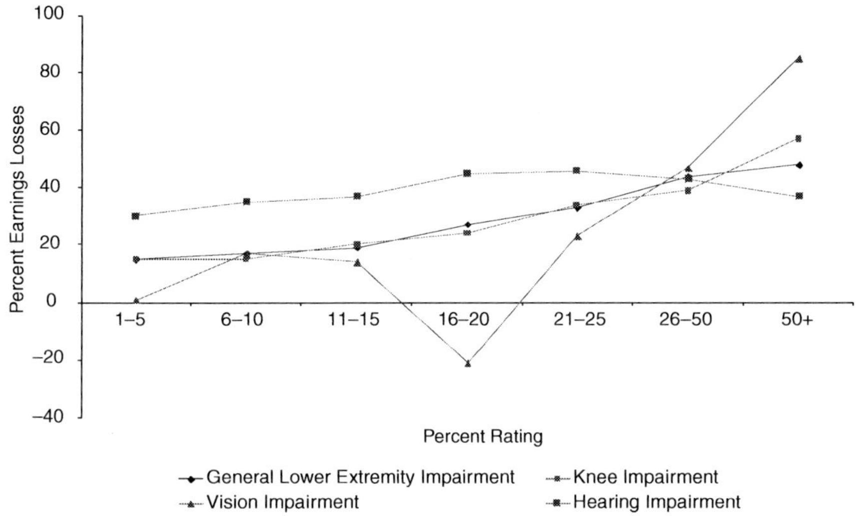

FIGURE C-11 Percentage earnings losses for California workers with four types of injuries.

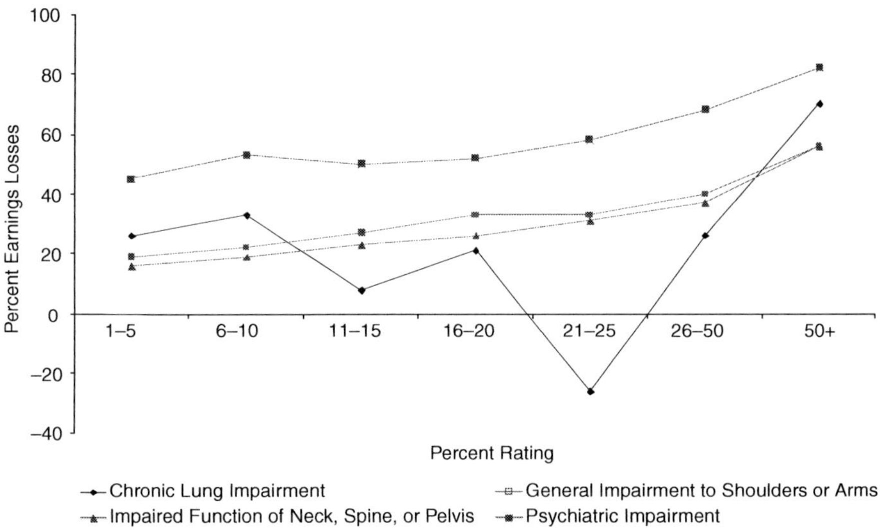

FIGURE C-12 Percentage earnings losses for California workers with four types of injuries.

(general impairment to shoulder or arm) and 16 (impaired function of neck, spine, or pelvis) in Figure C-12. With one or two exceptions, the earnings losses increase with higher disability ratings for condition 6 (vision impairment) and condition 7 (hearing impairment) in Figure C-11 and condition 18 (psychiatric impairment) in Figure C-12. (The vertical equity for psychiatric impairment must be qualified, however, since workers with a 1 to 5 percent rating experienced a 45 percent loss of earnings, which increases very little until the condition receives a disability rating of at least 21 percent.) The condition for which vertical equity for ratings is clearly lacking is condition 10 (chronic lung impairment) in Figure C-12.

Vertical Equity for Ratings—Revisited

Shall we look at the trees (represented by Figures C-11 and C-12) or the forest (represented by Figure C-13)? As shown in Figure C-13, for all California workers, there is a monotonic relationship between rating categories and percentage earnings losses: They consistently increase together. However, the magnitudes of the ratings and the losses are not particularly close. The dashed line represents an exact correspondence between ratings and losses (for example, an 8 percent disability rating equals an 8 percent earnings loss). For the three lowest rating categories, earnings losses clearly exceed the ratings, while for the 21–25 and 26–50 percent rating categories, the earnings losses are clearly less than the ratings. At this level of aggrega-

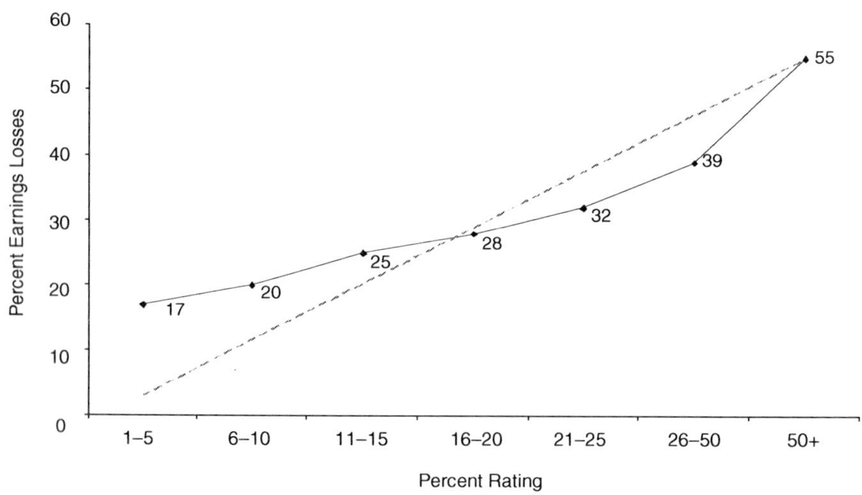

FIGURE C-13 Percentage earnings losses for all California workers.

tion, the California rating system does a moderately good job of providing vertical equity.

Intra-Injury Horizontal Equity for Ratings

Intra-injury horizontal equity for ratings requires that the actual wage losses for workers with the same disability ratings and the same type of injury should be the same or similar. This test cannot be used for the California workers' compensation program because we lack information on the extent of variation within each cell (which is why Table C-2 does not contain Panel D).

Inter-Injury Horizontal Equity for Ratings

Inter-injury horizontal equity for ratings requires that the actual wage losses for workers with the same disability ratings and different types of injuries should be the same or similar. The results in Figures C-11 and C-12 suggest there are significant differences among the types of injuries concerning the relationships between ratings and lost earnings. For example, for the five lowest rating categories, hearing impairment (condition 7) has the highest earnings losses for each rating category in Figure C-11, and without exception, psychiatric impairment has the highest earnings losses for each rating category in Figure C-12.

Observations on the California Results

1. We confine our observations to the ability of the disability rating system to accurately predict earnings losses, because we do not have the data necessary to assess the ability of the benefit system to match benefits to earnings losses.

2. We have data on disabled workers with 22 medical conditions, which constitute a significant portion, but not the universe, of California workers who received permanent partial disability benefits during the years covered by our study.

3. At the most aggregate level—the total experience of workers with all 22 conditions—the California rating system did a moderately good job of providing vertical equity. As shown in Figure C-13, the earnings losses increase monotonically with higher disability ratings, but the correspondence between the magnitudes of the disability ratings and the earnings losses is far from perfect. For lower disability ratings, the earnings losses are much higher than the ratings.

4. We selected eight medical conditions for particular scrutiny and, at this level, the California system also does a moderately good job of providing vertical equity. As shown in Figures C-11 and C-12, earnings losses generally increase with higher ratings for most medical conditions, but there are serious vertical equity problems for two conditions.

5. There are serious problems with the California rating system in terms of inter-injury horizontal equity. As shown in Figures C-11 and C-12, there are significant differences among the eight types of injuries in the relationships among disability ratings and lost earnings.

6. As previously noted, the results in this section involve injuries that occurred well before the 2004 reforms to the California workers' compensation program. These reforms introduced a new method for rating the severity of permanent disability, beginning with the use of the *Guides*. However, the new disability rating system continued to use proxies to predict the loss of earning capacity or actual loss of earnings. A distinctive feature of the new California system is a provision designed to incorporate empirical data on wage losses into revisions of the permanent disability rating system in order to reduce the types of horizontal and vertical inequities discussed in this section. This adjustment feature bears watching, although currently there are insufficient data on post-injury outcomes for workers who were recently injured to evaluate whether the 2004 reforms have been successful.

THE 1971 REPORT ON THE ECONOMIC VALIDATION OF THE [VA] RATING SCHEDULE STUDY

The Veterans Disability Compensation Program

Disability compensation is a cash benefit paid to veterans who are disabled by injuries or diseases incurred or aggravated during active military service. The benefit amount is graduated according to the degree of the veteran's disability rated on a scale from 10 to 100 percent (in increments of 10 percent). The monthly benefit depends on the veteran's disability rating and dependency status. As of December 2006, the monthly benefit for a veteran with no dependents ranged from $115 for a 10 percent rating to $712 for a 50 percent rating to $2,471 for a 100 percent rating. The monthly benefit is higher for veterans with dependents; for example, as of December 2006, a veteran with a 50 percent disability rating with a spouse and one child received $832 per month.

Purpose of the Cash Benefits in the Veterans Disability Compensation Program

As discussed above, the sole purpose of the cash benefits specified by §4.1 of the *Code of Federal Regulations* dealing with the VA's Rating Schedule is to compensate for work disability (as that term is used in this study):

> The percentage ratings represent as far as can practicably be determined the average impairment in earning capacity resulting from such diseases and injuries and their residual conditions in civil occupations.

The Operational Basis for the Cash Benefits in the Veterans Disability Compensation Program

While the purpose of the cash benefits in the veterans disability compensation program is to compensate for work disability, the program is similar to the Wisconsin and California programs in the use of a proxy or proxies for work disability as the operational basis for the benefits. The Rating Schedule used for the program is contained in the *Code of Federal Regulations* (38 CFR Ch.1). The general guidance for the basis of the ratings is contained in

> §4.10 Functional impairment.
>
> The basis of disability evaluations is the ability of the body as a whole, or of the psyche, or of a system or organ of the body to function under the ordinary conditions of daily life including employment. Whether the upper or lower extremities, the back or abdominal wall, the eyes or ears, or the cardiovascular, digestive, or other systems, or psyche are affected, evaluations are based upon lack of usefulness, of these parts or systems, especially in self-support. This imposes upon the medical examiner the responsibility of furnishing, in addition to the etiological, anatomical, pathological, laboratory and prognostic data required for ordinary medical classification, full description of the effects of disability upon the person's ordinary activity. In this connection, it will be remembered that a person may be too disabled to engage in employment although he or she is up and about and fairly comfortable at home or upon limited activity.

This paragraph appears to direct that ratings should be based on at least two concepts in Figure C-2, including limitations in activities of daily living (II) and loss of earning capacity (IIIA). The paragraph also appears to contain an admonition to not consider loss of capacity for nonwork experiences (IVA) in determining the rating.

Despite the language of § 4.10 that mandates consideration of a broad array of factors in determining the disability rating, the instructions for the ratings of specific injuries contained in the *Code of Federal Regulations* appear to rely on more constricted criterion. For example, the rating for medical condition 5120 (arm, amputation of: above insertion of deltoid) is 90 percent for the major arm and 80 percent for the minor arm. The basis for rating medical condition 5120 appears to correspond to medical impairment: anatomical loss (IA) in Figure C-2. Another example is the ratings for medical condition 5201 (arm, limitation of motion of), which are 40 percent for limitation to 25° from side, 30 percent for limitation to midway between side and shoulder level, and 20 percent for limitation at shoulder level. The basis for rating medical condition 5201 appears to correspond to medical impairment: functional loss (IB) in Figure C-2.

Summary of the Economic Validation of the Rating Schedule Study

In 1971, VA conducted a study of the 1967 earnings of disabled veterans called *Economic Validation of the Rating Schedule* or ECVARS. The results were tabulated by the diagnostic codes used in the Rating Schedule and by the rating degrees for the veterans' medical conditions. We examined the results for disabled veterans with 10 medical conditions. These conditions were chosen because (1) they were among the 21 medical conditions selected by the IOM committee for special scrutiny; (2) there are results from the 1971 study for the medical conditions being scrutinized by the IOM committee;[16] and (3) the 1971 results include at least two levels of disability rating for the medical condition.[17]

The results from the ECVARS study are included in the panels in Table C-3. The panels correspond to those used in Tables C-1 (Wisconsin) and C-2 (California) in order to facilitate comparisons. However, some panels are omitted from Table C-3 because data are not available for the veterans with disabilities.

Panel A. There are no data on the number of veterans in each cell; therefore, this panel is missing in Table C-3. Because we do not have the number of veterans with disabilities in each cell, we cannot calculate a weighted average for all veterans in the tables.[18]

[16]For example, there are no 1971 results for diagnostic code 6351 (HIV-related illness), so this condition is not included in Table C-3.

[17]For example, there is only one rating level for diagnostic code 6350 (Lupus) in the 1971 results, so this condition is not included in Table C-3.

[18]According to the ECVARS study, the number of cases in each cell was at least 200, except for a small number of cells with fewer than 200 that were included "because of unique problems associated with them [i.e., those particular conditions]." If the population in a cell was greater than 500, it was sampled. Overall, there were approximately 500,000 cases in a little more than the 1,000 cells.

Panel B. The potential earnings for veterans with disabilities in each cell were based on the actual median earnings of the veterans without disabilities in the control group, as reported on a survey questionnaire administered by the Census Bureau. The *control group* consisted of 14,000 veterans not receiving disability compensation from VA or the Department of Defense (DoD).[19] The veterans without disabilities in the control group were matched to the veterans with disabilities on the basis of age, education, and region.[20] The potential earnings in Panel B correspond to the potential earnings in Figure C-3 for 1967 and represent the estimate of what the veterans in the study would have earned had they not been injured. For veterans with injuries that resulted in an amputation of an upper extremity, the median potential earnings were $7,444.

Panel C. The actual median earnings of the veterans in each cell in 1967 were determined based on the survey conducted by the Census Bureau. The actual earnings used to calculate the results in Panel C correspond to the actual earnings shown in Figure C-3. The actual earnings were subtracted from the potential earnings to determine the earnings losses in Panel C. For veterans with injuries that resulted in an amputation of an upper extremity, the median of the earnings losses was $335.

Panel D. There are no data on the standard deviation of the earnings losses for the veterans with disabilities: therefore, this panel is missing in Table C-3.

Panel E. The proportional earnings losses are shown in Panel E. These figures represent the median earnings losses in Panel C divided by the median potential earnings in Panel B. For veterans with injuries that resulted in an amputation of an upper extremity, the proportional earnings loss was 0.045 ($335 divided by $7,444), which means that the earnings losses for disabled veterans with this type of injury were 4.5 percent of potential earnings.

Panel F. The median disability benefits for veterans are shown in Panel F. Because the benefits are a function of the rating category, there are no variations in benefits among veterans with the same percentage disability

[19]Military personnel separated from the service because of disability are eligible for disability compensation from the Department of Defense (DoD). They also may receive disability compensation from VA, although the amount is offset, except in certain circumstances. Unlike disability compensation from DoD, VA compensation is not taxed.

[20]VA used four age groups (under 30, 30–49, 50–64, and 65 and older); three education classes (less than high school graduate; high school graduate; and one or more years more than a high school graduate); and two regions (South and all other regions).

TABLE C-3 Veterans with Disabilities in 1967

	Medical Conditions	Percent Rating 10	20	30	40	50	60	70	80	90	100
Panel B		Median potential earnings (in dollars)[a]									
1	Amputation, upper extremity	7,444	7,135	7,176	6,743	7,016	7,003	7,272	7,412	7,517	
2	Spine disorders	8,119	7,559		7,413		7,108				
3	Impairment of knee (other than ankylosis)	7,955	7,699	7,550							
4	Defective visual acuity	7,576	8,262	7,241	7,439	7,018	6,993	7,209	7,243	7,008	7,507
5	Hearing impairment	7,821	7,425	7,293	7,223		7,263		7,203		
6	Chronic respiratory diseases	7,844		7,069			6,605				6,502
7	Hypertensive vascular disease	7,672	7,519		7,275						
8	Gastrointestinal ulcers	7,287	7,023		6,691						
9	Scars	7,692		7,592		7,447			7,215		
10	Diabetes mellitus	7,547	7,617		7,709		7,500				7,035
11	Average	7,696	7,530	7,320	7,213	7,160	7,079	7,241	7,268	7,263	7,015
Panel C		Median earnings losses (in dollars)[a]									
1	Amputation, upper extremity	335	899	775	1,733	1,747	2,500	2,269	2,283	1,977	
2	Spine disorders	479	703		1,401		4,144				
3	Impairment of knee (other than ankylosis)	700	1,047	755							
4	Defective visual acuity	500	694	1,231	1,964	2,000	2,930	3,691	4,838	5,599	6,013
5	Hearing impairment	219	891	547	809		1,271		2,096		
6	Chronic respiratory diseases	753		1,633			5,046				5,533
7	Hypertensive vascular disease	468	1,421		1,746						
8	Gastrointestinal ulcers	634	927		1,559						
9	Scars	300		782		700			2,720		
10	Diabetes mellitus	800	815		1,457		2,700				5,565
11	Average	519	925	954	1,524	1,482	3,099	2,980	2,984	3,788	5,704

Panel E		Proportional earnings losses[a]									
1	Amputation, upper extremity	0.045	0.126	0.108	0.257	0.249	0.357	0.312	0.308	0.263	
2	Spine disorders	0.059	0.093		0.189		0.583				
3	Impairment of knee (other than ankylosis)	0.088	0.136	0.100							
4	Defective visual acuity	0.066	0.084	0.170	0.264	0.285	0.419	0.512	0.668	0.799	0.801
5	Hearing impairment	0.028	0.120	0.075	0.112		0.175		0.291		
6	Chronic respiratory diseases	0.096		0.231			0.764				0.851
7	Hypertensive vascular disease	0.061	0.189		0.240						
8	Gastrointestinal ulcers	0.087	0.132		0.233						
9	Scars	0.039		0.103		0.094			0.377		
10	Diabetes mellitus	0.106	0.107		0.189		0.360				0.791
11	Average	0.068	0.123	0.131	0.212	0.209	0.443	0.412	0.411	0.531	0.814
Panel F		Median benefits (in dollars)[a]									
1	Amputation, upper extremity	252	480	720	984	1,356	1,632	1,932	2,232	2,508	
2	Spine disorders	252	480		984		1,632				
3	Impairment of knee (other than ankylosis)	252	480	720							
4	Defective visual acuity	252	480	720	984	1,356	1,632	1,932	2,232	2,508	3,600
5	Hearing impairment	252	480	720	984		1,632		2,232		
6	Chronic respiratory diseases	252		720			1,632				3,600
7	Hypertensive vascular disease	252	480		984						
8	Gastrointestinal ulcers	252	480		984						
9	Scars	252		720		1,356			2,232		
10	Diabetes mellitus	252	480		984		1,632				3,600
11	Average	252	480	720	984	1,356	1,632	1,932	2,232	2,508	3,600

continued

TABLE C-3 Continued

	Medical Conditions	Percent Rating									
		10	20	30	40	50	60	70	80	90	100
Panel G		Replacement rates: Benefits as proportion of earnings losses									
1	Amputation, upper extremity	0.752	0.534	0.929	0.568	0.776	0.653	0.851	0.978	1.269	
2	Spine disorders	0.526	0.683		0.702		0.394				
3	Impairment of knee (other than ankylosis)	0.360	0.458	0.954							
4	Defective visual acuity	0.504	0.692	0.585	0.501	0.678	0.557	0.523	0.461	0.448	0.599
5	Hearing impairment	1.151	0.539	1.316	1.216		1.284		1.065		
6	Chronic respiratory diseases	0.335		0.441			0.323				0.651
7	Hypertensive vascular disease	0.538	0.338		0.564						
8	Gastrointestinal ulcers	0.397	0.518		0.631						
9	Scars	0.840		0.921		1.937			0.821		
10	Diabetes mellitus	0.315	0.589		0.675		0.604				0.647
11	Average	0.572	0.544	0.858	0.694	1.130	0.636	0.687	0.831	0.858	0.632

[a]In 1967 dollars.

rating.[21] For veterans with injuries that resulted in an amputation of an upper extremity, the median of the disability benefits was $252.

Panel G. The replacement rates are shown in Panel G. For veterans with injuries that resulted in an amputation of an upper extremity, the replacement rate was 0.752 ($252 divided by $335), which means these veterans received benefits that replaced 75.2 percent of their earnings losses.

The Veterans Disability Rating System and Equity

The results from the study of disabled veterans can be used to illustrate the use of the equity and adequacy criteria to evaluate the performance of a system providing benefits to persons experiencing losses of earnings as a result of injuries or diseases. The balance of this section discusses several figures derived from the information in Table C-3. (The figures transform the proportions in Table C-3 into percentages.) Figures C-14 and C-15 each contain five of the medical conditions included in Table C-3.

Vertical Equity for Ratings

The data in Figures C-14 and C-15 suggest that the Rating Schedule performed reasonably well when evaluated using the vertical equity criteria. This test requires that actual wage losses generally increase as the disability ratings increase. In most instances, as the percentage disability ratings increase for a particular medical condition, the percentage earnings losses also increase. The major exception is for amputations to the upper extremity, where earnings losses increase as ratings increase over the 10 to 60 percent range, and then earnings losses decrease over the 60 to 90 percent range. There is a general tendency for earnings losses to increase less rapidly than the disability ratings, as shown by the location of the plots of the 10 conditions below the exact proportionate increase line (shown as a dashed line in Figures C-15 and C-16).

Vertical Equity for Ratings—Revisited

Shall we look at the trees (represented by Figures C-14 and C-15) or the forest (represented by Figure C-16)? As shown in Figure C-16, which represents an unweighted average of the 10 conditions shown in Figures C-14 and C-15, the relationship between rating categories and percentage earn-

[21]The compensation value is the basic compensation amount. It does not include compensation for dependents of veterans rated 50 through 100 percent or additional special monthly compensation for physical loss or loss of use of limbs or body functions.

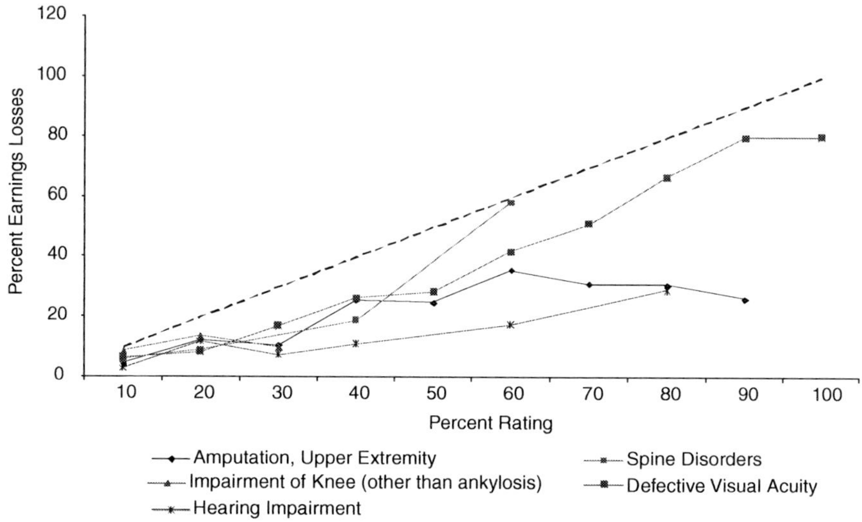

FIGURE C-14 Percentage earnings losses for veterans with five types of injuries.

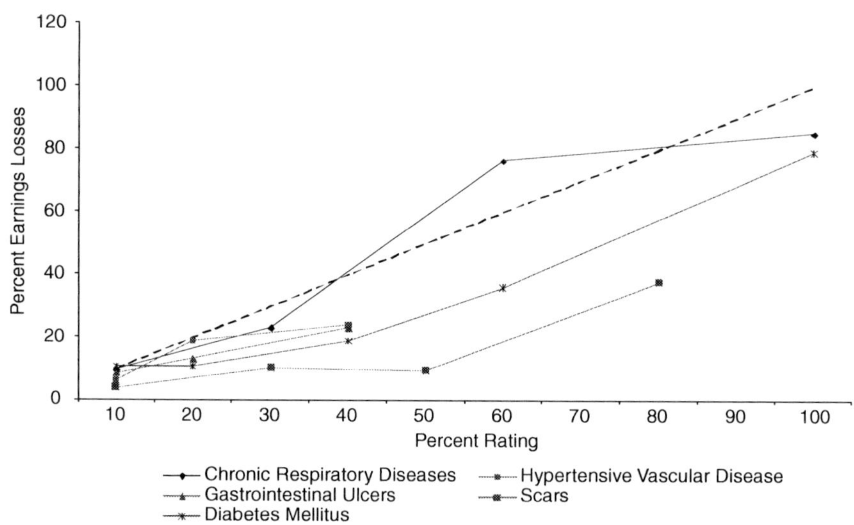

FIGURE C-15 Percentage earnings losses for veterans with five types of injuries.

ings losses is not monotonic: They do not consistently increase together. For example, the earnings losses decline as ratings increase from 60 to 70 to 80 percent. Moreover, the magnitudes of the ratings and the losses are not particularly close. The dashed line represents an exact correspondence between ratings and losses (for example, a 40 percent disability rating equals a 40 percent earnings loss). For every level of rating, ratings clearly exceed the earnings losses. For example, for veterans with a 40 percent rating, earnings losses are 21.2 percent of potential earnings. At this level of aggregation, the VA rating system does a fairly poor job of providing vertical equity.

Intra-Injury Horizontal Equity for Ratings

Intra-injury horizontal equity for ratings requires that the actual wage losses for veterans with the same disability ratings and the same types of injury should be the same or similar. This test cannot be applied to the Rating Schedule because we lack information on the extent of variation within each cell (which is why Table C-3 does not contain Panel D.)

Inter-Injury Horizontal Equity for Ratings

Inter-injury horizontal equity for ratings requires that the earnings losses for veterans with the same disability ratings and different types of

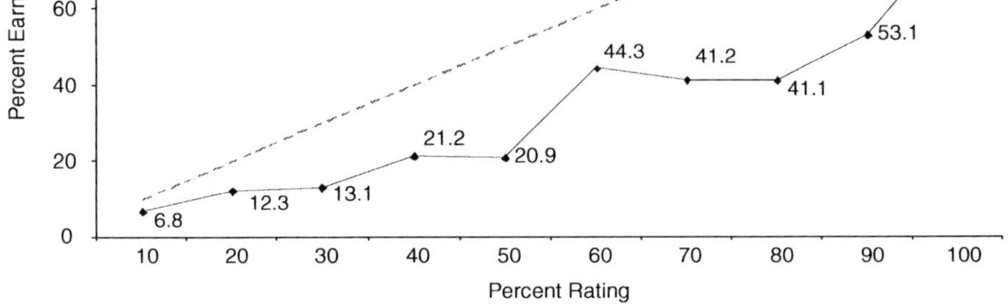

FIGURE C-16 Percentage earnings losses for veterans: averages for ten types of injuries.

injuries should be the same or similar. The results in Figures C-14 and C-15 suggest that the earnings losses for the various types of injuries with ratings from 10 to 40 percent are similar. However, there are significant differences among the types of injuries concerning the relationships between disability ratings and lost earnings for more serious injuries. For example, defective visual acuity (condition 4) has higher earnings losses than upper extremity amputations (condition 1) and hearing impairments (condition 5) for disability ratings between 40 and 90 percent in Figure C-14. In addition, without exception, veterans with scars have the lowest earnings losses for each rating category in Figure C-15.

Replacement Rates and Adequacy for Veterans with Disabilities

The relationships between disability ratings and replacement rates for each of the 10 types of injuries in Table C-3 are shown in Figures C-17 and C-18. The relationship between disability ratings and replacement rates for the average of the 10 types of injuries are shown in Figure C-19.

Adequacy of Benefits

The data in Figures C-17 through C-19 could be used to assess the adequacy of benefits provided by the veterans disability compensation pro-

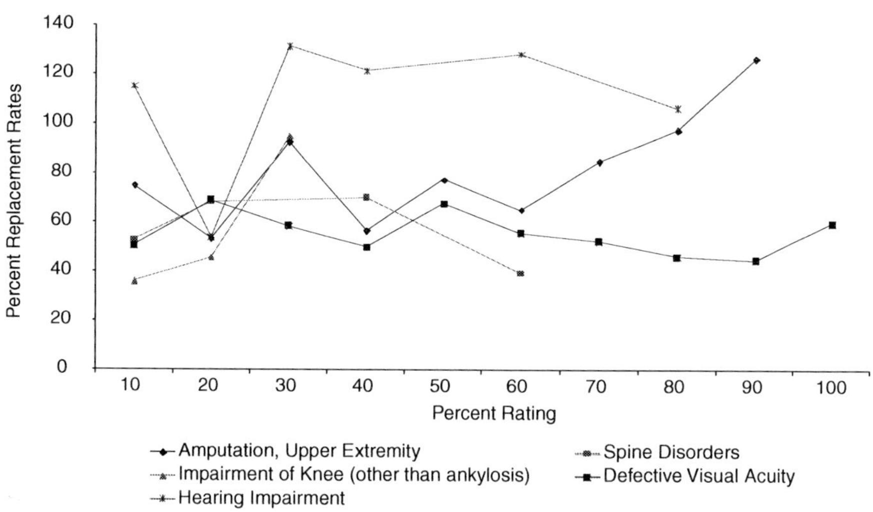

FIGURE C-17 Replacement rates (benefits as a percentage of earnings losses) for veterans with five types of injuries.

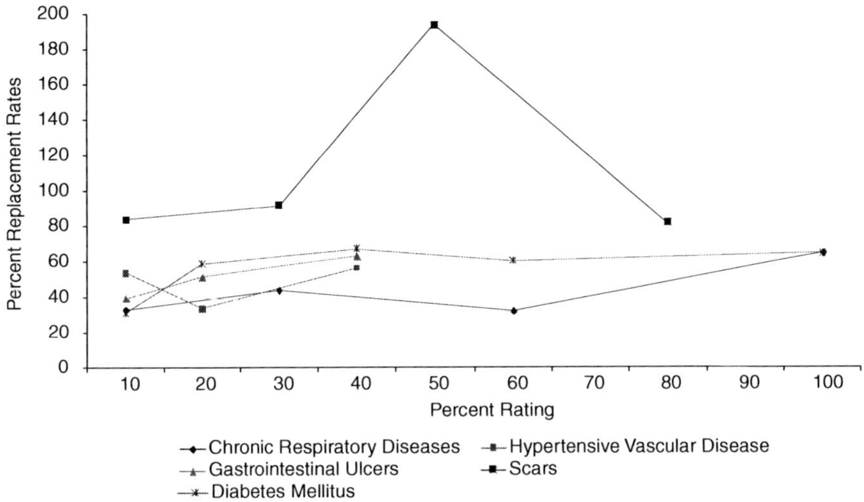

FIGURE C-18 Replacement rates (benefits as a percentage of earnings losses) for veterans with five types of injuries.

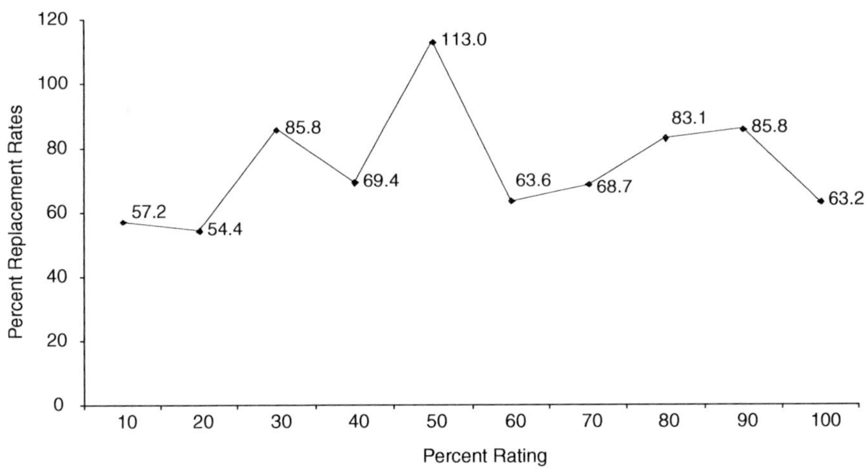

FIGURE C-19 Replacement rates (benefits as a percentage of earnings losses) for veterans: averages for 10 types of injuries.

gram. However, the decision about what constitutes adequate benefits is not part of the charge for the IOM committee for whom this report is being prepared. We therefore will not discuss that topic other than to note that the contributions of veterans to the security of the United States provides a special justification for adequate benefits.

Replacement Rates and Equity for Veterans with Disabilities

Vertical Equity for Benefits

The data in Figures C-17 through C-19 can also be used to examine the vertical equity of benefits for veterans with disabilities. Vertical equity requires that the same proportion of lost wages should be replaced for veterans at all disability ratings, which would require the lines for an injury to be flat in these figures. In this instance, there is fairly good vertical equity for the benefits for the five conditions included in Figure C-18, with the obvious exception of the spike in the replacement rate for veterans with scars rated at 50 percent. There is less vertical equity for the five conditions shown in Figure C-17. For the average of the 10 types of injuries, shown in Figure C-17, the replacement rates vary between roughly 55 and 85 percent for all the rating categories, except the 50 percent rating category, which indicates there is reasonable degree of vertical equity for the benefits in the veterans disability benefit program.

Inter-Injury Horizontal Equity for Benefits

Inter-injury horizontal equity for benefits requires that the replacement rates for veterans with the same disability ratings and different types of injuries should be the same or similar. The results in Figures C-17 and C-18 suggest there are significant differences among the types of injuries concerning the relationships between benefits and lost earnings.

Observations on the Veterans Disability Compensation Program

1. We again note it is important to distinguish between the ability of the disability rating system to accurately predict earnings losses (discussed in entries 3 through 5 below) and the ability of the benefit system to match benefits to earnings losses (discussed in entries 6 and 7). The former is of particular relevance to this study because the IOM committee has been asked to assess the accuracy of the disability ratings produced by the Rating Schedule.

2. We have analyzed data on veterans with 10 medical conditions, which constitute a small portion of veterans who received disability benefits during the year covered by the ECVARS study.

3. At the most aggregate level—the average for the 10 medical conditions—the disability rating system for veterans does a fairly poor job of providing vertical equity. As shown in Figure C-16, the earnings losses decline with higher ratings for several levels of severity. In addition, the earnings losses are consistently less than the ratings levels.

4. When the veterans are separated into the 10 injury types, the rating system appears to do a better job of providing vertical equity. In general, as shown in Figures C-14 and C-15, earnings losses increase as ratings increase, although there are exceptions. Of interest is that earnings losses are less than the disability ratings for almost all entries in the figures.

5. There are serious problems with the rating system for veterans with disabilities in terms of inter-injury horizontal equity. As shown in Figures C-14 and C-15, there are significant differences among the 10 types of medical conditions in the relationships between disability ratings and lost earnings.

6. The veterans disability system does a reasonably good job of providing vertical equity for benefits. Vertical equity for benefits is better at the aggregate level (Figure C-16) than at the level of individual medical conditions (Figures C-17 and C-18).

7. Finally, the benefit system for veterans with disabilities has serious problems with inter-injury horizontal equity. As shown in Figures C-14 and C-19, there were significant differences among the types of medical conditions in the relationships between benefits and lost earnings.

CONCLUSIONS

Purpose of This Study

The primary purpose of this study is to provide a framework for examining the relationship between disability ratings and earnings losses in order to help the IOM committee formulate a response to the first task assigned to the committee. We use that framework to examine three different programs that provide cash benefits to persons with disabilities. We realize that the three programs—the Wisconsin and California workers' compensation programs and the veterans disability compensation program—are quite different in many aspects. However, the three programs all have a common goal—compensating persons with earnings losses resulting from injuries or diseases—and a common procedure—using a proxy or proxies for actual earnings losses as the basis for predicting earnings losses rather than relying on direct measurement of each person's actual earnings losses.

Our study provides a useful framework and several empirical findings important for our understanding of VA's Rating Schedule and other disability rating systems. However, we did not have access to current data concerning the earnings losses for veterans who are receiving benefits from the compensation program. A study being conducted by the Center for Naval Analyses (CNA) should provide data that can be used in connection with our framework to revise the Rating Schedule and related rating regulations.

Use of the Equity Criteria

We used several variants of equity criteria to assess the performance of the three programs. *Vertical equity* requires that actual wage losses increase in proportion to increases in disability ratings. At the aggregate level (the entire sample of workers or veterans), we concluded that the Wisconsin rating system did an excellent job, the California rating system did a moderately good job, and the VA rating system did a fairly poor job using the vertical equity criterion. When the samples were disaggregated by type of injury (or medical condition), Wisconsin did not do as well as at the aggregate level, California did a moderately good job (similar to the performance at the aggregate level), and the VA rating system did reasonably well (and better than at the aggregate level). Overall, we conclude that the three ratings did a reasonably good job on the vertical equity criterion.

Inter-injury horizontal equity requires that workers or veterans with similar disability ratings but different types of injuries should experience similar earnings losses. We concluded there were serious inter-injury equity problems in the ratings systems used by the Wisconsin and California workers' compensation programs, as well as the veterans disability compensation program. Each of the programs systematically treated some injuries or medical conditions different from other injuries in terms of the extent of earnings losses associated with similar disability ratings.

Intra-injury horizontal equity requires that workers or veterans with the same injuries or medical conditions and the same ratings should experience similar earnings losses. We only have data for the Wisconsin workers' compensation program to apply this criterion, and we found serious equity problems.

Our overall conclusion is that the three programs do a reasonably good job on vertical equity—especially at the aggregate level—but that there are serious horizontal equity problems in each of the programs. As a result, we conclude that the various factors in Figure C-1 (such as medical impairment or loss of earning capacity) currently used by various workers' compensation programs and VA do a reasonably good job in serving as proxies for actual wage loss.

Distinguishing Between the Purpose of Benefits and the Operational Basis for Benefits

We distinguish between the purpose of benefits and the operational basis for benefits. The purpose of the two workers' compensation programs we examined and the current purpose of the veterans disability compensation program is to compensate for work disability (loss of earnings). However, all three programs use proxies (or predictors) for losses of earnings as the operational basis for benefits. For example, the amount of benefits is determined for some medical conditions by rating the severity of the permanent impairment (a medical concept) because the severity of the impairment is assumed to be a good predictor of the loss of earnings resulting from the impairment.

The Use of Proxies to Predict Earnings Losses

We conclude that the various factors in Figure C-1 (such as medical impairment or loss of earning capacity) currently used by various workers' compensation programs and VA do a reasonably good job in serving as proxies for actual wage loss. If the factors in Figure C-1 can be used as rough proxies for actual wage loss, what can be done to improve the match between the proxies and the actual wage loss? We have several observations and suggestions.

One issue we have considered is whether the disability rating systems would do a better job of predicting actual wage loss if they placed less emphasis on impairment as the proxy for wage loss and more emphasis on functional limitations and loss of earning capacity as proxies. That is, should we be "shifting to the right" in the factors in Figure C-1 to find better proxies for actual wage loss? The answer—based on the comparison of Wisconsin and California results—is no! Wisconsin at the time the data shown in Table C-2 were collected relied strictly on assessments of medical impairment to determine the amount of PPD benefits, while California relied on a variety of the consequences shown in Figure C-2 as proxies for work disability. Wisconsin did a better job in terms of vertical equity than California and a comparable job in terms of horizontal equity. We therefore tentatively conclude based on the workers' compensation data that there is no reason to incorporate consequences of injuries and disease other than medical impairment in order to improve the accuracy of the predictions of actual earnings losses. We want to make clear that this tentative conclusion needs to be carefully examined in subsequent research, especially in studies of the veterans disability compensation program. The forthcoming data from CNA, for example, should be studied to compare the ability to predict earnings losses for (1) medical conditions for which the ratings are based on permanent impairment with (2) medical conditions for which ratings are based on limitations in the activities of daily living or other "intermediate" concepts in Figure C-2.

One policy change recommended by RAND for California workers' compensation was to periodically assess the actual earnings losses associated with workplace injuries and to determine if there were systematic overestimates or underestimates of the earnings losses associated with the disability ratings for both the system as a whole and for particular injuries or medical conditions. This information could then be used to recalibrate the rating system.[22] A similar procedure could be adopted for the VA disability compensation program. For example, if mental disorders were found to have greater earnings losses than would be expected based on the disability ratings, the rating system could be revised. This could be done either by changing the rating system directly (so that a given level of mental impairment would now be rated at 40 percent rather than 20 percent) or indirectly by producing a set of "modifiers" (so that the medical impairment ratings for mental impairments would be multiplied by two to produce a "disability rating" used for determining the amount of benefits). This policy change could help improve the vertical equity and the inter-injury horizontal equity for the ratings in the veterans disability program.

Intra-Injury Horizontal Equity and Outliers

The preceding discussion essentially pertains to the virtues and deficiencies in the rating system for disabilities in two workers' compensation programs and in the veterans disability program using the criteria of vertical equity and inter-injury horizontal equity, and to some possible policies to deal with the deficiencies. Another topic we want to examine is intra-injury horizontal equity for ratings, which requires that workers or veterans with the same disability rating and same type of injury or medical condition should experience the same or similar levels of earnings losses. The evidence from Wisconsin in Panels C and D of Table C-2, as summarized in Figure C-5, suggest that lack of intra-injury equity is a pervasive phenomenon.

[22]The implications of periodically recalibrating the rating schedule based on empirical studies of actual wage loss is discussed in Reville et al. (2005).

We are skeptical that any disability rating system—no matter how refined—can accurately predict the actual earnings losses resulting from medical conditions for substantial numbers of workers or veterans. Most systems can accommodate those cases in which the earnings losses are much less than is predicted based on the disability rating. The challenge is to deal with the other type of "outliers"—the worker or veteran who has earnings losses far in excess of the amount predicted based on the person's disability rating.

There are four possible responses to this challenge. First, the disability program can assert that in a system of social insurance (or social justice), outliers should be ignored in order to reduce administrative costs and to avoid excessive costs to the system. This is the approach used in most workers' compensation programs for the vast majority of workers with permanent disabilities.

Second, the disability program can treat every worker or veteran as an individual and determine benefits based on his or her own labor market experience. This comes close to the "wage-loss" approach (which bases the benefits solely or primarily on the worker's own labor market experience) that has been tried in several workers' compensation programs and generally rejected as unworkable or too expensive. The "wage-loss" approach foregoes the use of proxies as the basis for benefits, which have generally been incorporated into disability compensation systems because of administrative convenience and to avoid the incentive effects that occur if higher earnings result in reduced benefits.

Third, the disability program may be able to identify variables that increase the accuracy of the rating system but that do not cause inappropriate incentives for beneficiaries. For example, if after controlling for the type and severity of injury, the addition of age to the disability rating system increases the accuracy of the predictions of loss of actual earnings, intra-injury horizontal equity will be improved. However, whether there are such variables that improve the accuracy of the rating system is an empirical question where logic is probably a poor guide.[23]

Fourth, the disability program can use the disability rating system to determine the amount of benefits for the majority of beneficiaries, but provide a safety valve for "outliers" who have earnings losses far in excess of the amount of losses predicted by the rating system. This approach is used

[23]The age adjustments in the California workers' compensation program are discussed by Reville et al. (2005). The baseline age is 39; individuals receive higher permanent partial disability ratings if they are older than age 39, and lower ratings if they are younger than age 39. The adjustments are presumably based on an assumption that older persons find it more difficult to adapt to permanent disabilities than do younger persons with equally severe impairments. However, when workers were placed into four age categories, the youngest workers (ages 18–29) had the highest proportional earnings losses in the three years after their injuries.

in some workers' compensation programs in which workers with relatively low "impairment ratings" can receive additional benefits either because they are reclassified from PPD to permanent total disability (using the "odd lot" doctrine[24]) or because they are workers in a state with hybrid benefits (where workers who exhaust their benefits based on the rating schedule qualify for additional benefits because they have continuing wage losses due to their workplace injuries[25]).

The counterpart to this provision of additional benefits for extraordinary wage loss in some workers' compensation programs is the veterans disability compensation program provision of "individual unemployability" (IU) benefits, which serve as the program's safety valve for those veterans who have much greater earnings losses than the disability rating system predicts. Without endorsing the specific aspects of the IU benefits in the veterans disability compensation program, we endorse the general concept of a special benefit for those veterans who are outliers in terms of their actual earnings losses compared with their expected earnings losses. The reason is that the best of all possible disability rating systems will seriously underpredict the earnings losses of some disabled persons.

The Difference Between Rating Systems and Benefit Systems

We have distinguished between the rating systems for permanent disability and the benefits systems for permanent disability. The former measures the seriousness of an injury or disease in terms of the consequences, such as permanent impairment, limitations in activities of daily living, and loss of earning capacity. The latter uses the disability rating, perhaps in connection with other information, such as the disabled person's age or education, to determine the amount of disability benefits.

We have focused on disability rating systems because that is the domain of the IOM committee. We have provided criteria for evaluating the rating system—horizontal and vertical equity. We have also briefly discussed benefits systems, and provided criteria for evaluating such systems—horizontal equity, vertical equity, and adequacy. While we have concluded that the disability rating systems for the two workers' compensation programs and the veterans disability compensation program do a reasonably good job of providing equity, we have not attempted to make any judgment about the adequacy of the veterans disability benefits.

[24]The "odd lot" doctrine is discussed by Larson and Larson (2006).

[25]The hybrid approach to permanent partial disability benefits is discussed by Burton (2005). States that recently used or currently use the hybrid approach for permanent partial disability benefits include Connecticut, Texas, and Florida. Section 15(3)(v) of the New York workers' compensation law also utilizes the hybrid approach for a limited number of permanent partial disability cases.

Methodological Limitations

There are several methodological issues that sophisticated examinations of disability ratings systems must consider, and that are beyond the scope of the current study. We will briefly comment on two of them.

First, there is a question concerning the proper level of aggregation for examining the relationship between disability ratings and loss of earnings. In our tables, we have divided the mean (or median) earnings losses for all workers in a cell (defined by medical condition and age) by the mean (or median) earnings losses for all workers in the cell. Thus, in Table C-1, we divided the mean earnings losses for workers with upper extremity injuries rated 1–2 percent in Panel C ($1,535) by the mean potential earnings for those workers shown in Panel B ($42,740) to produce the proportional earnings losses shown in Panel E (0.036 or 3.6 percent). An alternative approach would be to calculate the proportional earnings losses for individual workers by using each worker's earnings losses and potential earnings. The approach we used may be affected by a few outliers, that is, by workers whose experience was much different than most workers in the cell. Using the distribution of proportional earnings losses for individual workers might show, for example, that the rating system accurately predicted the earnings losses for the vast majority of workers in the cell. We did not use this alternative procedure to assess the equity of the rating systems we examined because the necessary data were unavailable for the Wisconsin workers' compensation program and the veterans disability compensation program. We suggest that subsequent examinations of disability rating systems consider this alternative approach.

Second, there is a difficult methodological problem caused by the possible comingling of disability ratings and earnings losses, as discussed by Greenberg and Rosenheck (2007). This can occur for two reasons. In some disability systems, such as the Disability Insurance (DI) component of the Social Security program, eligibility for the benefits depends on demonstrating an inability to engage in gainful activity. If DI benefits increase, some workers may limit the amount of time they work in order to qualify for benefits. If there were no DI program (or if the DI benefits were lower) the workers would have higher earnings. Thus, the disability benefits system induces higher earnings losses than would have occurred in the absence of the system.

The permanent partial disability benefits provided by most workers' compensation programs and the veterans disability compensation program do not in general link eligibility for the cash benefits to a demonstration of earnings losses and, consequently, the possible inducement to reduce earnings in order to qualify for benefits is muted.[26] There is, however, another possible effect on earnings resulting from the cash benefits provided by these programs. The benefits received by injured workers and injured veterans increase their wealth, and the wealth effect (as it is termed by economists) may induce the beneficiaries to reduce their supply of labor. Thus, a higher disability rating may lead to higher disability benefits and, in turn, to lower earnings than would have occurred if there were no disability benefits system, with the result that part of the lower earnings associated with higher ratings may be due to the inducements provided by the disability benefits system. Ideally, an empirical study of the relationship between disability benefits and earnings losses would separate the effects of the severity of the consequence of the injury from the effects of the benefits provided by the disability benefits system.[27]

We do not think these methodological issues detract from the primary conclusions of the current study.

REFERENCES

Berkowitz, M., and J. F. Burton, Jr. 1987. *Permanent disability benefits in workers' compensation*. Kalamazoo, MI: W. E. Upjohn Institute for Employment Research.

Boden, L. I., R. T. Reville, and J. Biddle. 2005. The adequacy of workers compensation benefits. In *Workplace injuries and diseases: Prevention and compensation: Essays in honor of Terry Thomason*, edited by K. Roberts, J. F. Burton, Jr., and M. M. Bodah. Kalamazoo, MI: W. E. Upjohn Institute for Employment Research. Pp. 37–68.

Burton, J. F., Jr. 2005. Permanent partial disability benefits. In *Workplace injuries and diseases: Prevention and compensation: Essays in honor of Terry Thomason*, edited by K. Roberts, J. F. Burton, Jr., and M. M. Bodah. Kalamazoo, MI: W. E. Upjohn Institute for Employment Research, Pp. 69–116.

Cocchiarella, L., G. B. J. Andersson. 2001. *Guides to the evaluation of permanent impairment*, Fifth Edition. Chicago, IL: American Medical Association.

Greenberg, G. A., and R. A. Rosenheck. 2007. Compensation of veterans with psychiatric or substance abuse disorders and employment and earnings. *Military Medicine* 172:162–168.

Hunt, H. A. 2004. *Adequacy of earnings replacement in workers compensation programs*. Kalamazoo, MI: W. E. Upjohn Institute for Employment Research.

Larson, A., and L. K. Larson. 2006. *Larson's workers' compensation, desk edition*. Newark, NJ: LexisNexis.

Musgrave, R. A. 1959. *The theory of public finance*. New York: McGraw-Hill.

The National Commission (National Commission on State Workmen's Compensation Laws). 1972. *The report of the National Commission on State Workmen's Compensation Laws*. Washington, DC: Government Printing Office.

[26]One exception is individual unemployability benefits, which require the veteran to demonstrate lack of significant earnings.

[27]Greenberg and Rosenheck (2007) examine the determinant of employment and earnings of veterans, and attempt to separate the effects of the severity of the injury from the effects of benefits from the veterans disability compensation program and from other programs.

Peterson, M. A., R. T. Reville, R. K. Stern, and P. S. Barth. 2001. *Compensating permanent workplace injuries: A study of California's system*. Santa Monica, CA: RAND Corporation.

Reville, R. T. 1999. The impact of a disabling workplace injury on earnings and labor participation. In *The creation and analysis of linked employer-employee data, contributions to economic analysis*, edited by J. C. Haltiwanger, J. I. Lane, J. R. Spletzer, J. J. M. Theeuwes, and K. R. Troske. New York: Elsevier Science, North-Holland. Pp. 147–173.

Reville, R. T., J. Bhattacharya, and L. Sager. 2001. New methods and data sources for measuring the economic consequences of workplace injuries. *American Journal of Industrial Medicine* 40:452–463.

Reville, R. T., S. A. Seabury, F. W. Neuhauser, J. F. Burton, Jr., and M. D. Greenberg. 2005. *An evaluation of California's permanent disability rating system*. Santa Monica, CA: RAND Institute for Civil Justice.

Willborn, S. L., S. J. Schwab, J. F. Burton, Jr., and G. L. L. Lester. 2007. *Employment law: Cases and material*, Fourth Edition. Newark, NJ: LexisNexis.

Appendix D

The Role of Medical Personnel in Selected Disability Benefit Programs

This appendix describes some of the major features of five major disability benefit programs:

1. Veterans disability compensation
2. Social Security Disability Insurance (SSDI) and Supplemental Security Income (SSI) Disability
3. Disability retirement from the U.S. Military
4. Federal Civilian Disability Retirement under the Civil Service Retirement (CSRS) and Federal Employee Retirement Systems (FERS)
5. Workers' compensation and other benefits under the Federal Employee Compensation Act (FECA)

Table D-1, at the end of the appendix, summarizes and compares the role of medical personnel in these disability benefit programs.

VETERANS DISABILITY COMPENSATION

The veterans disability compensation program pays monthly cash benefits to veterans to compensate for loss of earning capacity resulting from injuries or diseases that occurred while in the military, or that became worse during military service. Disability rating (from 10 to 100 percent, in increments of 10 percent) determines the monthly benefit amount.

Program Administration

The Veterans Benefits Administration within the Department of Veterans Affairs administers the veterans disability compensation program.

Program References

Program rules and operating procedures are primarily contained in 38 U.S.C 1100ff; 38 CFR Parts 3 and 4; VA's *Compensation and Pension Adjudication Manual* M21-1MR; and various program guides and worksheets.

Disability Definition or Other Qualifying Criteria

Qualifying disability is defined as follows:

> *For disability resulting from personal injury suffered or disease contracted in line of duty, or for aggravation of a preexisting injury suffered or disease contracted in line of duty, in the active military, naval, or air service, . . . the United States will pay to any veteran thus disabled and who was discharged or released under conditions other than dishonorable from the period of service in which said injury or disease was incurred, or preexisting injury or disease was aggravated, compensation as provided in this subchapter, but no compensation shall be paid if the disability is a result of the veteran's own willful misconduct or abuse of alcohol or drugs.*[1]

Health-Care Professional Role

The primary role of the health-care professional is as the provider of medical records used in making the eligibility decision and impairment rating. The initial rating is based on medical records obtained from the applicant's own heath-care providers, including the veteran's service medical record (SMR). In most circumstances, this evidence is supplemented by a medical examination from a VA medical center or a contract examination provider. These examinations may be conducted by a physician or by a registered nurse (RN) or physician's assistant (PA) (reports of RN or PA examinations must be reviewed and countersigned by a physician). In limited circumstances, a specialist conducts the examination. This might be a physician specializing in a certain area of medicine, or a nonphysician health-care provider skilled in a particular kind of examination (e.g., audiologist, psychologist).

Health-care professionals are not involved in claim adjudication (including the disability rating). Initial compensation claim ratings are made by

[1]38 U.S.C. § 1110 and § 1131.

a rating veterans service representative (RVSR), a layperson trained in rating principles and VA's Schedule for Rating Disabilities (Rating Schedule). Although the RVSR may obtain a medical opinion or an independent medical opinion from a physician to assist with the case evaluation, the physician does not participate in the rating decision. Physicians may also be involved in training RVSRs.

The Board of Veterans' Appeals (BVA) handles appeals of denied claims. Members of the BVA are attorneys. Health-care professionals are not involved, although BVA may also request a medical opinion or independent medical opinion from a physician.

SSDI AND SSI DISABILITY

These programs provide monthly cash payments to individuals who are unable to work due to a disability. SSDI pays monthly benefits to disabled individuals who are "insured" for these benefits by having paid Federal Insurance Contributions Act (FICA) taxes. Benefits are also available to certain dependents of retired, disabled, or deceased workers. SSI payments are made to disabled individuals who have limited income and financial resources.

Program Administration

The Social Security Administration administers both the SSDI and SSI programs.

Program References

Program rules and operating instructions are primarily in 42 U.S.C. 421, 423, 1382, and 1382c; 20 CFR Part 404, Subparts J, P, and Q; 20 CFR Part 416, Subparts I, J, and N; Social Security Rulings; and the agency's Program Operations Manual System.

Disability Definition or Other Qualifying Criteria

"Disability" is defined as follows:

> *The term 'disability' means . . . inability to engage in any substantial gainful activity by reason of any medically determinable physical or mental impairment which can be expected to result in death or which has lasted or can be expected to last for a continuous period of not less than 12 months. . . . An individual shall be determined to be under a disability only if his physical or mental impairment or impairments are of such severity that he is not only unable to do his previous work but cannot, considering his age,*

> *education, and work experience, engage in any other kind of substantial gainful work which exists in the national economy, regardless of whether such work exists in the immediate area in which he lives, or whether a specific job vacancy exists for him, or whether he would be hired if he applied for work.*[2]

Health-Care Professional Role

SSA's rules require that the existence of a "medically determinable impairment" (in other words, a diagnosis) be established by evidence from an "acceptable medical source," generally a physician or, for specific kinds of impairments, a psychologist, optometrist, podiatrist, or speech-language pathologist. These medical professionals must meet appropriate licensure or certification requirements, but need not be board certified. The claimant's own medical sources are the preferred sources of this evidence, as well as additional evidence of the severity of the impairment, which may come from a variety of medical and nonmedical sources.

If evidence from the claimant's own medical sources is insufficient, SSA may obtain a consultative examination from another medical source. These examinations may be obtained from the claimant's own medical sources, but they are usually obtained from contract medical examination providers. These providers may be physician or nonphysician medical sources, depending on the information being sought. They must be licensed in the state in which they practice, and have the appropriate training and experience to perform the type of examination or test requested.

Initial case adjudications are generally performed by two-person teams. One team member is the "medical consultant," usually either a physician or psychologist. The other team member is the disability examiner, a lay person who is trained by the agency. In limited circumstances, the medical consultant may be a nonphysician optometrist, podiatrist, or speech-language pathologist. There are no requirements that the medical consultant be board certified, although the Institute of Medicine (IOM) Committee on Improving the Social Security Disability Decision Process recently recommended that all physician medical consultants be board certified.

First-level appeals, called "reconsiderations," are generally decided by a different, but identically composed, two-person team (with one lay person and a medical consultant). Second-level appeals are decided by administrative law judges in a nonadversarial administrative proceeding. Administrative law judges may request the presence of a medical expert at the hearing, which is done about 12 percent of the time. Third-level appeals are to the

[2]42 U.S.C. § 423(d)(1)(A). There is a similar definition of disability for the SSI program in 42 U.S.C. § 1382c(a)(3)(b).

Appeals Council, a panel of judges that reviews administrative law judge decisions. After exhausting these administrative appeals, claimants may seek further relief in the federal courts.

SSA has tested several variations on this adjudication process in recent years, and is now in the process of implementing a variation that replaces the reconsideration process with a federal review officer (nonmedical) as the first level of appeal, and an alternative review board as the final step in the administrative review process in place of the Appeals Council.

DISABILITY RETIREMENT FROM THE U.S. MILITARY

This program provides early retirement benefits to servicemembers who are unable to perform their military duties due to a disability that occurred during service (referred to as a "physical disability," although the disability may be either a physical or mental disorder). To qualify, the disability must be permanent, must not be the result of intentional misconduct or willful neglect, and must not have been incurred during a period of unauthorized absence. The servicemember must have at least 20 years of service or have a service-connected disability rating (using the VA Rating Schedule) of 30 percent or more.

Program Administration

The Department of Defense (DoD) and individual U.S. military services administer the program.

Program References

Program rules and operating instructions are in 10 U.S.C. 1200ff; Department of Defense Directive 1332.18, DoD Instructions 1332.38 and 1332.39; Army Regulations (AR) 635-40 and (AR) 40-501; Secretary of the Navy Instruction 1850.4E; Coast Guard Commandant Instruction M1850.2; and Air Force Instructions (AFI) 36-3212 and (AFI) 48-123.

Disability Definition or Other Qualifying Criteria

Qualifying disability is defined as

> . . . *unfit to perform the duties of the member's office, grade, rank, or rating because of physical disability* . . . [3]

[3] 10 U.S.C § 1201(a).

Health-Care Professional Role

The military services rely on a multistep process, referred to as the DoD Disability Evaluation System, to evaluate fitness for duty when there has been an illness or injury that may affect a servicemember's ability to perform his or her job. The process begins with a referral to a medical evaluation board (MEB), which is convened at the local medical treatment facility when a servicemember has been treated for a medical condition and has reached maximum medical improvement but may still be unfit for duty. Generally, when an individual's disability may prevent him or her from meeting service retention standards, the unit commander or a physician at the pertinent medical treatment facility makes the MEB referral. An MEB is composed of 2–3 medical officers (physicians) who determine whether the servicemember's medical condition calls into question his or her fitness for continued military service or ability to meet retention standards. If not, the MEB returns the servicemember to duty.

If the MEB concludes that the servicemember's disability significantly interferes with the ability to carry out his or her duties, the case is referred to an informal physical evaluation board (PEB), which will make the initial determinations of fitness for duty. The PEB is generally a three-member board consisting of a senior military officer, a personnel officer, and a medical officer (physician). The PEB relies on reports from the applicant's own health-care professionals (generally, the medical treatment facility at the servicemember's duty station) and the findings of the MEB. If the PEB decides that the individual is not fit for duty, a disability rating (percentage) based on the VA Rating Schedule also will be assigned.

A servicemember who is not satisfied with the PEB decision may request a hearing before a formal PEB. A formal PEB also is a three-member panel with one medical officer (physician). As the name implies, formal PEBs conduct more formal proceedings (hearings at which additional medical evidence and testimony may be presented).

FEDERAL CIVILIAN DISABILITY RETIREMENT UNDER CSRS OR FERS

Federal Civilian Disability Retirement provides monthly cash benefits to federal employees who are unable to perform their job or a comparable job because of a disability.

Program Administration

The Office of Personnel Management (OPM) administers the CSRS and FERS programs.

Program References

Program rules and operating instructions are in 5 U.S.C. 8337 and 8451, and 5 CFR 831 and 844.

Disability Definition or Other Qualifying Criteria

Qualifying disability is defined as follows:

> *Any employee shall be considered to be disabled only if the employee is found by the Office of Personnel Management to be unable, because of disease or injury, to render useful and efficient service in the employee's position and is not qualified for reassignment, under procedures prescribed by the Office, to a vacant position which is in the agency at the same grade or level and in which the employee would be able to render useful and efficient service.*[4]

Health-Care Professional Role

The primary health-care professional's role is as the provider of medical records used in case adjudication. Medical documentation is obtained from the federal employee's own medical source(s). OPM has the authority to request that an applicant undergo examination by an OPM-designated physician; however, such referrals are rare.

Initial disability decisions are made by a legal administrative specialist, who is a trained lay person. The disability decision is based on the report(s) of the applicant's own medical sources, which have to conform to specific report content requirements. Although decision makers have the authority to obtain medical advice from physicians when conducting case adjudication, physicians are not involved in the decision-making process.

Second-level appeals are decided by administrative law judges at the Merit System Protection Board. No health-care professionals are involved.

BENEFITS UNDER FECA

FECA provides for workers' compensation benefits to civilian federal employees who are not covered by state-run workers' compensation programs for work-related illnesses and injuries. Benefits include cash compensation, medical coverage, and vocational rehabilitation.

Permanent disability may be total or partial. For permanent total disability, claimants receive compensation based on their preinjury earnings.

---

[4]5 U.S.C. § 8337(a).

Claimants are rarely found to have total disability, which is considered only in catastrophic injuries or long-standing chronic conditions after all attempts at rehabilitation have failed. This is true even for impairments that the law states are "prima facie" evidence of permanent total disability (loss of both hands, arms, feet, or legs, or the loss of sight of both eyes).

Permanent partial disability compensation is based on the difference between the wages earned at the time of injury and the wages the claimant is capable of earning after the injury.

For schedule awards, the degree of impairment is established solely by medical evidence and expressed as a percentage of loss of the body part involved. For permanent disability, the determination is considered economic, rather than just medical, and based on both medical and non-medical factors.

Although FECA rules distinguish between impairment (as a medical concept) and disability (as an economic concept), both require a medical evaluation. Case adjudication is performed primarily by nonmedical claims examiners, but with close medical scrutiny.

Program Administration

The Department of Labor's (DOL's) Office of Workers' Compensation Programs (OWCP) administers the FECA program.

Program References

Program rules and procedures are in 5 U.S.C. 8101 and 8123; 20 CFR part 10; FECA Procedural Manual Parts 2 and 3; and FECA Program Memoranda.

Disability Definition or Other Qualifying Criteria

Under FECA, injured workers receive compensation in one of two ways:

- If the illness or injury involves a limb or organ on a statutory list, they receive compensation according to a fixed schedule, meaning for so many weeks, according to the schedule (referred to as "schedule awards" or permanent impairment).[5]
- For permanent disability, they receive compensation for loss of earnings, either on the basis of total or partial disability.[6]

[5]The schedule is in 5 U.S.C. § 8107(c).

[6]5 U.S.C. § 8105 and § 8106.

Health-Care Professional Role

OWCP administers the FECA program nationally through a network of 12 district offices, each of which has a significant medical staff:

- The district medical director is a physician[7] employed by OWCP who has administrative oversight of the medical functions of the district office, and also serves as liaison with the medical community and federal employers within the district office's jurisdiction. The district medical director administers the district office's network of district medical advisors (discussed below) and second opinion medical specialists; provides training to staff regarding medical issues; and provides medical opinions and advice on complex claims.
- At least one district medical advisor, also a physician, is responsible for interpreting medical reports; performing medical evaluations; performing ratings on schedule awards; and providing guidance to staff on medical issues. District medical advisors are usually part-time contract employees.
- The staff nurse manages the work of a staff of field nurses who are responsible for case management, including monitoring claimants' medical progress and assisting their efforts to return to work.
- The medical management assistant assists the district medical director in the administration of the medical unit and performs associated support functions (e.g., referrals to second opinion and referee specialists).

Initial case adjudication is performed by claims examiners based on evidence provided by physicians who have examined the claimant, as well as employment and other records. For cases involving schedule awards, a district medical advisor performs the rating. Permanent total disability determinations must be based on not only the reports of the attending physician and other physicians who have examined the claimant, but also on the opinion of a district medical advisor.

If the evidence provided by the treating physician is not sufficient, the claims examiner may request a "second opinion examination" by another physician. Each district office uses a commercial medical examination service, chosen through competitive bidding, to provide second opinion examinations.

If the second opinion differs from the treating physician's, the claims examiner may order a third examination, called a "referee examination." In this case, the physician is chosen from a directory of physicians maintained

[7]By statute, the term *physician* includes surgeons, podiatrists, dentists, clinical psychologists, optometrists, osteopathic practitioners, and chiropractors within the scope of their practice as defined by state law.

by the American Board of Medical Specialties. Consequently, most referee examiners are board certified, although this is not a requirement.

Claimants who are dissatisfied with the initial decision on their claim may appeal. They may request reconsideration by the district office within one year. Reconsideration determinations are made by senior claims examiners.

The employee may also request either an oral hearing before a Branch of Hearings and Review representative or a review of the written record (but not both), as long as the request is made within 30 days of the formal decision and a reconsideration has not already been requested. Claimants are allowed to submit new evidence when requesting an oral hearing or review of the written record. If the claimant requests a review of the written record, he or she will not be asked to attend or testify. At an oral hearing, the claimant can testify in person or through a designated representative. For either a hearing or review of the record, the hearing representative decides whether to affirm the initial decision, reverse the initial decision and administer benefits to the claimant, or remand the claim to the district office for a new decision.

The final appeal option available to claimants is through the Employee's Compensation Appeals Board (ECAB). The ECAB was created within DOL, but outside of OWCP, to give federal employees the same administrative due process of law and appellate review that nongovernmental workers enjoy under workers' compensation laws in most states. Each case on appeal is reviewed by three members of the ECAB. ECAB members are appointed by the secretary of Labor. Regulations prohibit the claimant from submitting new evidence during this phase, but the ECAB is not limited by previous "finding of fact" by the district office or Branch of Hearings and Review and can, therefore, reevaluate the evidence and determine if the law was appropriately applied. The ECAB represents the end of the appeal process; claimants may not obtain review through a state or federal court system.

TABLE D-1 Summary of the Role of Medical Personnel in Selected Disability Benefit Programs

	VA	SSA
Treating physician[a] provides medical evidence?	Treating physicians are a source of evidence.	Treating physicians are usually the main source of evidence.
Specific examination required?	Generally, yes. Compensation and Pension (C&P) examination is required in most cases.	No, but an examination may be required if treating physician records are incomplete or inconsistent.
Examination required if treating physician and agency medical examiner disagree?	No	No
Medical professionals involved in making initial decisions?	No. The decision is made by a rating veterans service representative (RVSR).	Yes. The decision is made jointly by a medical consultant and claims examiner.
Adjudicator access to medical expertise?	No, although the RVSR may refer the case back to the C&P examiner in the Veterans Health Administration for further information.	Yes. The medical consultant deciding a case may consult other medical consultants.
Health-care professionals involved in the appeal process?	No, although administrative law judges may remand a case to the field office for development of additional medical evidence.	No, although administrative law judges may request the presence of a medical expert at hearings.

[a]The term "treating physician" may include nonphysician health-care practitioners.

DoD	CSRS, FERS	FECA
Treating physicians are a source of evidence.	Treating physicians are usually the main source of evidence.	Treating physicians are usually the main source of evidence.
No. A medical evaluation board reviews the applicant's medical treatment records and recommends whether to refer the case to a physical evaluation board.	No, but in rare instances, the Office of Personnel Management (OPM) may require examination by an OPM-designated physician.	No, but if the evidence provided by the treating physician is not sufficient, the claims examiner may request a "second opinion examination."
No	No	Yes. Examination is by a physician selected from the American Board of Medical Specialties directory.
Yes. At least one member of the physical evaluation board is a physician, who also determines the rating.	No. The decision is made by a legal administrative specialist.	Yes, in cases involving a schedule award. Then the rating is determined by a district medical adviser, usually a contract physician.
Yes. The medical officer on the physical evaluation board may consult other medical officers.	No	Yes. Each district office has a district medical director and one or more district medical advisers with whom the claims examiner can consult.
Yes, although the services differ somewhat in their approach to appeals.	No. Appeal is to the Merit System Protection Board.	No

Appendix E

Diagram: Assessing Impairment and Functional Disability

The purpose of this diagram is to illustrate a process for compensating veterans for impairment and functional limitations resulting from service-connected injury or disease. (It does not include compensation for loss of quality of life [QOL], because the methodology for determining loss of QOL remains to be determined based on a research and development effort.)

In addition to distinguishing between the criteria appropriate for determining impairment severity, such as the New York Heart Association (NYHA) classification of cardiovascular limitations and failure and the METS (metabolic equivalents of task) measure of congestive heart failure, and those appropriate for determining functional capacity, such as activities of daily living (ADLs) and instrumental activities of daily living (IADLs), the diagram shows how evaluation of disability could be connected directly to rehabilitation services.